Central Nervous System Infections

Editor

GAURANG SHAH

NEUROIMAGING CLINICS OF NORTH AMERICA

www.neuroimaging.theclinics.com

Consulting Editor

SURESH K. MUKHERJI

November 2012 • Volume 22 • Number 4

ELSEVIER

1600 John F. Kennedy Boulevard ● Suite 1800 ● Philadelphia, Pennsylvania 19103-2899

http://www.theclinics.com

NEUROIMAGING CLINICS OF NORTH AMERICA Volume 22, Number 4
November 2012 ISSN 1052-5149, ISBN 13: 978-1-4557-1109-3

Editor: Pamela M. Hetherington
Developmental Editor: Donald Mumford

Neuroimaging Clinics of North America (ISSN 1052-5149) is published quarterly by Elsevier Inc., 360 Park Avenue South, New York, NY 10010-1710. Months of issue are February, May, August, and November. Business and editorial offices: 1600 John F. Kennedy Blvd., Suite 1800, Philadelphia, PA 19103-2899. Business and editorial offices: 6277 Sea Harbor Drive, Orlando, FL 32887-4800. Periodicals postage paid at New York, NY, and additional mailing offices. Subscription prices are USD 342 per year for US individuals, USD 471 per year for US institutions, USD 172 per year for US students and residents, USD 396 per year for Canadian individuals, USD 590 per year for Canadian institutions, USD 502 per year for international individuals, USD 590 per year for international institutions and USD 246 per year for Canadian and foreign students and residents. To receive student/resident rate, orders must be accompanied by name of affiliated institution, date of term, and the *signature* of program/residency coordinator on institution letterhead. Orders will be billed at individual rate until proof of status is received. Foreign air speed delivery is included in all *Clinics* subscription prices. All prices are subject to change without notice. POSTMASTER: Send address changes to *Neuroimaging Clinics of North America*, Elsevier Health Sciences Division, Subscription Customer Service, 3251 Riverport Lane, Maryland Heights, MO 63043. Telephone: 1-800-654-2452 (U.S. and Canada); 314-447-8871 (outside U.S. and Canada). Fax: 314-447-8029. E-mail: journalscustomerservice-usa@elsevier.com (for print support); journalsonlinesupport-usa@elsevier.com (for online support).

Reprints. For copies of 100 or more of articles in this publication, please contact the Commercial Reprints Department, Elsevier Inc., 360 Park Avenue South, New York, NY 10010-1710. Tel.: 212-633-3812; Fax: 212-462-1935; E-mail: reprints@elsevier.com.

Neuroimaging Clinics of North America is covered by *Excerpta Medical/EMBASE,* the RSNA Index of Imaging Literature, *MEDLINE/PubMed (Index Medicus),* MEDLINE/MEDLARS, SciSearch, Research Alert, and Neuroscience Citation Index.

Printed and bound by CPI Group (UK) Ltd, Croydon, CR0 4YY

Transferred to digital print 2012

GOAL STATEMENT

The goal of *Neuroimaging Clinics of North America* is to keep practicing radiologists and radiology residents up to date with current clinical practice in radiology by providing timely articles reviewing the state of the art in patient care.

ACCREDITATION

The *Neuroimaging Clinics of North America* is planned and implemented in accordance with the Essential Areas and Policies of the Accreditation Council for Continuing Medical Education (ACCME) through the joint sponsorship of the University of Virginia School of Medicine and Elsevier. The University of Virginia School of Medicine is accredited by the ACCME to provide continuing medical education for physicians.

The University of Virginia School of Medicine designates this enduring material activity for a maximum of 15 *AMA PRA Category 1 Credit*(s)™ for each issue, 60 credits per year. Physicians should claim only the credit commensurate with the extent of their participation in the activity.

The American Medical Association has determined that physicians not licensed in the US who participate in this CME enduring material activity are eligible for a maximum of 15 *AMA PRA Category 1 Credit*(s)™ for each issue, 60 credits per year.

Credit can be earned by reading the text material, taking the CME examination online at http://www.theclinics.com/home/cme, and completing the evaluation. After taking the test, you will be required to review any and all incorrect answers. Following completion of the test and evaluation, your credit will be awarded and you may print your certificate.

FACULTY DISCLOSURE/CONFLICT OF INTEREST

The University of Virginia School of Medicine, as an ACCME accredited provider, endorses and strives to comply with the Accreditation Council for Continuing Medical Education (ACCME) Standards of Commercial Support, Commonwealth of Virginia statutes, University of Virginia policies and procedures, and associated federal and private regulations and guidelines on the need for disclosure and monitoring of proprietary and financial interests that may affect the scientific integrity and balance of content delivered in continuing medical education activities under our auspices.

The University of Virginia School of Medicine requires that all CME activities accredited through this institution be developed independently and be scientifically rigorous, balanced and objective in the presentation/discussion of its content, theories and practices.

All authors/editors participating in an accredited CME activity are expected to disclose to the readers relevant financial relationships with commercial entities occurring within the past 12 months (such as grants or research support, employee, consultant, stock holder, member of speakers bureau, etc.). The University of Virginia School of Medicine will employ appropriate mechanisms to resolve potential conflicts of interest to maintain the standards of fair and balanced education to the reader. Questions about specific strategies can be directed to the Office of Continuing Medical Education, University of Virginia School of Medicine, Charlottesville, Virginia.

The faculty and staff of the University of Virginia Office of Continuing Medical Education have no financial affiliations to disclose.

The authors/editors listed below have identified no professional/financial affiliations for themselves or their spouse/partner:

Ayca Akgoz, MD; Mohammad Arabi, MD, FRCR; John L. Go, MD; Amogh N. Hegde, MBBS, MD, FRCR; Jason A. Heth, MD; Pamela Hetherington, (Acquisitions Editor); Marion Hughes, MD; Mohannad Ibrahim, MD; Krishan K. Jain, MD, PDCC; Carl E. Johnson, MD; Malini Lawande, MD; Thomas C. Lee, MD; Alexander Lerner, MD; Mahan Mathur, MD; Paul E. McKeever, MD, PhD; Suyash Mohan, MD, PDCC; Jayant Narang, MD; Amit Pandya, MD; Hemant Parmar, MD; Deepak Patkar, MD; Ashley Prosper, MD; Tanya J. Rath, MD; James Riddell IV, MD; Stephen Rothman, MD; Gaurang V. Shah, MD (Guest Editor); Lubdha M. Shah, MD (Test Author); Emily K. Shuman, MD; Richard Silbergleit, MD; Gordon Sze, MD; Rama Yanamandala, MD; and Chi-Shing Zee, MD.

The authors listed below have identified the following professional/financial affiliations for themselves or their spouse/partner:

Meng Law, MD, MBBS is on the Speakers' Bureau for Toshiba America Medical, is on the Advisory Board for Siemens Medical, iCAD Inc, and Fuji Inc, and receives research support from Bayer Healthcare.

Suresh K. Mukherji, MD, FACR (Consulting Editor) is a consultant for Philips.

Srini Mukundan, MD receives research support from Tashiba and Siemens, and is a consultant for and owns stock in Marval Biosciences.

Mark S. Shiroishi, MD is a consultant for Bayer Healthcare.

Disclosure of Discussion of Non-FDA Approved Uses for Pharmaceutical Products and/or Medical Devices.

The University of Virginia School of Medicine, as an ACCME provider, requires that all faculty presenters identify and disclose any off-label uses for pharmaceutical and medical device products. The University of Virginia School of Medicine recommends that each physician fully review all the available data on new products or procedures prior to clinical use.

TO ENROLL

To enroll in the Neuroimaging Clinics of North America Continuing Medical Education program, call customer service at 1-800-654-2452 or sign up online at http://www.theclinics.com/home/cme. The CME program is available to subscribers for an additional annual fee of USD 196.

NEUROIMAGING CLINICS OF NORTH AMERICA

Contributors

CONSULTING EDITOR

SURESH K. MUKHERJI, MD, FACR
Director of Neuroradiology, Professor and
Chief of Neuroradiology and Head & Neck
Radiology; Professor of Radiology,
Otolaryngology Head Neck Surgery, Radiation
Oncology, Periodontics and Oral Medicine,
University of Michigan Health System,
Ann Arbor, Michigan

GUEST EDITOR

GAURANG V. SHAH, MD
Associate Professor, Department of Radiology,
University of Michigan Health System,
Ann Arbor, Michigan

AUTHORS

AYCA AKGOZ, MD
Department of Radiology, Brigham & Women's
Hospital, Harvard Medical School, Boston,
Massachusetts

MOHAMMAD ARABI, MD, FRCR
Department of Radiology, University of Michigan
Health System, Ann Arbor, Michigan; Presently,
Riyadh military hospital, Prince Sultan Medical
Military city, Riyadh, Saudi Arabia

JOHN L. GO, MD
Assistant Professor of Radiology and
Otolaryngology, Division of Neuroradiology,
Department of Radiology, Keck School of
Medicine, University of Southern California,
Los Angeles, California

AMOGH N. HEGDE, MBBS, MD, FRCR
Associate Consultant, Department of
Radiology, Singapore General Hospital,
Singapore

JASON A. HETH, MD
Assistant Professor, Department of
Neurosurgery, University of Michigan,
Ann Arbor, Michigan

MARION HUGHES, MD
Assistant Professor, Department of Radiology,
University of Pittsburgh Medical Center,
Pittsburgh, Pennsylvania

MOHANNAD IBRAHIM, MD
Associate Professor of Radiology, Division
of Neuroradiology, Department of Radiology,
University of Michigan Health System,
Ann Arbor, Michigan

KRISHAN K. JAIN, MD, PDCC
Department of Neuroradiology, National
Neuroscience Institute, Singapore

CARL E. JOHNSON, MD
Department of Radiology, New York-
Presbyterian Hospital, New York, New York

MENG LAW, MD, MBBS
Professor of Radiology and Neurological
Surgery, Department of Radiology, Keck
School of Medicine, University of Southern
California, Los Angeles, California

MALINI LAWANDE, MD
MRI Center, Dr Balabhai Nanavati Hospital,
Mumbai, India

THOMAS C. LEE, MD
Staff Neuroradiologist, Department of
Radiology, Brigham & Women's Hospital,
Instructor in Radiology, Harvard Medical
School, Boston, Massachusetts

ALEXANDER LERNER, MD
Assistant Professor of Radiology, Division of
Neuroradiology, Department of Radiology,
Keck School of Medicine, University of
Southern California, Los Angeles, California

MAHAN MATHUR, MD
Department of Radiology, Yale University
Medical Center, New Haven, Connecticut

PAUL E. MCKEEVER, MD, PhD
Professor of Pathology, Department of
Pathology, University of Michigan Medical
Center, Ann Arbor, Michigan

SUYASH MOHAN, MD, PDCC
Assistant Professor of Radiology, Division of
Neuroradiology, Department of Radiology,
University of Pennsylvania School of Medicine,
Philadelphia, Pennsylvania

SRINI MUKUNDAN, MD
Department of Radiology, Brigham & Women's
Hospital, Harvard Medical School, Boston,
Massachusetts

JAYANT NARANG, MD
MRI Center, Dr Balabhai Nanavati Hospital,
Mumbai, India; Department of Neuroradiology,
Henry Ford Health System, Detroit, Michigan

HEMANT PARMAR, MD
Associate Professor of Radiology, Division of
Neuroradiology, Department of Radiology,
University of Michigan Health System,
Ann Arbor, Michigan

AMIT PANDYA, MD
Department of Radiology, University of
Michigan Health System, Ann Arbor, Michigan

DEEPAK PATKAR, MD
MRI Center, Dr Balabhai Nanavati Hospital,
Mumbai, India

ASHLEY PROSPER, MD
Radiology Resident, Department of Radiology,
Keck School of Medicine, University of
Southern California, Los Angeles, California

TANYA J. RATH, MD
Assistant Professor and Director of Head and
Neck Imaging, Department of Radiology,
University of Pittsburgh Medical Center,
Pittsburgh, Pennsylvania

JAMES RIDDELL IV, MD
Clinical Associate Professor, Department of
Internal Medicine, Division of Infectious
Diseases, University of Michigan Health
System, Ann Arbor, Michigan

STEPHEN ROTHMAN, MD
Clinical Professor of Radiology, Department
of Radiology, Keck School of Medicine,
University of Southern California,
Los Angeles, California

GAURANG V. SHAH, MD
Associate Professor, Department of Radiology,
University of Michigan Health System,
Ann Arbor, Michigan

MARK S. SHIROISHI, MD
Assistant Professor, Department of Radiology,
Keck School of Medicine, University of
Southern California, Los Angeles, California

EMILY K. SHUMAN, MD
Instructor in Medicine, Workforce Health and
Safety Clinic, New York Presbyterian Hospital/
Weill Cornell Medical College, New York,
New York

RICHARD SILBERGLEIT, MD
Professor of Radiology, Vice Chief, Diagnostic
Radiology, William Beaumont Hospital,
Oakland University William Beaumont School
of Medicine, Royal Oak, Michigan

GORDON SZE, MD
Department of Radiology, Yale University
Medical Center, New Haven, Connecticut

RAMA YANAMANDALA, MD
MRI Center, Dr Balabhai Nanavati Hospital,
Mumbai, India

CHI-SHING ZEE, MD
Professor of Radiology and Neurosurgery,
Department of Radiology, Keck School of
Medicine, University of Southern California,
Los Angeles, California

Contents

In cases of central nervous system infection, it is crucial for the neuroradiologist to provide an accurate differential diagnosis of the possible pathogens involved so that treating physicians can be aided in the choice of empiric therapy. This approach requires the radiologist to be aware of local epidemiology and have knowledge of infectious agents that are endemic to their area of practice. This article reviews and discusses the changing epidemiology of pathogens most often observed in meningitis, brain abscess, epidural abscess, postoperative infections, and human immunodeficiency virus infection.

Central nervous system infections account for 1% of primary hospital admissions and 2% of nosocomial infections and when encountered require prompt diagnosis and initiation of specific treatment. Imaging findings are mostly nonspecific with respect to the causative pathogen. This article describes the anatomy of cranial meninges and extra-axial spaces of the brain. Characteristic findings and recent advances in neuroimaging of meningitis and its complications and ventriculitis are summarized, and certain noninfectious causes of meningitis and meningitis mimics are described.

Imaging plays an important role in the diagnosis and treatment of brain abscess, pyogenic infection, and encephalitis. The role of CT and MRI in the diagnosis and management of pyogenic brain abscess and its complications is reviewed. The imaging appearances of several common and select uncommon infectious encephalitides are reviewed. Common causes of encephalitis in immunocompromised patients, and their imaging appearances, are also discussed. When combined with CSF, serologic studies and patient history, imaging findings can suggest the cause of encephalitis.

Fungal infections of the central nervous system (CNS) frequently occur in the immunocompromised or debilitated host. Imaging findings are non-specific but may be organized into extra-axial, parenchymal, and vascular categories. Furthermore, knowledge of fungal morphology may predict the imaging manifestations with large, hyphal species having a predilection for brain parenchymal involvement, while small, unicellular organisms typically result in meningitis. Advanced imaging techniques such as diffusion-weighted imaging, MR perfusion and MR spectroscopy, when combined with clinical findings, may help in differentiating fungal disease from other mimckers such as pyogenic infection or cystic metastases.

This article is an update and literature review of the clinical and neuroimaging findings of the commonly known rickettsial, spirochetal, and eukaryotic parasitic infections. Being familiar with clinical presentation and imaging findings of these infections is crucial for early diagnosis and treatment especially in patients who live in or have a travel history to endemic regions or are immunocompromised.

Neurocysticercosis (NCC) is an infection of the central nervous system by the Taenia solium larvae, and is the most common cause of acquired epilepsy in endemic regions. The natural history of parenchymal NCC lesions can be divided into 4 stages with unique imaging and clinical features. Evaluation of cysticerci is challenging on conventional magnetic resonance (MR) imaging and computed tomography, and is significantly improved with MR cysternography techniques. Differentiation of NCC lesions from metastatic disease and pyogenic abscesses can be improved with advanced MR imaging including ^{1}H nuclear MR spectroscopy, diffusion-weighted imaging, and MR perfusion imaging.

With the onset of the human immunodeficiency virus pandemic, the incidence of tuberculosis, including central nervous system (CNS) tuberculosis, has increased in developed countries. It is no longer a disease confined to underdeveloped and developing countries. The imaging appearance has become more complex with the onset of multidrug-resistant tuberculosis. Imaging plays an important role in the early diagnosis of CNS tuberculosis and may prevent unnecessary morbidity and mortality. This article presents an extensive review of typical and atypical imaging appearances of intracranial tuberculosis, and discusses pathogenesis, patterns of involvement, and advances in imaging of intracranial tuberculosis.

Infection of the central nervous system (CNS) in children is an important entity and early recognition is paramount to avoid long-term brain injury, especially in very young patients. The causal factors are different in children compared with adults and so are the clinical presentations. However, imaging features of CNS infection show similar features to those of adults. This article reviews some of the common types of pediatric infections, starting with the congenital (or in utero) infections followed by bacterial infections of the meninges and brain parenchyma.

Contents

Infections of the head and neck vary in their clinical course and outcome because of the diversity of organs and anatomic compartments involved. Imaging plays a central role in delineating the anatomic extent of the disease process, identifying the infection source, and detecting complications. The utility of imaging to differentiate between a solid phlegmonous mass and an abscess cannot be overemphasized. This review briefly describes and pictorially illustrates the typical imaging findings of some important head and neck infections, such as malignant otitis externa, otomastoiditis, bacterial and fungal sinusitis, orbital cellulitis, sialadenitis, cervical lymphadenitis, and deep neck space infections.

Acute infections of the spine represent a rare but potentially debilitating and neurologically devastating condition for patients. Early diagnosis, imaging, and intervention may prevent some of the more critical complications that may ensue from this disease process, including alignment abnormalities, central canal compromise, nerve root impingement, vascular complications, and spinal cord injury. This article reviews the underlying pathophysiologic basis of infection, clinical manifestations, and imaging modalities used to diagnose infections of the spine and spinal cord.

Radiology provides valuable gross pathologic information about central nervous system (CNS) infections. Major categories of infectious lesions of the brain and spinal cord are recognized by imaging such as diffuse, focal, or multifocal. This article discusses the pathologic basis of these radiographic findings. It illustrates examples with gross and microscopic photographs of CNS infections, and the tissue reactions in these infections. Where the organism can spread within the CNS, and cellular responses to the organism underlie both the radiographic and pathologic findings.

Infections of the central nervous system (CNS) can be severe, disabling, and potentially fatal. Infections of the central nervous system (CNS) can be severe, disabling, and potentially fatal. Appropriate recognition of symptoms facilitates expeditious evaluation, prompt diagnosis, and timely treatment. Further work-up may include cranial or spinal imaging, lumbar puncture, and invasive biopsy. Therapy involves antibiotic, antiviral, or antifungal treatment. Surgical treatment for debridement, decompression, or reconstruction may also be required. This review explores the presentation, pathogenesis, evaluation, and treatment of the most common infections of the CNS. Discussion of treatment options also includes possible neurosurgical interventions. The infections considered are cerebral abscess, subdural empyema, meningitis, encephalitis, toxoplasmosis, neurocysticercosis, discitis, and spinal epidural abscess.

Foreword

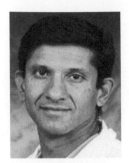

Suresh K. Mukherji, MD, FACR
Consulting Editor

There is no one more qualified to edit this edition of *Neuroimaging Clinics* on infections of the central nervous system than Gaurang Shah. I have known Dr Shah for nearly 20 years and am very familiar with his background, expertise, and academic drive. Gaurang was a very prominent radiologist in India and worked with one of the first MRI units ever installed in India in the 1990s. He decided to immigrate to the United States to advance his career, has had extraordinary success, and is currently Associate Professor of Radiology and in charge of both clinical fMRI and clinical trials within the University of Michigan Neuroradiology Division.

Gaurang is a highly sought-after lecturer on the international circuit and continues to be an iconic figure in his home country. He has assembled an extraordinary group of contributors for this edition, which I am sure will become an instant classic, and I thank all of the contributors for their wonderful contributions.

Even more importantly, Gaurang is one of the nicest and most humble people you will ever meet. He has a beautiful family and his wife, Kinnari, is a lovely person and a terrific cook! His oldest son, Sharvil, is beginning his first year of dental school in the fall of 2013 and I hope that his youngest son, Sahil, is destined to be a head and neck radiologist! On behalf of all us at *Neuroimaging Clinics*, I wish to personally thank Dr Gaurang Shah for creating this wonderful edition of *Neuroimaging Clinics*.

Suresh K. Mukherji, MD, FACR
Department of Radiology
University of Michigan Health System
1500 East Medical Center
Ann Arbor, MI 48109-0030, USA

E-mail address:
mukherji@med.umich.edu

Neuroimag Clin N Am 22 (2012) xi
http://dx.doi.org/10.1016/j.nic.2012.08.002
1052-5149/12/$ – see front matter © 2012 Elsevier Inc. All rights reserved.

neuroimaging.theclinics.com

Preface

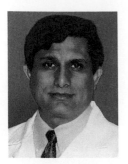

Gaurang Shah, MD
Guest Editor

In this day and age it is hard to imagine that septicemia following a toe blister caused by a chafing tennis shoe can result in the death of a presidential progeny. However, it happened less than 90 years ago, in 1924, to the 16-year-old son of President Calvin Coolidge. The advent of antibiotics in 1940s revolutionized the treatment of infections and was responsible for the biggest jump in life expectancy in human history: 8 years within a decade. Apart from the epithelial barrier system and mucosal immune system, the presence of the blood brain barrier creates a unique defense mechanism in the pathophysiology of neuroinflammation. Unlike other body parts, the relative inaccessibility of the brain and spine to traditional methods of clinical assessment creates a unique role for neuroimaging in the diagnosis of craniospinal infections.

We all are privileged to be the healer physicians to the highest form of life on earth—the human beings. However our existence is in a finely balanced symbiotic, harmonious, and synchronous relationship with ingenious human microbiota, which astonishingly contains 100 times the number of genes than the 20,000 contained in the human genome. The human microbiome is involved in many aspects of our physiology and is integrated with our immune system–based defense mechanisms. The NIH has launched an ambitious $115 million Human Microbiome Project to identify and characterize the microorganisms that are found in association with both healthy and diseased humans to test if changes in the human microbiome are associated with human health or disease. In this context, it is important to understand the spectrum of infectious conditions that continues to haunt us.

I am lucky to have a fine team of brilliant global contributors stretching from Singapore and India in the east to California in the west! The various articles encompass a wide variety of infectious conditions of the pediatric and adult population affecting the entire central nervous system, including the brain, the spine, and the head and neck. The volume also includes individual articles on the epidemiology, neuropathology, and neurosurgical treatment and, proudly, is a comprehensive compendium for infectious conditions of the central nervous system.

I express my sincere gratitude to all the authors for their outstanding contributions. The success of this edition is a reflection of their efforts and expertise. I would also like to thank Joanne Husovski and Sarah Barth from Elsevier for their patience and encouragement. I thank Michelle Wang and Caroline Novak for their beautiful illustrations. I am grateful to Suresh Mukherji for inviting me to be the guest editor of this volume. Last, I thank my caring parents, my beautiful and supportive wife, and my wonderful sons for their love and encouragement—they make it all worthwhile.

Gaurang Shah, MD
Department of Radiology
University of Michigan System Health System
1500 E. Medical Center Drive; Room B2A209F
Ann Arbor, MI 48109-5030, USA

E-mail address:
gvshah@med.umich.edu

neuroimaging.theclinics.com

Epidemiology of Central Nervous System Infection

James Riddell IV, MD[a],*, Emily K. Shuman, MD[b]

KEYWORDS

- Central nervous system infection • Epidemiology • Meningitis • Brain abscess

KEY POINTS

- The rapid recognition and diagnosis of central nervous system (CNS) infection is critical to achieving a favorable clinical outcome.
- Pathogens vary based on the location of infection within the CNS, geographic exposures, vaccination status, age, surgical intervention, and immune suppression.
- Knowledge of the organisms that are most commonly present in various types of CNS infection is important in the selection of appropriate empiric antimicrobial therapy.
- Treatment of most CNS infections should be initiated promptly with the guidance of an infectious diseases specialist.

INTRODUCTION

Central nervous system (CNS) infections remain an important cause of morbidity and mortality worldwide. In 2004, globally there were 340,000 deaths estimated by the World Health Organization to be related to meningitis, with an incidence of 700,000.[1] In the Americas there were approximately 13,000 deaths attributed to meningitis, which disproportionately affects those of low and middle income 12:1 when compared with individuals with high income.[1] There are many infectious pathogens known to cause CNS infection, including the broad categories of bacteria, viruses, fungi, mycobacteria, and parasites. In most cases, it is impossible for the radiologist with certainty to identify a specific organism as the cause of an observed radiographic abnormality in the CNS. However, the geography, exposures, season, and clinical information supplied in the medical record can significantly aid in developing a more specific differential diagnosis. This review discusses the epidemiology and typical pathogens associated with infection of the CNS including meningitis, brain abscess, epidural abscess, and postoperative complications of neurologic surgery, as well as human immunodeficiency virus HIV/AIDS.

MENINGITIS

Bacteria

When bacteria infect the CNS, in most cases an acute syndrome of headache, fever, nuchal rigidity, and change of mental status occurs. Meningitis caused by bacteria continues to be a significant clinical syndrome that requires rapid recognition and treatment by clinicians to prevent associated life-threatening complications. With the introduction of vaccination for certain pathogens, the epidemiology of bacterial meningitis has changed dramatically over the past 2 decades.

Financial disclosures: None.
[a] Division of Infectious Diseases, Department of Internal Medicine, University of Michigan Health System, 1500 East Medical Center Drive, 3120 Taubman Center, Ann Arbor, MI 48109-5378, USA; [b] Workforce Health and Safety Clinic, New York Presbyterian Hospital/Weill Cornell Medical College, 1319 York Avenue, New York, NY 10021, USA
* Corresponding author.
E-mail address: jriddell@med.umich.edu

Neuroimag Clin N Am 22 (2012) 543–556
doi:10.1016/j.nic.2012.05.003

The number of cases of meningitis caused by *Haemophilus influenzae* type B decreased by 94% after 1988 when the vaccine was introduced to a rate of 0.2 cases per 100,000.[2] Unvaccinated adults with nontypable *H influenzae* now make up the majority of cases. Meningitis caused by *Streptococcus pneumoniae* has decreased 30%, from 1.1 cases per 100,000 in the late 1990s to 0.79 per 100,000 in the period 2004 to 2005.[3] This decrease occurred after the introduction of the 7-valent conjugate pneumococcal vaccine for children, which was licensed in 2000. This decrease in incidence has extended to not only children but also adults, presumably secondary to herd immunity. However, other pneumococcal serotypes not covered in the vaccine are now being seen with increased frequency in certain locations.[4] Mortality rates attributable to pneumococcal meningitis have remained the same at around 21% for adults[2,3] and 8% for children. Other pathogens such as *Neisseria meningitidis* (0.6/100,000), Group B streptococcus (0.3/100,000), and *Listeria monocytogenes* (0.2/100,000) occur less frequently.

The patient's age and immune status affects the organism most likely to be present in bacterial meningitis (**Table 1**). While pneumococcus remains the most common in all age groups, organisms such as *Listeria* are more likely to be observed in older and immune-compromised patients. Group B streptococcus and gram-negative organisms such as *Escherichia coli* are most common in neonates who develop meningitis related to exposure to urogenital flora at the time of birth. Outbreaks of meningococcal meningitis occur under conditions of crowding. Clusters of cases have been reported on college campuses and with religious gatherings such as the Hajj.[5,6] For the Hajj, vaccination programs have been initiated such that visitors are required to have received the quadrivalent meningococcal vaccine, which has decreased the incidence of invasive infection substantially.[7] However, pilgrims often can still become colonized with *N meningitidis* and can therefore transmit the organism to household contacts on their return home, which has led to outbreaks in several European countries.[8] In 2000 there were 25 cases per 100,000 pilgrims to the Hajj from Singapore.[9] In addition, there was a subsequent attack rate of 18 cases per 100,000 in household contacts who were exposed to returning pilgrims. Therefore, there are now recommendations for household contacts of at-risk travelers to also receive the meningococcal vaccine.

The performance of a lumbar puncture is the first step in the evaluation of any patient suspected of meningitis or encephalitis. Imaging of the brain is often indicated in patients with neurologic deficits, immune-compromising conditions, or decreased level of consciousness. In one study, 45% of patients with bacterial meningitis met criteria for CNS imaging.[10] If a mass lesion is present, there is risk for brain herniation at the time of cerebrospinal fluid (CSF) withdrawal.

Viruses

CNS infections caused by viruses are often referred to as aseptic meningitis because traditional bacterial cultures from the CSF are negative. Patients tend to present in a subacute fashion with headache and fever. There are many viruses that can cause aseptic meningitis (**Table 2**). A study performed in Finland analyzing consecutive adult patients with aseptic meningitis found that 26% of cases were related to enteroviruses, 17% to herpes simplex virus (HSV)-2, and 8% related to varicella zoster virus (VZV).[11] Of patients with

Table 1
Bacterial/mycobacterial pathogens that commonly cause meningitis

Pathogen	Risk Factor	Incidence
Streptococcus pneumoniae	Day care, HIV infection	Most common
Neisseria meningitidis	Crowded conditions	Outbreaks
Haemophilus influenzae		Significantly less common after vaccination
Listeria monocytogenes	Immune compromise, elderly	Less common
Group B streptococcus	Neonates	Decreased with antenatal detection of group B streptococcus
Escherichia coli	Neonates	Less common
Mycobacterium tuberculosis	Exposure, older age, immune compromise	Rare

Table 2
Viral pathogens that commonly cause meningitis

Pathogen	Risk Factor	Incidence
Enteroviruses	Warm weather	Most common
Herpes simplex virus	Presence of latent virus	Common
Varicella zoster virus	Presence of latent virus, immune compromise	Occasional
West Nile virus	Mosquito borne	Outbreaks, declining in USA
La Crosse virus	Mosquito borne	Rare
Dengue	Mosquito borne	Regional outbreaks
Human herpesvirus 6	Immune compromise	Rare
Lymphocytic choriomeningitis	Exposure to contaminated rodent excreta	Rare
Powassan virus	Regional tick exposure	Very rare
Chikungunya virus	Regional mosquito exposure	Regional outbreaks
Rabies	Exposure to infected animals	Rare
Japanese encephalitis	Summer, Southeast Asia	Regional
Mumps	Setting of outbreak	Very rare
HIV	Unprotected sexual exposure	Rare
Adenovirus	Outbreaks	Rare
Influenza	Seasonal epidemics	Rare

encephalitis, VZV was found in 12% of cases and HSV-1 in 9%, with tick-borne viruses identified in 9%.[11] In 44% of patients, a specific cause was not confirmed. Because viral culture is difficult and insensitive, molecular testing via the polymerase chain reaction (PCR) from CSF has greatly aided in the diagnosis of meningitis caused by viruses.[12,13] With these techniques it has been shown that more than 90% of cases of aseptic meningitis are caused by enteroviruses in other studies.[14] Enterovirus infection typically occurs in the summer to fall months and is most common in children, although it is also the most common cause of aseptic meningitis in adults.[15] Outbreaks have been identified in various locations globally, including a large outbreak described in Taiwan in patients who also had associated hand-foot-and-mouth disease.[16]

Viral CNS infections often also can cause encephalitis. This situation occurs when there is infection of the brain parenchyma with associated inflammation, which is accompanied by changes in mental status and behavior, and sometimes reduced level of consciousness. Overall, it is estimated that there are 10.5 to 13.8 per 100,000 hospitalizations for children and 2.2 per 100,000 hospitalizations for adults for acute encephalitis syndrome.[17] In one review, from 1950 to 1981 in Minnesota, there were 7.4 per 100,000 hospitalizations for encephalitis, with

a specific virus identified in 25% of the cases.[18] Early in the study period mumps and arboviruses were most common. The epidemiology of viral meningitis and encephalitis has been significantly altered by vaccination. In the 1940s and 1950s, mumps virus was encountered as a cause of viral meningitis in 15% of cases.[19] Occasional outbreaks of mumps still occur; however, meningitis caused by this virus is now rare.[20] In the Minnesota study, no cases of mumps-related encephalitis occurred after 1972.[18]

Viruses transmitted by arthropod vectors that cause encephalitis and meningitis have become more common in recent years. During the summer of 1999, West Nile virus was recognized as having caused a widespread epidemic that began in New York City[21] and eventually spread across the United States along bird-migratory routes. In 2002 there were 2942 cases of neuroinvasive West Nile disease, which represented 71% of the cases of viral meningoencephalitis reported.[22] The incidence of West Nile–associated meningitis peaked in the late summer months during the years of increased incidence. As immunity has developed and the susceptible reservoir of bird populations has decreased, the incidence of West Nile encephalitis has decreased substantially in recent years. In 2009 there were only 373 cases of encephalitis or meningitis reported.[23]

There are a variety of other arthropod-transmitted viruses that can cause meningitis and that have certain geographic distributions. St. Louis encephalitis, La Crosse virus, and Eastern Equine encephalitis are endemic within the United States and are observed to cause disease sporadically, from 0.01 to 0.04 cases per 100,000.[24] Dengue is caused by a group of 4 viruses transmitted by mosquitoes and is a common cause of viral meningitis in tropical areas, particularly in South and Central America. The World Health Organization estimates that 50 million people are infected by dengue yearly. In the Americas in 2007 there were 890,000 cases reported, with 26,000 cases complicated by dengue hemorrhagic fever.[25] In recent history dengue has not been endemic in the United States; however, in 2009 28 cases of dengue were identified in individuals who either traveled to or lived in Key West, Florida.[26] Thus, as with West Nile virus, emerging pathogens are able to become endemic in new geographic locations including the United States.

Reactivation or new infection with herpes viruses can also lead to infection in the CNS. The diagnosis of these infections has also been transformed by the ability to apply molecular techniques such as the PCR, although occasional false-negative results may be obtained.[27] HSV-2 most commonly causes meningitis and can be associated with primary infection while HSV-1 can cause necrotizing encephalitis with significant neurologic sequelae. In a study performed in Sweden, there were 2.2 cases per million population of HSV-1–related encephalitis per year.[28] Attributable mortality was 14%, with 21% of surviving patients having developed a seizure disorder as sequelae. HSV-1 has also been linked to a recurrent, benign lymphocytic meningitis known as Mollaret meningitis, which is considered to be rare. In this syndrome patients present with recurrent aseptic meningitis in which HSV-1 DNA has been found in some patients.[29] In immune-compromised patients with solid organ transplantation or stem cell transplantation, human herpesvirus 6 (HHV-6) can cause meningitis or encephalitis when latent virus reactivates. Similarly, VZV can cause meningitis or encephalitis in immune-compromised patients when reactivation occurs in the setting of zoster or disseminated disease in those who are susceptible to primary infection.

Other less commonly encountered viruses are listed in Table 2 and include lymphocytic choriomeningitis virus, which can occur after exposure to contaminated rodent excreta. HIV infection can cause an aseptic meningitis–type syndrome at the time of acute infection and should be considered in patients with risk factors such as recent high-risk sexual contact. Neurologic disorders including aseptic meningitis have been described in up to 12% of patients who develop the acute retroviral syndrome associated with the acquisition of HIV infection.[30] The clinician also must be aware of outbreaks that are occurring in various geographic areas to which patients may have traveled or where they reside. Powassan virus is transmitted by ticks and can cause encephalitis.[31] This rare virus has been found to cause disease mostly in Maine, Vermont, and New York, where 7 cases were reported between 1999 and 2005.[32,33] In an outbreak of Chikungunya virus on La Reunion Island from 2005 to 2006, out of 274 patients evaluated 70% had symptoms of headache.[34] CNS symptoms have been reported rarely, but CNS pleocytosis has not been observed with this infection. Meningitis has rarely been reported as a complication of influenza. A large study conducted in Great Britain identified only 0.01% (21) of more than 141,000 patients with influenza-like illness who had developed this complication.[35]

Infection with the rabies virus leads to severe encephalitis and carries a very high mortality rate. The incidence of human infection with rabies has declined substantially in the United States, from 33 cases in 1946 to 3 cases in 2006.[36] Most cases of rabies occur after exposure to infected wild animals such as bats, skunks, raccoons, or foxes. In other locations globally, unvaccinated domestic dogs remain a significant reservoir for transmission.[37] Postexposure prophylaxis can be life-saving in circumstances of high-risk animal bites. Japanese encephalitis is another serious viral infection that is transmitted by mosquitoes in South East Asia during the late summer and fall months. The annual incidence is estimated to be 30,000 to 50,000 cases in endemic areas, with 10,000 to 15,000 associated deaths.[38] Vaccination is available to travelers who are at particularly high risk during times of peak transmission.

Fungi

CNS infections caused by fungi are generally considered to be rare and are mostly restricted to immune-compromised patients (Table 3). Fungal organisms tend to cause chronic lymphocytic meningitis with a prolonged course of symptoms. The most common fungal organism encountered that causes CNS infection is *Cryptococcus neoformans*. This organism is a form of yeast with a large characteristic polysaccharide capsule that has a particular predilection for infection of the CNS. Patients infected with HIV with $CD4^+$ T-cell counts of less than 100/μL have a reported incidence of infection of 6% to 13%.[39]

Table 3
Fungal organisms that commonly cause meningitis

Pathogen	Risk Factor	Incidence
Cryptococcus neoformans	Immune compromise, older age	Most common
Coccidioides immitis	Regional exposure	Regional
Blastomyces dermatitidis	Regional exposure, immune compromise	Rare
Histoplasma capsulatum	Regional exposure, immune compromise	Rare
Candida spp	Systemic infection	Rare
Aspergillus spp	Immune compromise, infection of structures adjacent to central nervous system	Rare
Zygomycetes	Immune compromise, infection of structures adjacent to central nervous system	Rare

Prolonged corticosteroid use consisting of greater than 20 mg prednisone per day also is a risk factor, particularly for those with solid organ transplantation. It has been estimated that 20% of patients who develop cryptococcal meningitis have no underlying risk factor.[40]

The second most common fungal organism to cause meningitis is *Coccidioides immitis*. This endemic fungal organism is found only in certain areas of the Sonoran desert in the southwestern United States and in certain areas of southern California. One-third to one-half of patients who have disseminated infection will develop meningitis.[41] Immune-compromised patients are at higher risk for CNS infection. In one study from Tucson, Arizona, 27% of patients who had *Coccidioides* meningitis were found to have HIV infection complicated by AIDS.[42]

Other fungal organisms are much less commonly observed to cause meningitis. *Candida* spp rarely invade the CNS in cases of intravenous drug use or in cases of systemic candidiasis in the setting of neutropenia. Other endemic fungi-related conditions such as blastomycosis or histoplasmosis also rarely invade the CNS and can lead to chronic meningitis or intraparenchymal CNS lesions. Finally, filamentous fungi such as *Aspergillus*, Zygomycetes, dematiaceous molds, and others all have been reported to cause CNS disease, mostly in instances of direct inoculation from trauma or direct extension from infection in adjacent structures such as the sinuses in patients with underlying diabetes or severe immune compromise.

Mycobacteria

Tuberculosis (TB) is the most common cause of CNS infection by mycobacteria. Meningitis caused by *Mycobacterium tuberculosis* tends to be characterized as a chronic process with chronic headache and a lymphocytic pleocytosis on CSF analysis. Tuberculosis cases increased substantially on a global scale when the HIV/AIDS epidemic began. In South Africa, of 60 patients presenting with meningitis type symptoms, 66% were infected by HIV and 9 had tuberculous meningitis.[43] Since the 1990s in the United States, cases of TB have declined from 25,000 per year to 12,000 in 2008.[44] 2000 of those cases were documented to be extrapulmonary TB, of which a fraction are cases of CNS infection. In a study from Denmark performed between 1988 and 2000 there were 20 patients with tuberculous meningitis,[45] more than half of whom had come from countries of high TB endemicity. CNS infection with other atypical mycobacteria has not been commonly reported.

Parasites

Meningitis caused by parasitic organisms is rare. The organism most often associated is *Strongyloides stercoralis*, which can occasionally cause meningitis as part of the hyperinfection syndrome (Table 4). Free-living amoeba such as *Naegleria*

Table 4
Parasites that can cause meningitis

Pathogen	Risk Factor	Incidence
Strongyloides stercoralis	Regional exposure, immune compromise	Rare
Naegleria fowleri	Warm fresh water	Very rare
Angiostrongylus cantonensis	Regional exposure	Rare

fowleri or Acanthamoeba can cause a rapidly fatal granulomatous meningoencephalitis. Although uncommon, occasional clusters of cases can be associated with children or young adults who swim in contaminated warm freshwater lakes. One study in Florida documented only 5 cases over 14 years, even though 58% of lakes were found to be contaminated with the organism.[46,47] The larvae of the rat lungworm Angiostrongylus cantonensis, which is endemic to the tropics and southeast Asia, can cause an eosinophilic meningitis when humans become an accidental host, usually through ingesting contaminated mollusks. Worms that migrate through the CNS cause brain inflammation, resulting in neurologic sequelae such as cranial nerve paralysis. The epidemiology has not been systematically studied; however, approximately 2500 cases have been reported in the literature from various geographic locations including Hawaii and New Orleans, Louisiana.[48]

Other Organisms

A variety of organisms in other categories have also been associated with CNS infection (Table 5). In the United States there are approximately 15,000 cases of Lyme disease, caused by infection with Borrelia burgdorferi, which is transmitted by ticks primarily in the northeastern states. Up to 15% of patients who are untreated will develop acute neuroborreliosis, which leads to chronic lymphocytic meningitis. Chronic CNS infection can occur in up to 5% of patients if left untreated.[49] Syphilis can infect almost any organ including the CNS. Meningitis should be suspected particularly in patients with HIV infection with secondary syphilis. Most experts recommend lumbar puncture even in asymptomatic HIV-infected patients, because

treatment strategies differ in patients with CNS involvement.[50] Leptospirosis is one of the most common zoonoses. The spirochete is transmitted from animals to humans, usually by exposure to fresh water contaminated with infected animal urine. The organism can cause a multisystem illness in the first phase. In the second phase, an immune-mediated aseptic meningitis can develop in up to 80% of patients with a CSF lymphocytic pleocytosis.[51] Over a 4-year period, 18 cases of CNS leptospirosis were identified in California when serology was retrospectively performed on patients with aseptic meningitis.[52] Meningitis can also occur in the setting of infection with various rickettsial organisms. Rocky Mountain spotted fever, a tick-borne illness caused by Rickettsia rickettsii, can cause symptoms of meningismus in up to 18% of affected patients. Long-term neurologic sequelae were commonly detected, suggesting frequent CNS infection with this organism.[53] Murine typhus, which is caused by Rickettsia typhi and is transmitted by fleas, can also rarely present with meningitis.[54]

BRAIN ABSCESS AND MASS LESIONS
Bacteria

Bacteria, mycobacteria, fungi, or parasites may invade the parenchyma of the brain, either from direct spread from adjacent sites of infection, trauma, or surgery, or through hematogenous seeding in the setting of bacteremia (Table 6). Direct spread of bacteria typically results in a solitary brain abscess, whereas bacteremia more often results in multiple abscesses. Direct spread from adjacent sites of infection accounts for 20% to 70% of cases of brain abscess, depending on the case series.[55,56] The most common primary

---

Table 5
Other organisms that can cause meningitis

Pathogen	Risk Factor	Incidence
Borrelia burgdorferi (Lyme)	Regional tick exposure	Regional
Treponema pallidum (syphilis)	Sexual transmission	Common with HIV coinfection
Leptospirosis	Contaminated fresh water	Regional
Rickettsia rickettsii	Tick borne	Regional
Rickettsia typhi	Fleas	Regional
Rickettsia prowazekii	Lice	Regional, epidemic
Rickettsia tsutsugamushi	Mites	Regional
Ehrlichia spp	Tick borne	Regional
Bartonella henselae	Cat-scratch	Rare
Coxiella burnetii	Contact with infectious material from infected animals	Rare

Table 6
Microorganisms that can cause brain abscess or mass lesion

Pathogen	Risk Factor	Incidence
Anaerobic bacteria: anaerobic streptococci, *Prevotella melaninogenica*, *Propionibacterium* spp, *Fusobacterium* spp, *Eubacterium* spp, *Veillonella* spp, *Actinomyces* spp, *Bacteroides* spp	Oral or otolaryngologic infection (contiguous spread) or intra-abdominal or pelvic infection (hematogenous spread)	Isolated in culture in >50% of patients with brain abscess in some case series
Gram-positive aerobic bacteria: Viridans streptococci, *Streptococcus milleri*, microaerophilic streptococci, *Staphylococcus aureus*, *Rhodococcus equi*, *Listeria monocytogenes*, *Nocardia asteroides*	Endocarditis, thoracic or abdominal infection, surgery, trauma, immunosuppression (*Rhodococcus*, *Listeria*, and *Nocardia*)	Most common aerobic organisms isolated from culture
Gram-negative aerobic bacteria: *Klebsiella* spp, *Pseudomonas* spp, *Escherichia coli*, *Proteus* spp, *Haemophilus* spp	Otogenic infection, trauma, surgery, liver abscess (*Klebsiella*)	Much less common than anaerobes or gram-positive aerobes
Mycobacteria: *Mycobacterium tuberculosis*	Residence in region with high incidence of tuberculosis	Exceedingly rare in developed world
Fungi: *Aspergillus* spp, *Mucor* spp, *Rhizopus* spp, *Candida* spp, *Cryptococcus neoformans*, *Coccidioides immitis*	Immunosuppression	
Parasites: *Toxoplasma gondii*, *Taenia solium* (pork tapeworm), *Schistosoma* spp, *Paragonimus* spp, *Echinococcus* spp	HIV infection (*Toxoplasma*), residence in endemic area (other parasites)	Incidence of *Toxoplasma* infection declining with use of antiretroviral therapy; neurocysticercosis due to *Taenia solium* most common cause of brain infection and seizures in some endemic areas

bacterial infections that may spread directly to the brain include subacute or chronic otitis media or mastoiditis, frontal or ethmoid sinusitis, and dental infection. Otitis media and mastoiditis have become less common sources of brain abscess in developing countries with increasing use of antimicrobials, with only 0.24% of individuals in a large series of patients with suppurative otitis media developing intracranial infection (meningitis or brain abscess).[57] Trauma to the face or skull can occasionally result in brain abscess, particularly when there is involvement of a foreign body such as a bullet. Delayed abscess formation has been reported with retained foreign bodies such as pencil tips that have penetrated the dura as a result

of orbital penetration.[58] Brain abscess may also occur as a complication of neurosurgical procedures, discussed in more detail in a later section.

Hematogenous spread of infection is presumably responsible for the remainder of brain abscesses caused by bacteria. Bacterial endocarditis is a common cause of brain abscess, which complicates 2% to 4% of cases.[59] Other underlying infections that may lead to development of hematogenous brain abscesses include chronic pulmonary infections, particularly in patients with underlying cystic fibrosis or bronchiectasis, skin infections, and intra-abdominal and pelvic infections.[60,61] Certain underlying conditions, including cyanotic congenital heart disease and pulmonary arteriovenous malformations, predispose to development of hematogenous brain abscesses.[62,63] In patients with pulmonary arteriovenous malformations, the incidence of brain abscess may be as high as 10%. Certain procedures, such as gastrointestinal endoscopy, which may produce transient bacteremia, can result in development of brain abscesses.[64] In 20% to 40% of cases of apparent hematogenous brain abscess, no primary source of infection is apparent.[65]

The bacterial pathogens most commonly associated with brain abscess are anaerobes, which typically arise from the normal microbiota of the mouth and upper respiratory tract and cause brain abscess by contiguous spread of infection. In one case series, anaerobes were isolated in culture from 52.4% of patients with brain abscess, either alone or in combination with aerobic bacteria.[66] The most commonly isolated anaerobes isolated from brain abscesses include anaerobic streptococci, *Prevotella melaninogenica*, *Propionibacterium* species, *Fusobacterium* species, *Eubacterium* species, *Veillonella* species, and *Actinomyces* species.[66,67] *Bacteroides* species are also isolated relatively frequently from brain abscesses, and can be associated with intraabdominal or pelvic infection.

Many aerobic bacteria are also commonly isolated from brain abscesses. Frequently identified aerobic gram-positive cocci include viridians streptococci, *Streptococcus milleri*, microaerophilic streptococci, and *Staphylococcus aureus*. *S milleri* is a particularly common cause of brain abscess, with hematogenous spread to the brain often arising from the thoracic or abdominal cavities.[68] *S aureus* is a frequently identified pathogen in brain abscesses that form after neurosurgical procedures or trauma.[69] The gram-positive rod *Rhodococcus equi* can cause brain abscess in immunocompromised hosts but has also been reported in an immunocompetent host.[70] Another gram-positive rod, *Listeria monocytogenes*, a common contaminant of food products, can cause single or multiple brain or brainstem abscesses. This lesion primarily occurs in patients who are immunocompromised because of use of corticosteroids, and is associated with high mortality.[71] A gram-positive, partially acid-fast soil organism, *Nocardia asteroides*, initially causes pulmonary infection and then often can cause brain abscesses via hematogenous spread in immunocompromised patients.[72]

Gram-negative bacilli are typically isolated from brain abscesses in the setting of otogenic infection, trauma, or prior surgery.[73] Commonly isolated pathogens in this category include *Klebsiella*, *Pseudomonas*, *E coli*, *Proteus*, and *Haemophilus*. *Klebsiella pneumoniae* brain abscess can occur as metastatic infection related to a primary liver abscess.[74] This phenomenon has primarily been reported in patients in Southeast Asia, and often manifests with ocular involvement of infection as well.

Mycobacteria

Although tuberculous meningitis is more common, *M tuberculosis* can also cause intracranial mass lesions known as tuberculomas. Intracranial tuberculomas are rare in the developed world but are frequently encountered in regions where the incidence of TB is high. For example, in some parts of Asia tuberculomas account for 20% to 30% of intracranial space-occupying lesions in children.[75] Intracranial tuberculomas develop as a result of hematogenous dissemination in primary infection or reactivation of infection, and typically present with focal neurologic deficits. As with meningitis, mass lesions of the brain caused by atypical mycobacteria have not been commonly reported.

Fungi

Aspergillus species, which are ubiquitous environmental molds, can cause intracranial mass lesions in immunocompromised patients. Risk factors include prolonged corticosteroid use, prolonged neutropenia, hematopoietic stem cell transplantation, and solid organ transplantation.[76] Infection typically results from hematogenous dissemination from the lungs but may also occur as a complication of fungal sinusitis, particularly in neutropenic patients.[77] Similarly, fungi in the order Mucorales (*Rhizopus*, *Mucor*, and *Rhizomucor*) can cause intracranial mass lesions in the setting of chronic sinusitis, most commonly in patients with underlying diabetes mellitus.[78] Other molds such as *Scedosporium apiospermum* have been reported to cause brain abscess in the setting of underlying immunosuppression.[79] In one series of 1620 transplant patients, there were 17 cases of fungal brain abscess, most commonly attributable to *Aspergillus* species.[79] Altered mental status was the most common presenting feature, and prognosis was very poor.

Candida species more often cause meningitis in immunosuppressed patients, but multiple small intracranial abscesses can occur as a result of disseminated infection.[80] Risk factors for CNS candidiasis (described earlier) also include recent surgery. Similarly, *Cryptococcus neoformans*, which causes meningitis in immunosuppressed patients, can also result in formation of intracranial mass lesions known as cryptococcomas, although this is uncommon. Most patients who develop intracranial cryptococcomas are immunosuppressed because of HIV/AIDS, corticosteroid use, malignancy, or chronic liver disease, but cases have been reported in immunocompetent patients.[81] Intracranial mass lesions have also been described rarely in patients with disseminated infection caused by *Coccidioides immitis*, with underlying diabetes mellitus identified as a possible risk factor.[82]

Parasites

The intracellular protozoan parasite *Toxoplasma gondii* is a common cause of intracranial mass lesions in HIV-infected individuals, and is primarily seen in those patients with CD4 counts of less than 100 cells/mm³. Primary infection with *Toxoplasma*, which is generally asymptomatic, typically occurs through contact with felines or ingestion of undercooked meat. Seropositivity ranges from 15% in the United States to more than 50% in parts of Europe. CNS infection typically involves reactivation of preexisting infection.[83] The incidence of CNS toxoplasmosis in HIV patients in the United States decreased from 3.8 cases per 1000 person-years in the early 1990s to 2.2 cases per 1000 person-years in the late 1990s, most likely as a result of widespread use of antiretroviral therapy.[84] Typical clinical manifestations of CNS toxoplasmosis include headache, confusion, fever, focal neurologic deficits, and seizures.

Other parasites account for the most common causes of brain abscess in patients who previously lived outside the United States. Neurocysticercosis, caused by infection with the larval stage of the pork tapeworm *Taenia solium*, is responsible for 85% of brain infections in Mexico City and is the most common cause of seizures in this population.[85] Many cases of neurocysticercosis likely remain asymptomatic, as it is common to find lesions consistent with this disease incidentally on neuroimaging.

Other parasitic infections in endemic areas may also have CNS involvement. Brain abscess caused by the protozoan intestinal parasite *Entamoeba histolytica* has been reported in the setting of concomitant liver abscess.[86] Infection with *Schistosoma* species can lead to mass lesions in the CNS when eggs enter the vertebral venous plexus and embolize to the brain or spinal cord, or when adult worms migrate to these locations.[87] Worldwide, more than 200 million individuals have schistosomiasis, but CNS infection is rare. *Schistosoma mansoni* and *Schistosoma haematobium*, which are endemic in Africa and the Middle East (as well as South America and the Caribbean for *S mansoni*), more commonly cause spinal cord lesions, whereas *Schistosoma japonicum*, which is endemic in Asia, is more commonly associated with brain lesions. The lung fluke *Paragonimus*, which is endemic in parts of Central and South America, West Africa, and Asia, is associated with brain abscess in fewer than 1% of symptomatic cases.[88] CNS involvement almost always occurs in patients younger than 30 years, and is caused by direct invasion of the meninges and brain parenchyma. Tapeworms belonging to the genus *Echinococcus*, which cause hydatid cyst disease in endemic areas including the Middle East and Central and South America, can occasionally cause intraparenchymal brain cysts in 1% to 3% of cases.[80]

EPIDURAL ABSCESS

The epidural space can become infected by 3 major pathways: hematogenous spread of bacteria, direct inoculation as a result of trauma or a surgical intervention, or direct extension of infection from an adjacent source. Of patients who suffered intracranial infection as a complication of sinusitis, epidural abscess was the most common complication, occurring in 23% of cases where an intracranial complication was identified.[90] Several studies have suggested that the incidence of epidural abscess has increased over the past 10 to 15 years. In one study from 1983 to 1992 there was a significant increase at one institution from fewer than 10 cases per year to more than 100,[91] which has been confirmed in other studies.[92] An incidence of 1.96 per 10,000 hospital admissions was found in another single-center study.[93] It has been postulated that the increasing incidence is likely a result of increased intravenous drug use during these periods as well as an increase in spinal surgical procedures. Based on the mechanism of entry, the organisms usually present in these types of infections consist of *S aureus* (30%–60%), coagulase-negative staphylococci (4%–60%), *E coli* (4%) and, less commonly, other gram-negative bacteria and mycobacteria such as TB.[91,94] Risk factors associated with the development of spinal epidural abscess include older age, prolonged epidural catheter usage, intravenous drug use, and diabetes. In one study of patients with cancer who received long-term epidural pain management with indwelling catheters, 11 of 91 patients developed epidural abscess as a complication of their treatment.[94] Prolonged use of epidural catheters and significant comorbidity likely contributed to the high rate of infection in this study. Others have reported much lower rates of infection complicating epidural catheter use, in the range of 4.3% to 0.6%.[94] In another report, none of 1062 patients who used epidural anesthesia for a brief period of less than 14 days developed a serious infectious complication.[95]

POSTOPERATIVE INFECTIONS OF THE CENTRAL NERVOUS SYSTEM

Infection of the CNS often occurs as a consequence of brain, spine, or otolaryngologic surgery. Postoperative wound infection after intracranial neurosurgery may manifest as meningitis, brain abscess, subdural empyema, or epidural abscess, with meningitis and brain abscess being most common.[96] Rates of postoperative wound infection after intracranial neurosurgery range from less than 1% to more than 6% in North America and Europe. Risk factors for postoperative wound infection after craniotomy include emergency surgery, contamination of the surgical field, prolonged operative duration, and recent neurosurgery.[97] In one large series, the most commonly identified causative organisms in wound infection after craniotomy were S aureus, coagulase-negative staphylococci, streptococci, Enterobacteriaceae, Acinetobacter species, and Pseudomonas aeruginosa.[97]

Intracranial infection may also occur after implantation of indwelling devices such as ventriculoperitoneal (VP) shunts. Infection rates after VP shunt placement have been reported to range from 5% to 15% and are highest in the first month after shunt placement.[98] Approximately one-half of VP shunt infections are caused by coagulase-negative staphylococci and an additional one-third by S aureus. The remainder is due to diphtheroids, gram-negative bacilli, anaerobes, and fungi.

The rate of postoperative infection after spinal surgery varies with the type of surgical procedure, and ranges from less than 1% with simple laminectomy to 7% to 20% with presence of spinal instrumentation.[99] Risk factors for infection are similar to those for other types of surgery and include obesity, smoking, diabetes, immunosuppression, prior spinal surgery, prolonged operative duration, and surgery in the setting of trauma. Most infections that occur after spinal surgery manifest as superficial wound infection, diskitis, or osteomyelitis, and do not involve the CNS. However, epidural abscess has been reported as a complication of spinal surgery.[100] The most common organism to cause postoperative infection after spinal surgery is S aureus, which is isolated in more than 50% of cases.[99] Other common causative organisms include coagulase-negative staphylococci and gram-negative bacilli (especially in cases of trauma). Meningitis and epidural abscess have also been reported after use of epidural analgesia.[101]

Meningitis and brain abscess may complicate otolaryngologic surgery, particularly if there is endoscopic instrumentation of the sinuses. CSF leak is common after sinus surgery and is associated with a risk of meningitis of 10% per year.[102] Meningitis may complicate sinus surgery as a result of dural tear or vascular or lymphatic migration of organisms. Brain abscess after sinus surgery is much less common, and is more likely to occur as a result of chronic sinusitis rather than surgical intervention. Responsible organisms include those typically associated with meningitis and brain abscess in the setting of sinusitis (see earlier discussion).

HIV/AIDS

Because of the specific defects in cell-mediated immunity as well as B-cell dysfunction that occurs with HIV/AIDS, this population of patients is at risk for certain CNS infections. This risk can be stratified by the CD4$^+$ T-cell count as well as other factors such as geography, exposures, and intravenous drug use. Patients infected with HIV but with CD4 counts that are in the normal range are at higher risk for pneumococcal infection, including meningitis, because of abnormalities that are present in humoral immunity. Infection with the encapsulated S pneumoniae organism remains the most common bacterial pathogen in this population.[103] Patients from TB-endemic areas or who have had exposures to individuals with pulmonary disease are at high risk for infection. Extrapulmonary disease is most often observed in HIV-infected patients when compared with those who are HIV seronegative.[104] Regardless of CD4 cell count, patients who inject intravenous drugs under nonsterile conditions are at risk for bacteremia, endocarditis, and brain abscess as well as epidural abscess. When the CD4 cell count drops below 100 cells/mL (<200 cells/mL defined as AIDS), patients are at higher risk for infection with Cryptococcus, which can cause meningitis or, less commonly, parenchymal mass lesions (cryptococcoma).[105] In this range, patients are also at risk for reactivation of toxoplasmosis in the CNS, which most often presents with multiple ring-enhancing lesions. Toxoplasmosis is the most common infection to cause a focal mass lesion in this population.[106] Patients with CD4 cell counts of less than 50 cells/mL are at risk for a host of opportunistic infections because of profound immune dysfunction. Infiltrative-type CNS lesions without mass effect observed in this population can include progressive multifocal leukoencephalopathy associated with the JC virus, AIDS-related dementia complex, and cytomegalovirus encephalitis. Mass lesions can be caused by CNS lymphoma, toxoplasmosis or, less commonly, endemic fungi such as *Histoplasma* or filamentous fungi such as *Aspergillus*.

SUMMARY

Infections of the CNS often lead to significant morbidity and mortality if not recognized and treated promptly. Therefore, it is imperative for appropriate therapy to be initiated quickly when CNS infection is suspected. Such therapy is often initially empiric and therefore requires knowledge of the types of organisms commonly present in such infections. The pathogens involved in CNS infections as well as the incidence is continually changing, based on a variety of factors including vaccination, international travel, and the increased use of immune-suppressive drugs. If the radiologist who observes a particular CNS lesion suspected to be related to infection can provide an inclusive differential diagnosis, this information can significantly aid the treating physicians who care for complex patients with CNS infection.

REFERENCES

1. Mathers C, Boerma T, Ma Fat D. The global burden of disease: 2004 update. World Health Organization 2008;1–146.
2. Schuchat A, Robinson K, Wenger JD, et al. Bacterial meningitis in the United States in 1995. Active Surveillance Team. N Engl J Med 1997;337(14): 970–6.
3. Hsu HE, Shutt KA, Moore MR, et al. Effect of pneumococcal conjugate vaccine on pneumococcal meningitis. N Engl J Med 2009;360(3):244–56.
4. Lehmann D, Willis J, Moore HC, et al. The changing epidemiology of invasive pneumococcal disease in aboriginal and non-aboriginal western Australians from 1997 through 2007 and emergence of non-vaccine serotypes. Clin Infect Dis 2010;50(11): 1477–86.
5. Butler KM. Meningococcal meningitis prevention programs for college students: a review of the literature. Worldviews Evid Based Nurs 2006;3(4):185–93.
6. al-Gahtani YM, el Bushra HE, al-Qarawi SM, et al. Epidemiological investigation of an outbreak of meningococcal meningitis in Makkah (Mecca), Saudi Arabia, 1992. Epidemiol Infect 1995;115(3): 399–409.
7. Ahmed QA, Barbeschi M, Memish ZA. The quest for public health security at Hajj: the WHO guidelines on communicable disease alert and response during mass gatherings. Travel Med Infect Dis 2009;7(4):226–30.
8. Aguilera JF, Perrocheau A, Meffre C, et al. Outbreak of serogroup W135 meningococcal disease after the Hajj pilgrimage, Europe, 2000. Emerg Infect Dis 2002;8(8):761–7.
9. Wilder-Smith A. W135 meningococcal carriage in association with the Hajj pilgrimage 2001: the Singapore experience. Int J Antimicrob Agents 2003;21(2):112–5.
10. van de Beek D, de Gans J, Spanjaard L, et al. Clinical features and prognostic factors in adults with bacterial meningitis. N Engl J Med 2004;351(18): 1849–59.
11. Kupila L, Vuorinen T, Vainionpaa R, et al. Etiology of aseptic meningitis and encephalitis in an adult population. Neurology 2006;66(1):75–80.
12. van Vliet KE, Glimaker M, Lebon P, et al. Multi-center evaluation of the Amplicor Enterovirus PCR test with cerebrospinal fluid from patients with aseptic meningitis. The European Union Concerted Action on Viral Meningitis and Encephalitis. J Clin Microbiol 1998;36(9):2652–7.
13. Archimbaud C, Chambon M, Bailly JL, et al. Impact of rapid enterovirus molecular diagnosis on the management of infants, children, and adults with aseptic meningitis. J Med Virol 2009;81(1):42–8.
14. Irani DN. Aseptic meningitis and viral myelitis. Neurol Clin 2008;26(3):635–55, vii–viii.
15. Peigue-Lafeuille H, Croquez N, Laurichesse H, et al. Enterovirus meningitis in adults in 1999-2000 and evaluation of clinical management. J Med Virol 2002;67(1):47–53.
16. Ho M, Chen ER, Hsu KH, et al. An epidemic of enterovirus 71 infection in Taiwan. Taiwan Enterovirus Epidemic Working Group. N Engl J Med 1999;341(13):929–35.
17. Jmor F, Emsley HC, Fischer M, et al. The incidence of acute encephalitis syndrome in Western industrialised and tropical countries. Virol J 2008; 5:134.
18. Beghi E, Nicolosi A, Kurland LT, et al. Encephalitis and aseptic meningitis, Olmsted County, Minnesota, 1950-1981: I. Epidemiology. Ann Neurol 1984;16(3): 283–94.
19. Meyer HM Jr, Johnson RT, Crawford IP, et al. Central nervous system syndromes of "vital" etiology. A study of 713 cases. Am J Med 1960;29:334–47.
20. Centers for Disease Control and Prevention (CDC). Update: mumps outbreak—New York and New Jersey, June 2009-January 2010. MMWR Morb Mortal Wkly Rep 2010;59(5):125–9.
21. Mostashari F, Bunning ML, Kitsutani PT, et al. Epidemic West Nile encephalitis, New York, 1999: results of a household-based seroepidemiological survey. Lancet 2001;358(9278):261–4.
22. O'Leary DR, Marfin AA, Montgomery SP, et al. The epidemic of West Nile virus in the United States, 2002. Vector Borne Zoonotic Dis 2004;4(1):61–70.

23. Centers for Disease Control and Prevention (CDC). Final 2009 West Nile virus activity in the United States. 2010.

24. Centers for Disease Control and Prevention (CDC). Summary of notifiable diseases, United States, 1998. MMWR Morb Mortal Wkly Rep 1999;47(53):1–85.

25. World Health Organization. DengueNet. 2010.

26. Centers for Disease Control and Prevention (CDC). Locally acquired dengue—Key West, Florida, 2009-2010. MMWR Morb Mortal Wkly Rep 2010; 59(19):577–81.

27. Weil AA, Glaser CA, Amad Z, et al. Patients with suspected herpes simplex encephalitis: rethinking an initial negative polymerase chain reaction result. Clin Infect Dis 2002;34(8):1154–7.

28. Hjalmarsson A, Blomqvist P, Skoldenberg B. Herpes simplex encephalitis in Sweden, 1990-2001: incidence, morbidity, and mortality. Clin Infect Dis 2007;45(7):875–80.

29. Yamamoto LJ, Tedder DG, Ashley R, et al. Herpes simplex virus type 1 DNA in cerebrospinal fluid of a patient with Mollaret's meningitis. N Engl J Med 1991;325(15):1082–5.

30. Niu MT, Jermano JA, Reichelderfer P, et al. Summary of the National Institutes of Health workshop on primary human immunodeficiency virus type 1 infection. AIDS Res Hum Retroviruses 1993;9(9):913–24.

31. Romero JR, Simonsen KA. Powassan encephalitis and Colorado tick fever. Infect Dis Clin North Am 2008;22(3):545–59, x.

32. Hinten SR, Beckett GA, Gensheimer KF, et al. Increased recognition of Powassan encephalitis in the United States, 1999-2005. Vector Borne Zoonotic Dis 2008;8(6):733–40.

33. From the Centers for Disease Control and Prevention. Outbreak of Powassan encephalitis—Maine and Vermont, 1999-2001. JAMA 2001;286(16):1962–3.

34. Staikowsky F, Talarmin F, Grivard P, et al. Prospective study of Chikungunya virus acute infection in the Island of La Reunion during the 2005-2006 outbreak. PLoS One 2009;4(10):e7603.

35. Meier CR, Napalkov PN, Wegmuller Y, et al. Population-based study on incidence, risk factors, clinical complications and drug utilisation associated with influenza in the United Kingdom. Eur J Clin Microbiol Infect Dis 2000;19(11):834–42.

36. Manning SE, Rupprecht CE, Fishbein D, et al. Human rabies prevention—United States, 2008: recommendations of the Advisory Committee on Immunization Practices. MMWR Recomm Rep 2008;57(RR-3):1–28.

37. Madhusudana SN, Sukumaran SM. Antemortem diagnosis and prevention of human rabies. Ann Indian Acad Neurol 2008;11(1):3–12.

38. Endy TP, Nisalak A. Japanese encephalitis virus: ecology and epidemiology. Curr Top Microbiol Immunol 2002;267:11–48.

39. Gottfredsson M, Perfect JR. Fungal meningitis. Semin Neurol 2000;20(3):307–22.

40. Pappas PG, Perfect JR, Cloud GA, et al. Cryptococcosis in Human Immunodeficiency Virus-negative patients in the era of effective Azole therapy. Clin Infect Dis 2001;33:690–9.

41. Bouza E, Dreyer JS, Hewitt WL, et al. Coccidioidal meningitis. An analysis of thirty-one cases and review of the literature. Medicine (Baltimore) 1981;60(3):139–72.

42. Bronnimann DA, Adam RD, Galgiani JN, et al. Coccidioidomycosis in the acquired immunodeficiency syndrome. Ann Intern Med 1987;106(3): 372–9.

43. Silber E, Sonnenberg P, Ho KC, et al. Meningitis in a community with a high prevalence of tuberculosis and HIV infection. J Neurol Sci 1999;162(1): 20–6.

44. CDC. Reported tuberculosis in the United States, 2008. Department of Health and Human Services, CDC; 2009.

45. Bidstrup C, Andersen PH, Skinhoj P, et al. Tuberculous meningitis in a country with a low incidence of tuberculosis: still a serious disease and a diagnostic challenge. Scand J Infect Dis 2002;34(11):811–4.

46. Wellings FM, Amuso PT, Chang SL, et al. Isolation and identification of pathogenic Naegleria from Florida lakes. Appl Environ Microbiol 1977;34(6): 661–7.

47. Wellings FM, Lewis AL, Amuso PT, et al. Naegleria and water sports. Lancet 1977;1(8004):199–200.

48. Kliks MM, Palumbo NE. Eosinophilic meningitis beyond the Pacific Basin: the global dispersal of a peridomestic zoonosis caused by Angiostrongylus cantonensis, the nematode lungworm of rats. Soc Sci Med 1992;34(2):199–212.

49. Steere AC. Lyme disease. N Engl J Med 2001; 345(2):115–25.

50. Workowski KA, Berman SM. Centers for Disease Control and Prevention sexually transmitted diseases treatment guidelines. Clin Infect Dis 2007;44(Suppl 3):S73–6.

51. Berman SJ, Tsai CC, Holmes K, et al. Sporadic anicteric leptospirosis in South Vietnam. A study in 150 patients. Ann Intern Med 1973;79(2):167–73.

52. Hubbert WT, Humphrey GL. Epidemiology of leptospirosis in California: a cause of aseptic meningitis. Calif Med 1968;108(2):113–7.

53. Archibald LK, Sexton DJ. Long-term sequelae of Rocky Mountain spotted fever. Clin Infect Dis 1995;20(5):1122–5.

54. Galanakis E, Gikas A, Bitsori M, et al. Rickettsia typhi infection presenting as subacute meningitis. J Child Neurol 2002;17(2):156–7.

55. Chun CH, Johnson JD, Hofstetter M, et al. Brain abscess. A study of 45 consecutive cases. Medicine (Baltimore) 1986;65(6):415–31.

56. Yen PT, Chan ST, Huang TS. Brain abscess: with special reference to otolaryngologic sources of infection. Otolaryngol Head Neck Surg 1995; 113(1):15–22.

57. Kangsanarak J, Fooanant S, Ruckphaopunt K, et al. Extracranial and intracranial complications of suppurative otitis media. Report of 102 cases. J Laryngol Otol 1993;107(11):999–1004.

58. Seider N, Gilboa M, Lautman E, et al. Delayed presentation of orbito-cerebral abscess caused by pencil-tip injury. Ophthal Plast Reconstr Surg 2006;22(4):316–7.

59. Corral I, Martin-Davila P, Fortun J, et al. Trends in neurological complications of endocarditis. J Neurol 2007;254(9):1253–9.

60. Fischer EG, Shwachman H, Wepsic JG. Brain abscess and cystic fibrosis. J Pediatr 1979;95(3): 385–8.

61. Kum N, Charles D. Cerebral abscess associated with an intrauterine contraceptive device. Obstet Gynecol 1979;54(3):375–8.

62. Takeshita M, Kagawa M, Yato S, et al. Current treatment of brain abscess in patients with congenital cyanotic heart disease. Neurosurgery 1997;41(6): 1270–8 [discussion: 1278–9].

63. White RI Jr, Lynch-Nyhan A, Terry P, et al. Pulmonary arteriovenous malformations: techniques and long-term outcome of embolotherapy. Radiology 1988;169(3):663–9.

64. Schlaeffer F, Riesenberg K, Mikolich D, et al. Serious bacterial infections after endoscopic procedures. Arch Intern Med 1996;156(5):572–4.

65. Yang SY, Zhao CS. Review of 140 patients with brain abscess. Surg Neurol 1993;39(4):290–6.

66. Le Moal G, Landron C, Grollier G, et al. Characteristics of brain abscess with isolation of anaerobic bacteria. Scand J Infect Dis 2003; 35(5):318–21.

67. Brook I. Aerobic and anaerobic bacteriology of intracranial abscesses. Pediatr Neurol 1992;8(3): 210–4.

68. Jacobs JA, Pietersen HG, Stobberingh EE, et al. Bacteremia involving the "Streptococcus milleri" group: analysis of 19 cases. Clin Infect Dis 1994; 19(4):704–13.

69. Schliamser SE, Backman K, Norrby SR. Intracranial abscesses in adults: an analysis of 54 consecutive cases. Scand J Infect Dis 1988;20(1):1–9.

70. Corne P, Rajeebally I, Jonquet O. Rhodococcus equi brain abscess in an immunocompetent patient. Scand J Infect Dis 2002;34(4):300–2.

71. Eckburg PB, Montoya JG, Vosti KL. Brain abscess due to Listeria monocytogenes: five cases and a review of the literature. Medicine (Baltimore) 2001;80(4):223–35.

72. Valarezo J, Cohen JE, Valarezo L, et al. Nocardial cerebral abscess: report of three cases and review

73. Rau CS, Chang WN, Lin YC, et al. Brain abscess caused by aerobic gram-negative bacilli: clinical features and therapeutic outcomes. Clin Neurol Neurosurg 2002;105(1):60–5.

74. Fang CT, Lai SY, Yi WC, et al. Klebsiella pneumoniae genotype K1: an emerging pathogen that causes septic ocular or central nervous system complications from pyogenic liver abscess. Clin Infect Dis 2007;45(3):284–93.

75. Harder E, Al-Kawi MZ, Carney P. Intracranial tuberculoma: conservative management. Am J Med 1983;74(4):570–6.

76. Segal BH, Walsh TJ. Current approaches to diagnosis and treatment of invasive aspergillosis. Am J Respir Crit Care Med 2006;173(7):707–17.

77. Artico M, Pastore FS, Polosa M, et al. Intracerebral Aspergillus abscess: case report and review of the literature. Neurosurg Rev 1997;20(2):135–8.

78. Roden MM, Zaoutis TE, Buchanan WL, et al. Epidemiology and outcome of zygomycosis: a review of 929 reported cases. Clin Infect Dis 2005;41(5): 634–53.

79. Baddley JW, Salzman D, Pappas PG. Fungal brain abscess in transplant recipients: epidemiologic, microbiologic, and clinical features. Clin Transplant 2002;16(6):419–24.

80. Sanchez-Portocarrero J, Perez-Cecilia E, Corral O, et al. The central nervous system and infection by Candida species. Diagn Microbiol Infect Dis 2000;37(3):169–79.

81. Gologorsky Y, DeLaMora P, Souweidane MM, et al. Cerebellar cryptococcoma in an immunocompetent child. Case report. J Neurosurg 2007; 107(Suppl 4):314–7.

82. Banuelos AF, Williams PL, Johnson RH, et al. Central nervous system abscesses due to Coccidioides species. Clin Infect Dis 1996;22(2): 240–50.

83. Kaplan JE, Benson C, Holmes KH, et al. Guidelines for prevention and treatment of opportunistic infections in HIV-infected adults and adolescents: recommendations from CDC, the National Institutes of Health, and the HIV Medicine Association of the Infectious Diseases Society of America. MMWR Recomm Rep 2009;58(RR-4):1–207 [quiz: CE201–4].

84. Sacktor N, Lyles RH, Skolasky R, et al. HIV-associated neurologic disease incidence changes: Multicenter AIDS Cohort Study, 1990-1998. Neurology 2001;56(2):257–60.

85. Correa D, Sarti E, Tapia-Romero R, et al. Antigens and antibodies in sera from human cases of epilepsy or taeniasis from an area of Mexico where Taenia solium cysticercosis is endemic. Ann Trop Med Parasitol 1999;93(1):69–74.

86. Ohnishi K, Murata M, Kojima H, et al. Brain abscess due to infection with *Entamoeba histolytica*. Am J Trop Med Hyg 1994;51(2):180–2.

87. Pittella JE. Neurocysticercosis. Brain Pathol 1997; 7(1):681–93.

88. Kusner DJ, King CH. Cerebral paragonimiasis. Semin Neurol 1993;13(2):201–8.

89. Guzel A, Tatli M, Maciaczyk J, et al. Primary cerebral intraventricular hydatid cyst: a case report and review of the literature. J Child Neurol 2008; 23(5):585–8.

90. Gallagher RM, Gross CW, Phillips CD. Suppurative intracranial complications of sinusitis. Laryngoscope 1998;108(11 Pt 1):1635–42.

91. Rigamonti D, Liem L, Sampath P, et al. Spinal epidural abscess: contemporary trends in etiology, evaluation, and management. Surg Neurol 1999; 52(2):189–96 [discussion: 197].

92. Nussbaum ES, Rigamonti D, Standiford H, et al. Spinal epidural abscess: a report of 40 cases and review. Surg Neurol 1992;38(3):225–31.

93. Hlavin ML, Kaminski HJ, Ross JS, et al. Spinal epidural abscess: a ten-year perspective. Neurosurgery 1990;27(2):177–84.

94. Smitt PS, Tsafka A, Teng-van de Zande F, et al. Outcome and complications of epidural analgesia in patients with chronic cancer pain. Cancer 1998;83(9):2015–22.

95. Burstal R, Wegener F, Hayes C, et al. Epidural analgesia: prospective audit of 1062 patients. Anaesth Intensive Care 1998;26(2):165–72.

96. McClelland S 3rd. Postoperative intracranial neurosurgery infection rates in North America versus Europe: a systematic analysis. Am J Infect Control 2008;36(8):570–3.

97. Korinek AM. Risk factors for neurosurgical site infections after craniotomy: a prospective multicenter study of 2944 patients. The French Study Group of Neurosurgical Infections, the SEHP, and the C-CLIN Paris-Nord. Service Epidemiologie Hygiene et Prevention. Neurosurgery 1997;41(5):1073–9 [discussion: 1079–1].

98. Rehman AU, Rehman TU, Bashir HH, et al. A simple method to reduce infection of ventriculo-peritoneal shunts. J Neurosurg Pediatr 2010;5(6): 569–72.

99. Sasso RC, Garrido BJ. Postoperative spinal wound infections. J Am Acad Orthop Surg 2008;16(6):330–7.

100. Tokuhashi Y, Ajiro Y, Umezawa N. Conservative follow-up after epidural abscess and diskitis complicating instrumented metal interbody cage. Orthopedics 2008;31(6):611.

101. Chan YC, Dasey N. Iatrogenic spinal epidural abscess. Acta Chir Belg 2007;107(2):109–18.

102. Schnipper D, Spiegel JH. Management of intracranial complications of sinus surgery. Otolaryngol Clin North Am 2004;37(2):453–72, ix.

103. Janoff EN, Breiman RF, Daley CL, et al. Pneumococcal disease during HIV infection. Epidemiologic, clinical, and immunologic perspectives. Ann Intern Med 1992;117(4):314–24.

104. Gilks CF, Brindle RJ, Otieno LS, et al. Extrapulmonary and disseminated tuberculosis in HIV-1-seropositive patients presenting to the acute medical services in Nairobi. AIDS 1990;4(10):981–5.

105. Jarvis JN, Harrison TS. HIV-associated cryptococcal meningitis. AIDS 2007;21(16):2119–29.

106. Luft BJ, Chua A. Central nervous system toxoplasmosis in HIV. Pathogenesis, diagnosis, and therapy. Curr Infect Dis Rep 2000;2(4):358–62.

Imaging of Meningitis and Ventriculitis

Suyash Mohan, MD, PDCC[a],*, Krishan K. Jain, MD, PDCC[b],
Mohammad Arabi, MD[c], Gaurang V. Shah, MD[c]

KEYWORDS

- Central nervous system • Infection • Magnetic resonance imaging • Meningitis • Ventriculitis
- Complications

KEY POINTS

- Meningeal enhancement is nonspecific and can be seen in meningitis of any cause, including noninfectious processes.
- Imaging helps in noninvasive differentiation of infective from the noninfective conditions and helps in better clinical decision making.
- In acute meningitis, meningeal enhancement is located over the cerebral convexity, whereas in chronic meningitis it is most prominent in the basal cisterns.
- The role of neuroimaging is to confirm suspected meningitis, rule out meningitis mimics, evaluate for complications, and rule out increased intracranial pressure before lumbar puncture.
- Magnetic resonance imaging is critical in evaluating complications of meningitis (eg, ventriculitis, extra-axial collections, cerebritis and abscess, herniations, cranial neuropathy, and vasculopathy).

INTRODUCTION

Central nervous system (CNS) infections account for 1% of primary hospital admissions and 2% of nosocomial infections[1,2] and when encountered, require prompt diagnosis and initiation of specific treatment. The brain has some unique peculiarities like absence of lymphatics, lack of capillaries in the subarachnoid space, and presence of cerebrospinal fluid (CSF), which is an excellent culture medium for dissemination of infectious processes, in the subarachnoid space and into the ventricular system. The normal brain responds to these insults in a limited and stereotypical fashion, and in most cases there is concomitant abnormality of the blood-brain barrier, with associated enhancement. Therefore, the imaging findings are mostly nonspecific with respect to the causative pathogen.

However, imaging techniques are sensitive for detecting an abnormality, localizing it, and in many cases categorizing the lesion into infectious or inflammatory disease versus neoplastic. Contrast enhancement is generally useful, and in the light of clinical history and examination findings the radiologist can provide a probable differential diagnosis. Whereas analysis of CSF remains the gold standard to identify the infectious agent, neuroimaging plays a pivotal role not only in diagnosis but also in monitoring therapeutic response. This article begins by briefly describing the anatomy of cranial meninges and extra-axial spaces of the brain. Characteristic findings and recent advances in neuroimaging of meningitis and its complications and ventriculitis are then summarized, and certain noninfectious causes of meningitis and meningitis mimics are described.

[a] Division of Neuroradiology, Department of Radiology, University of Pennsylvania School of Medicine, 219 Dulles Building, 3400 Spruce Street, Philadelphia, PA 19104, USA; [b] Department of Neuroradiology, National Neuroscience Institute, 11 Jalan Tan Tock Seng, Singapore 308433; [c] Department of Radiology, University of Michigan Health System, 1500 East Med Center Dr, Ann Arbor, MI 48109, USA
* Corresponding author.
E-mail addresses: drsuyash@gmail.com; suyash.mohan@uphs.upenn.edu

Neuroimag Clin N Am 22 (2012) 557–583
doi:10.1016/j.nic.2012.04.003
1052-5149/12/$ – see front matter © 2012 Elsevier Inc. All rights reserved.

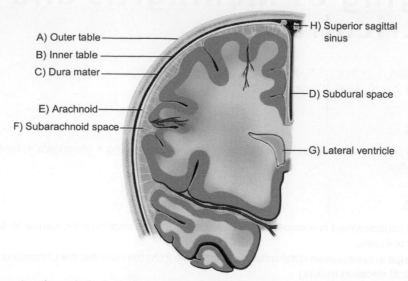

Fig. 1. Coronal section through the brain shows the meningeal layers and spaces. (A) Outer table, (B) inner table, (C) dura mater, (D) subdural space, (E) arachnoid, (F) subarachnoid space, (H) superior sagittal sinus, (G) lateral ventricle.

CRANIAL MENINGES AND EXTRA-AXIAL SPACES: NORMAL ANATOMY

Three membranes of connective tissue cover the brain, which are collectively called the meninges. They are named, from the outermost layer inward, the dura mater (also called pachymeninx [literally, "tough mother"]), arachnoid mater, and pia mater, which together constitute the leptomeninges. The space between the inner table of the skull and the dura mater is the epidural space. The space between the dural covering and the arachnoid is the subdural space (Fig. 1), which is a potential space containing bridging veins and arachnoid villi. The arachnoid is a delicate outer layer that parallels the dura and is separated from the pia by the subarachnoid space, which contains the CSF (Fig. 2). The pia is closely applied to the brain surface and carries a vast network of blood vessels.

NORMAL AND ABNORMAL MENINGEAL ENHANCEMENT

In normal meninges, enhancement is visualized as a thin, markedly discontinuous rim covering the surface of the brain, which is typically most prominent parasagittally. The enhancement is primarily in the dura and venous structures, along the inner table, falx, and tentorium, related to absent blood-brain barrier (Fig. 3). The arachnoid is thin and avascular. However, vascular enhancement of the normal, delicate pia is too subtle to visualize.[3] Thin, linear, well-demarcated and symmetric enhancement may sometimes be seen in the sulci, because of enhancing veins. Abnormal meningeal enhancement is usually not symmetric and is usually not so sharply demarcated and more importantly it extends deep into the base of the sulci (Fig. 4).[4] Quint and colleagues[5] reported that when meningeal enhancement was present

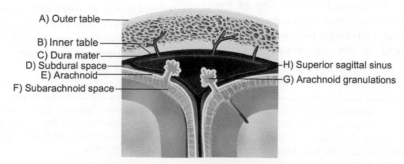

Fig. 2. The brain at the level of the superior sagittal sinus shows the meningeal layers and spaces and the relationship to the dural venous sinus. (A) Outer table, (B) inner table, (C) dura mater, (D) subdural space, (E) arachnoid, (F) subarachnoid space, (H) superior sagittal sinus, (G) arachnoid granulation.

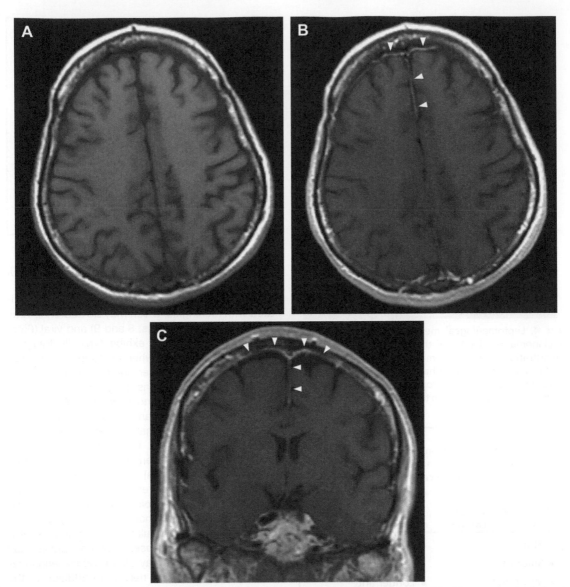

Fig. 3. Axial T1WI before (*A*) and after (*B*) contrast administration show normal, mild, thin, parasagittal dural enhancement (*arrowheads*). The enhancement is primarily in the dura and venous structures along the inner table and anterior falx. (*C*) Coronal T1WI after contrast shows the smooth, nonnodular, parasagittal dural enhancement.

on more than 3 contiguous 1.5-T spin-echo (SE) magnetic resonance (MR) images, it was highly correlated with substantial intracranial abnormality. Thicker, longer, or more intensely enhancing segments, as well as nodular meningeal enhancement, are abnormal (**Box 1**).

PATTERNS OF MENINGEAL ENHANCEMENT

Extra-axial meningeal enhancement may be classified as either pachymeningeal or leptomeningeal (**Box 2** and **Fig. 5**). Because the normal, thin arachnoid membrane is attached to the inner surface of

the dura mater, the pachymeningeal pattern of enhancement is also described as dura-arachnoid enhancement, whereas enhancement on the surface of the brain is called pial or pia-arachnoid enhancement, often referred to as leptomeningeal enhancement and usually described as having a gyriform or serpentine appearance.[6] The enhancement follows along the pial surface of the brain and fills the subarachnoid spaces of the sulci and cisterns. Combined dura-arachnoid and pia-arachnoid enhancement may coexist, typically focal in location and in association with vascularized extra-axial tumor, including metastases,

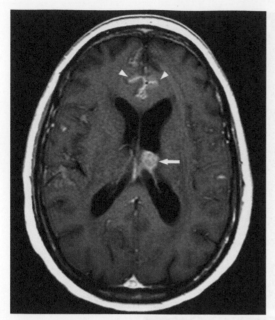

Fig. 4. Leptomeningeal metastasis in a patient with melanoma. Axial T1WI of the brain after contrast administration shows abnormal anterior frontal parasagittal leptomeningeal enhancement extending deep into the cerebral sulci (*arrowheads*). A subependymal enhancing nodule is seen in the lateral ventricle (*arrow*).

Box 1
Differentiation between normal meningeal vessels/cortical veins and abnormal leptomeningeal enhancement

Normal Meningeal Vessels/Cortical Veins	Abnormal Leptomeningeal Enhancement
• Thin	• Thick
• Smooth	• Nodular/irregular
• Short and discontinuous	• Longer and continuous
• Well-demarcated	• Poorly demarcated
• Symmetric	• Asymmetrical
• Superficial, and most prominent parasagittally	• Extends deep into the base of the sulci
• Short-segment convexity meningeal enhancement	• Long-segment (>3 cm) or diffuse convexity meningeal enhancement
• Isolated fine linear falcine and tentorial meningeal enhancement	• If meningeal enhancement was present on more than 3 contiguous 1.5-T SE MR images
• No enhancement of suprasellar cistern and ventricular walls	

Box 2
Conditions that produce pachymeningeal and leptomeningeal enhancement

Pachymeningeal	Leptomeningeal
• Intracranial hypotension	• Acute stroke
• Idiopathic	• Infection
• Infection	• Inflammatory diseases (eg, sarcoidosis)
• Inflammatory diseases (eg, sarcoidosis)	• Metastases
• Metastases	
• Shunting	
• SAH	

---

lymphoma, focal tuberculous meningitis (TBM), and sarcoidosis (**Figs. 6** and **7**).[7]

Leptomeningeal enhancement is usually associated with meningitis, which may be bacterial, viral, or fungal. Bacterial (**Figs. 8** and **9**) and viral (**Figs. 10** and **11**) meningitis exhibit typically thin and linear enhancement, whereas fungal meningitis usually produces thicker, lumpy, or nodular enhancement.[8] Neoplasms may spread into the subarachnoid space and produce enhancement of the brain surface and subarachnoid space, a pathologic process that is often called carcinomatous meningitis (**Fig. 12**). Both primary tumors (medulloblastoma, ependymoma, glioblastoma, and oligodendroglioma) and secondary tumors (eg, lymphoma and breast cancer) may spread through the subarachnoid space. Neoplastic disease in the subarachnoid space may produce thicker, lumpy, or nodular enhancement, similar to that of fungal disease. Viral encephalitis (as well as sarcoidosis) may also produce enhancement along the cranial nerves, in addition to the brain surface. Normal cranial nerves never enhance within the subarachnoid space, and such enhancement is always abnormal (**Fig. 13**).[6]

Pachymeningeal enhancement may arise from various benign or malignant processes, including transient postoperative changes, intracranial hypotension (**Figs. 14** and **15**), neoplasms such as meningioma, metastatic disease (from breast and prostate cancer), secondary CNS lymphoma, and granulomatous disease. Postoperative meningeal enhancement occurs in most patients and may be dura-arachnoid or pia-arachnoid (**Fig. 16**).[9] In patients who have not undergone surgery, other causes of this enhancement pattern should be considered. Although such enhancement has been reported after uncomplicated lumbar puncture, this observation is rare, occurring in less than 5% of patients (see **Fig. 14**).[10]

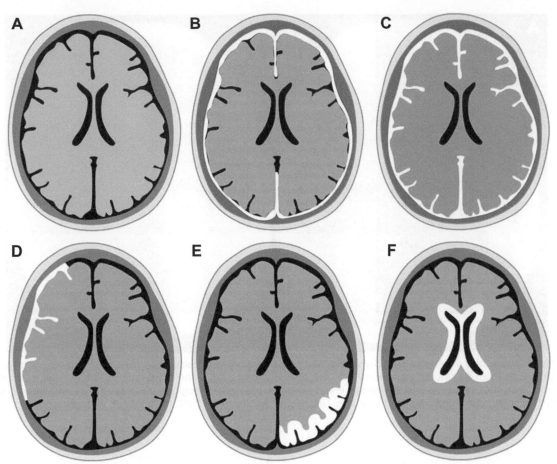

Fig. 5. The patterns of meningeal enhancement. (*A*) Normal meninges, (*B*) diffuse pachymeningeal enhancement, (*C*) diffuse leptomeningeal enhancement, (*D*) localized leptomeningeal enhancement, (*E*) gyriform cortical enhancement, and (*F*) ependymal enhancement.

SUMMARY OF CAUSES OF MENINGEAL THICKENING AND ENHANCEMENT

- Infectious: meningitis (bacterial, fungal, tuberculous, viral, or parasitic)
- Neoplastic meningitis: carcinoma, lymphoma, leukemia, primary CNS neoplasia
- Sarcoidosis: most common form is leptomeningitis; however, it also can present as a pachymeningitic process affecting predominantly the dura mater. Sarcoidosis is the most common cause of chronic meningitis in the Western world, whereas tuberculosis is the most common cause in the developing world
- Chemical meningitis: subarachnoid hemorrhage (SAH), dermoid cyst rupture, methotrexate instillation, and other neurotoxic substances
- Drug-induced aseptic meningitis: many antimicrobials, xanthine oxidase inhibitor allopurinol, nonsteroidal antiinflammatory

drugs, ranitidine, carbamazepine, vaccines against hepatitis B and mumps, immunoglobulins, OKT3 monoclonal antibodies, cotrimoxazole, radiographic agents, and muromonab-CD3 have also been associated. A high index of suspicion is needed to make an accurate diagnosis of drug-induced meningitis. Diagnostic accuracy in clinical care depends on a complete history and physical examination
- Collagen vascular disorders: pachymeningitis is occasionally seen in Wegener granulomatosis and rheumatoid arthritis. Aseptic meningitis is occasionally seen in systemic lupus erythematosus and Behçet disease
- Intracranial hypotension

CLINICAL FEATURES

Clinical features are related to patient's age (**Boxes 3** and **4**). In adults, meningitis presents with the classic triad of fever, neck stiffness, and

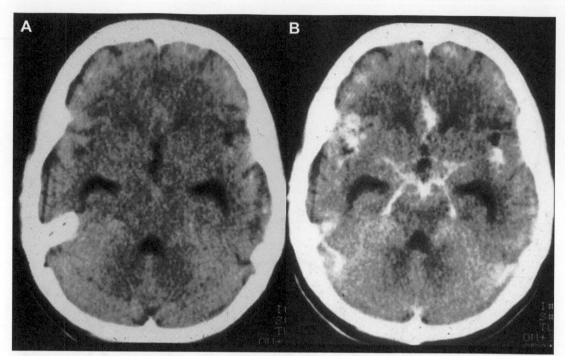

Fig. 6. Tubercular meningitis in a 45-year-old man who presented with seizures and fever. Axial plain CT image (*A*) shows dilated bilateral lateral ventricles with diffusely swollen gyri and obliteration of basal cisterns. Axial postcontrast CT (*B*) shows thick meningeal enhancement in basal cistern regions. (*From* Shah GV. Central nervous system tuberculosis: imaging manifestations. Neuroimaging Clin N Am 2000;10(2):355–74; with permission.)

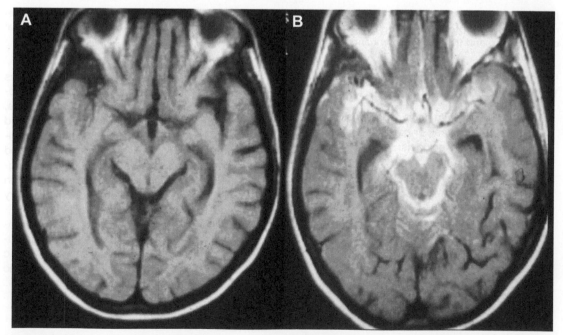

Fig. 7. Tubercular meningitis in a 45-year-old man who presented with seizures and fever. Axial plain T1WI (*A*) shows obliteration of basal cisterns with thick meningeal enhancement on contrast study (*B*). (*From* Shah GV. Central nervous system tuberculosis: imaging manifestations. Neuroimaging Clin N Am 2000;10(2):355–74; with permission.)

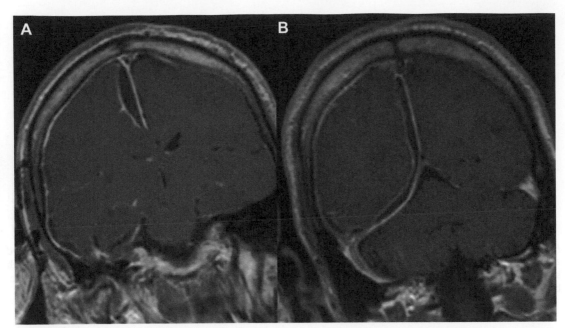

Fig. 8. Subdural empyema in a 34-year-old woman. Postcontrast T1WI (*A, B*) shows subdural collection abutting interhemispheric fissure and along the right tentorial leaf with peripheral enhancement.

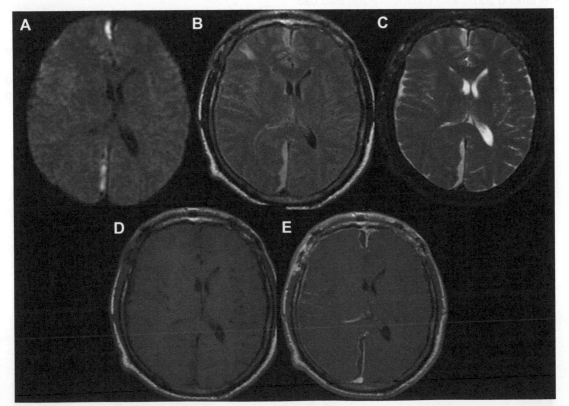

Fig. 9. Subdural empyema in a 34-year-old woman. Axial T2WI (*B*) and FLAIR imaging (*C*) shows concavo-convex hyperintense collection abutting anterior and posterior interhemispheric fissure, with presence of focal cortical hyperintensity in right frontal lobe. Collection is hypointense on T1WI (*D*) and showing restriction on axial DWI (*A*). Peripheral enhancement is seen on axial postcontrast T1WI (*E*), along with the presence of increased leptomeningeal enhancement.

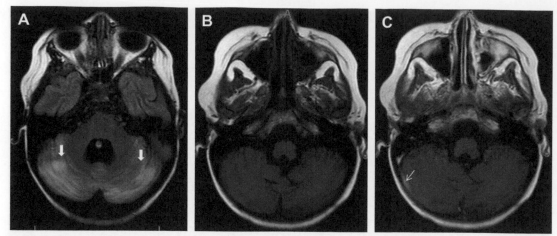

Fig. 10. Acute cerebellitis in a 9-year-old boy. Axial FLAIR imaging (*A*), plain axial T1WI (*B*) and contrast-enhanced axial T1WI (*C*) show diffuse hyperintense signal in bilateral cerebellar hemispheres (*white block arrows*), with some volume loss and increased leptomeningeal enhancement (*white arrow*), especially overlying the right cerebellar hemisphere.

an altered mental status.[11] However, it has been noted that the prevalence of this classic triad is low among adults with community-acquired bacterial meningitis. However, almost all patients (95%) present with at least 2 of the 4 symptoms of headache, fever, neck stiffness, and an altered mental status, and a high percentage of patients (33%) present with focal neurologic deficits at admission.[11]

ROUTES OF SPREAD AND PATHOPHYSIOLOGY

There are 4 common routes of entry infectious agents into the CNS.[1]

1. Hematogenous dissemination from a distant infectious focus is most common.
2. Direct implantation is usually traumatic and rarely iatrogenic when microbes are introduced

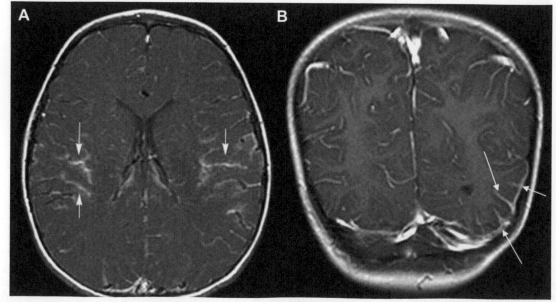

Fig. 11. Axial and coronal postcontrast T1WI (*A, B*) shows diffuse smooth increased meningeal enhancement along the cerebral sulci (*arrows*).

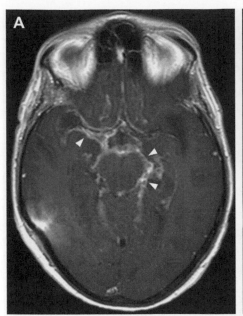
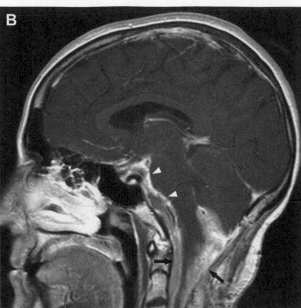

Fig. 12. Axial sagittal postcontrast T1WI (*A, B*) show diffuse meningeal thickening and enhancement along the basilar cisterns (*arrowheads*) and foramen magnum (*black arrows*), consistent with leptomeningeal metastasis from glioblastoma multiforme.

with a lumbar puncture needle or during surgery.

3. Local extension from sinusitis (**Fig. 17**), orbital cellulitis, mastoiditis (**Fig. 18**), otitis media, or an infected tooth is less common.

4. Spread of infection along the peripheral nervous system has also been described for certain viruses such as rabies and herpes simplex.

Other uncommon routes include inhalation, or rarely secondary to abscesses or infections in the epidural or subdural spaces. It is presumed that the infection enters the brain via the choroid plexus. Thereafter, the subarachnoid space is distended by purulent exudates that also extend into the perivascular spaces. Bacteria then stimulate the production of cytokines and other inflammatory compounds, which cause breakdown of the blood-brain barrier and allow contrast material to leak from vessels into the CSF, leading to meningeal enhancement, as seen on imaging studies.[12–15]

WHAT COMES FIRST: LUMBAR PUNCTURE OR COMPUTED TOMOGRAPHY?

Most patients who present with moderate or severe impairment of consciousness, neurologic deficits (not including cranial nerve abnormalities), or both, which are contraindications to performing lumbar puncture, should undergo computed tomography (CT) before lumbar puncture. Patients without these red flags can directly proceed to lumbar puncture if there is no clinical evidence to suggest raised intracranial pressure.[11,16]

ROLE OF IMAGING

Imaging studies are not used for the initial diagnosis of meningitis. Only 50% of patients with meningitis show subarachnoid space enhancement. Therefore, the role of neuroimaging is to confirm suspected meningitis, to rule out meningitis mimics and increased intracranial pressure before lumbar puncture, and to evaluate for complications. In cases of uncomplicated meningitis, cranial CT seems to be sufficient for clinical management to exclude acute brain edema, hydrocephalus, and disease of the base of the skull.[17] The most common signs of complicated meningitis are an enlarging head (in children) and increased intracranial pressure (persistent headache, nausea, vomiting, papilledema, and focal deficits).[12] These patients need imaging, preferably using MR imaging.

Although contrast-enhanced MR imaging has been used for many years in the evaluation of patients with complicated meningitis, during the last 5 years the introduction and widespread use of new imaging techniques have contributed significantly to the rapid and more specific diagnosis

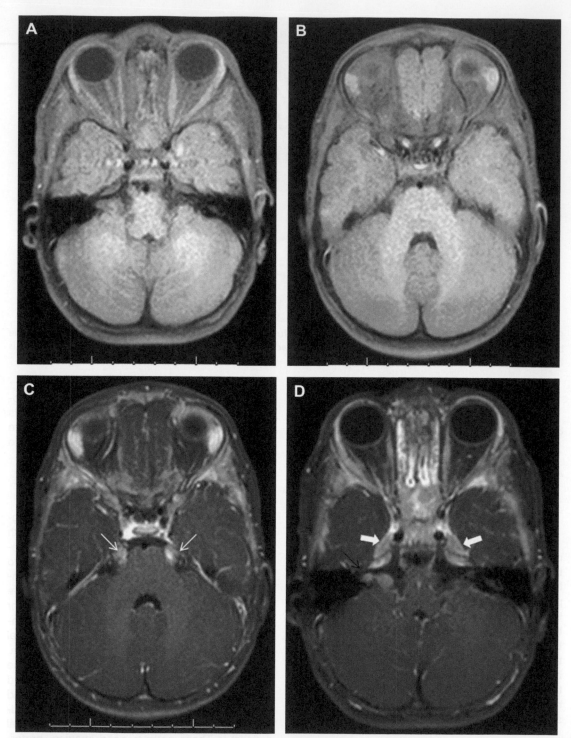

Fig. 13. Multiple cranial nerve involvement in a 1-year-old boy with acute lymphoblastic leukemia. Plain axial T1WI (*A, B*) and contrast-enhanced (*C, D*) images show enlarged, thickened and enhancing bilateral fifth (*white arrows*) and right ninth, 10th, and 11th nerve complex (*black arrow*), with expansion and enhancement of the bilateral cavernous sinus (*white block arrows*).

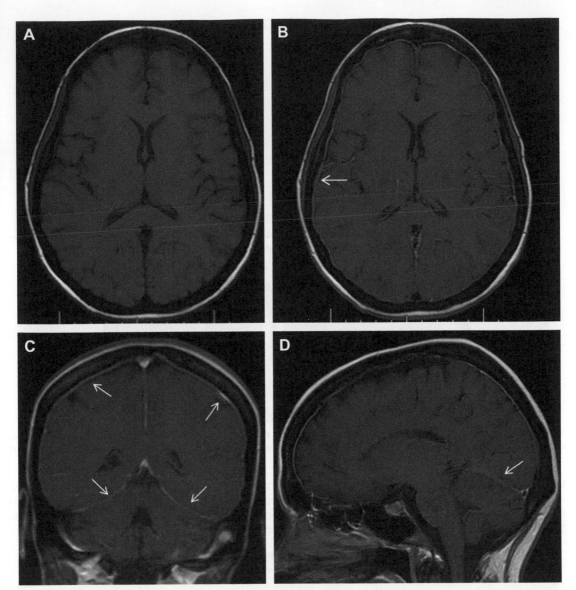

Fig. 14. Pachymeningeal enhancement in a 43-year-old man, 3 days after lumbar puncture. Pain axial T1WI (*A*) appears grossly normal; however, mildly increased pachymeningeal enhancement (*white arrows*) is seen on post-contrast axial, sagittal, and coronal T1WI (*B–D*). This enhancement resolved completely on the follow-up scan (*not shown*).

of the complications of meningitis and have helped in patient management.

INFECTIOUS MENINGITIS

Infectious meningitis is divided into the following general categories[14,15]:

1. Acute pyogenic meningitis
2. Acute lymphocytic meningitis
3. Chronic meningitis

Acute Pyogenic Meningitis

Acute pyogenic meningitis is a diffuse inflammation of the pia mater and arachnoid and is more common in children. The estimated incidence is 2.6 to 6 per 100,000 adults per year in developed countries and is up to 10 times higher in less-developed countries.[11] The diagnosis of meningitis is based on clinical and CSF analysis. CSF analysis shows neutrophilic pleocytosis and increased protein and low glucose levels. These

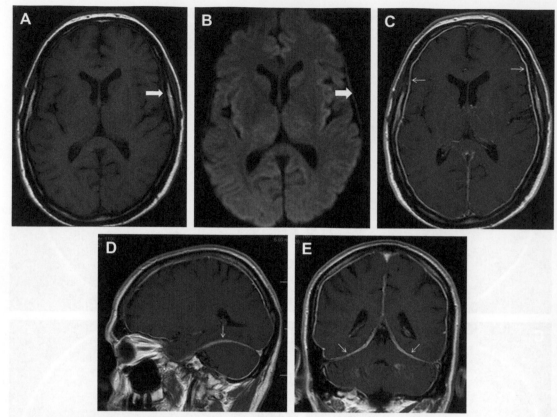

Fig. 15. Idiopathic pachymeningitis in a 46-year-old man. Axial T1WI (*A*) and DWI (*B*) show minimal dural thickening (*white block arrows*), with intense diffuse enhancement (*white arrows*) on postcontrast axial, sagittal, and coronal T1WI (*C–E*).

features suggest a pyogenic cause. The cause of meningitis varies according to the age of the patient and the status of their immune system. Common causative organisms of meningitis include group B streptococcus, and *Escherichia coli* (newborns), *Haemophilus influenzae* (children younger than 7 years), *Neisseria meningitidis* (older children and adolescents), and *Streptococcus*

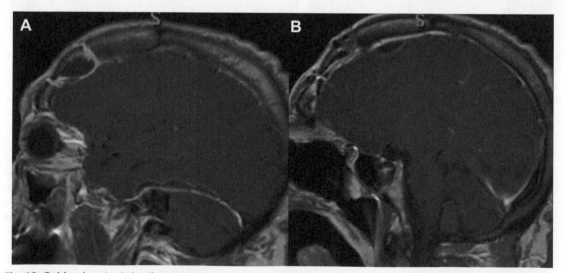

Fig. 16. Epidural and subdural empyemas in a 54-year-old woman. Postcontrast T1WI (*A, B*) shows epidural collection abutting frontal convexity and subdural collection along the tentorial leaf with peripheral enhancement. Increased leptomeningeal enhancement is also evident.

| Box 3 |
| Clinical features of leptomeningitis |

Infants	Adults
• Altered state of consciousness	• Fever
	• Kernig sign
• Anorexia	• Headache
• Bulging fontanelle	• Meningismus
• Constipation	• Photophobia
• Failure to thrive	
• Fever	
• Irritability	
• Kernig sign	
• Seizures	
• Vomiting	

pneumoniae (leading cause of bacterial meningitis in adults) (see **Fig. 9**). Immunocompromised patients are prone to infections caused by *E coli*, *Klebsiella, Pseudomona*s, and fungi. Iatrogenic infections are usually the result of gram-negative microorganisms. The epidemiology of bacterial meningitis has changed. Meningitis caused by *H influenzae* type b has been nearly eliminated in the Western world since vaccination against *H influenzae* type b was initiated, and the introduction of conjugate vaccines against *Streptococcus pneumoniae* is expected to reduce the burden of childhood pneumococcal meningitis significantly.[11] Pyogenic meningitis still remains a serious disease, with high potential for permanent neurologic impairment and high overall mortality (even with treatment) of up to 20%.[11,12]

Acute Lymphocytic Meningitis

Acute lymphocytic meningitis is usually a benign and self-limited condition. It is rare in adults and

| Box 4 |
| Imaging findings in leptomeningitis |

- Normal scan
- Enlargement of CSF spaces
- Poor visualization of basal cisterns
- Generalized cerebral swelling
- Diffuse meningeal enhancement
- ± Virchow-Robin spaces
- Communicating hydrocephalus
- Subdural effusion
- Focal high-signal parenchymal abnormalities secondary to infarction

is most commonly viral in origin. Common pathogens are enteroviruses and mumps viruses. Other agents include herpes simplex virus I and II, and human immunodeficiency virus (HIV).[15] Signs and symptoms such as headache, fever, and meningismus are similar to those of bacterial meningitis, but are often less severe. CSF studies show lymphocytic pleocytosis, moderate protein increase, and normal glucose.[14] Viral meningitis causes severe headache, but is usually self-limited. Imaging findings are usually normal unless coexisting encephalitis occurs (see **Fig. 10**).[14,15]

Chronic Meningitis

Chronic meningitis is a smoldering process usually caused by *Mycobacterium tuberculosis* and some fungi causing an indolent infection. Infection reaches the meninges generally by hematogenous spread.[15,18] It involves predominantly basal subarachnoid spaces, which are filled with thick, gelatinous exudates containing chronic inflammatory cells, fibrin, and hemorrhage. Chronic meningitis may also have more generalized disease.[19] Most children with TBM also have concomitant miliary brain infection, and 11% of all patients have combined parenchymal/meningeal lesions.[19,20] The clinical diagnosis of TBM may be difficult. Diagnosis is dependent on CSF cytology and biochemistry, detection of acid-fast bacilli in smear and culture; however, only 8% to 30% of cases show a positive result on smear and culture. CSF studies are also nonspecific and show moderate pleocytosis with monocytosis and neutrophils and increased protein and low glucose levels.[14] Moreover, because of the low sensitivity of laboratory tests, noninvasive imaging plays an important role in diagnosis (see **Figs. 6** and **7**). Sequelae of chronic meningitis include hydrocephalus, pachymeningitis, and infarctions caused by basal vascular occlusions, cranial nerve palsies, atrophy, and calcifications.[15,20]

IMAGING IN MENINGITIS

CT and MR imaging are normal in the early disease process in most cases of acute bacterial meningitis (see **Boxes 3** and **4**). Once the infection progresses, an unenhanced CT scan shows mild dilatation of the ventricular system and subarachnoid space with diffuse cerebral swelling. Obliteration of the basal or convexity cisterns by inflammatory exudates may be seen in some cases (see **Fig. 6** and **7**). Contrast-enhanced MR imaging has been shown to be more sensitive than contrast-enhanced CT in detection of abnormal meningeal enhancement in basal cistern, sylvian fissure region, and deep within the cortical sulci.[15,21,22]

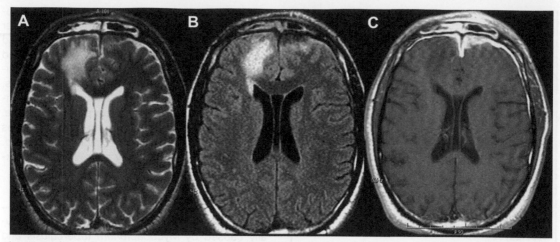

Fig. 17. Early cerebritis in a 34-year-old woman with meningitis. Axial T2WI (*A*) and FLAIR (*B*) images show focal area of hyperintensity in the right frontal lobe white matter along with the presence of mucosal hypertrophy of bilateral frontal sinuses. Axial postcontrast T1WI (*C*) shows increased pachymeningeal enhancement in bilateral frontal region, with enhancing mucosal thickening in bilateral frontal sinuses; no abnormal intraparenchymal enhancement was seen.

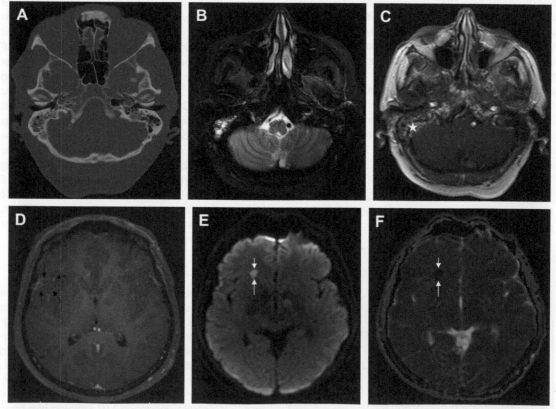

Fig. 18. Right-side mastoiditis in a 25-year-old man with meningitis and cerebritis. Axial CT (*A*), T2-weighted MR imaging (*B*) and postcontrast T1WI (*C, D*) showing right mastoiditis (*white asterisk*), with focal leptomeningitis in the right sylvian cistern region (*black arrows*). Focal area of cerebritis (*white arrows*) is seen in the right frontal lobe, with restricted diffusion on DWI (*E*) and ADC map (*F*); no obvious enhancement is seen on postcontrast image (*D*).

Enhancement can also be seen along the tentorium, falx, and the convexities.[22] MR imaging is superior to CT, not only in the evaluation of suspected meningitis, where precontrast T1-weighted imaging (T1WI) may show obliterated basal cisterns, but also in depicting complications such as subdural/epidural empyema and vasculitic complications, notably on fluid-attenuated inversion recovery (FLAIR) images.[17] FLAIR imaging shows leptomeningeal enhancement and CSF hyperintensity presumably caused by increased protein content (Fig. 19).[23] Sulcal hyperintensity on the FLAIR sequence has other differential diagnostic considerations, as listed in Box 5.[24]

In chronic meningitis, abnormal enhancement may be seen even years after the initial infection, and en plaque dural thickening and even popcorn-like dural calcification can be seen in some cases around the basilar cistern.[20] Sequelae of chronic meningitis include ischemic changes and atrophy, which in some cases may be striking.[21]

In acute meningitis, meningeal enhancement is preferentially located over the cerebral convexity, whereas in chronic meningitis enhancement is most prominent in the basal cisterns (Figs. 6,7,11).[1,25] Meningeal enhancement is a nonspecific finding, because it may be seen in meningitis of any cause, including noninfectious processes, such as carcinomatosis and chemical meningitis; however, carcinomatous meningitis typically presents with dural enhancement and thus may usually be differentiated from infectious cause.[15,26]

RECENT ADVANCES IN NEUROIMAGING OF MENINGITIS
Magnetization Transfer

The magnetization transfer (MT) technique has recently received attention as an additional sequence to differentiate TBM from meningitis with a nontuberculous cause. MT is reported to be superior to conventional SE sequences for imaging the abnormal meninges, which are seen as hyperintense on precontrast T1-weighted MT images and enhance further on postcontrast T1-weighted MT images.[27] In addition, quantification of MT ratio (MTR) helps in predicting the cause of meningitis. The MTR of these hyperintense meninges in TBM remains significantly higher than in viral meningitis. Fungal and pyogenic meningitis shows higher MTR compared with TBM.[27,28] It has also been reported that visibility of the inflamed meninges on precontrast T1-weighted MT images with low MTR is specific of TBM and differentiates it from other nontuberculous chronic meningitis.[28] The tuberculous bacteria remain laden with high lipid content, which is probably responsible for the low MTR in tubercular meningitis.

Diffusion-weighted Imaging

The newer technique of diffusion-weighted imaging (DWI) shows early parenchymal and certain extra-axial complications of meningitis earlier and with more clarity and is of help in differentiation

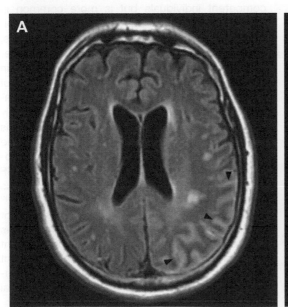
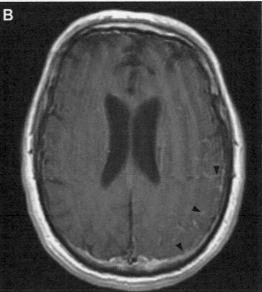

Fig. 19. (A) Axial FLAIR image through the brain shows increased signal along the left parietal cerebral sulci (arrowheads) in a patient with meningoencephalitis. (B) Corresponding axial T1WI shows localized pial enhancement along the parietal sulci and overlying meninges (arrowheads).

Box 5
Differential diagnosis of sulcal hyperintensity on FLAIR images

- Meningitis
- SAH
- Leptomeningeal carcinomatosis
- Leptomeningeal melanosis
- Fat-containing tumors
- Acute stroke
- Moyamoya disease
- Increased blood pool/CSF ratio
- Contrast media
- Supplemental oxygen
- CSF pulsation
- Vascular pulsation
- Magnetic susceptibility artifact
- Motion artifact

of pyogenic abscess from other ring-enhancing lesions.[17] Evidence of restricted diffusion on DWI with reduced apparent diffusion coefficient (ADC) is highly suggestive of brain abscess; however, in the absence of restriction, proton MR spectroscopy is useful to distinguish brain abscesses from cystic tumors.[29]

In Vivo Proton MR Spectroscopy

Although there is no published study of in vivo MR spectroscopy (MRS) in meningitis, ex vivo spectroscopy of CSF has been attempted in TBM.[30] High-resolution ex vivo MRS of CSF showed presence of Lac, acetate, and sugars along with the signals from cyclopropyl rings (–0.5 to +0.5 ppm) and phenolic glycolipids (7.1 and 7.4 ppm); these have not been observed with pyogenic meningitis. The combination of ex vivo MRS with MR imaging (possibly MT imaging) may be of value in the diagnosis of TBM.

Diffusion Tensor Imaging

Although conventional MR imaging is more sensitive to perceiving secondary complications of meningitis, it is insensitive to subtle changes in tissue microstructure. Diffusion tensor imaging (DTI) is a relatively new MR imaging technique, which has been shown to provide tissue microstructural information. The commonly used DTI-derived metrics are fractional anisotropy (FA) and mean diffusivity (MD). High FA values have been shown in enhancing as well as nonenhancing cortical ribbon in neonatal and adult patients with bacterial meningitis compared with age-matched controls.[31,32] These investigators have proposed that the oriented inflammatory cells in the subarachnoid space caused by upregulated immune response in meningitis are responsible for increased FA values. Increased FA values in the enhancing as well as nonenhancing cortical regions suggest diffuse inflammatory activity in the pia-arachnoid in patients with meningitis. They also suggest that FA may be a better indicator of active and diffuse meningeal inflammation than postcontrast T1WI. The inflammatory molecules like soluble intracellular adhesion molecules, tumor necrosis factor α, and interleukin 1β in the CSF of neonatal meningitis have shown strong correlation with FA values in the cortical region, confirming that the increased FA values may be used as a surrogate marker of inflammatory molecules in meningitis.[33] Periventricular white matter of neonatal brain is known to be vulnerable to oxidative and hypoxic/ischemic injury secondary to neuroinfections. A recent DTI study has reported decreased FA values in the periventricular white matter regions of neonates with bacterial meningitis compared with age-matched/sex-matched healthy controls, suggesting microstructural white matter injury.[34]

CRYPTOCOCCOSIS

Cryptococcus neoformans, an encapsulated yeastlike fungus infection, may occur in immunocompetent individuals but is more common in immunocompromised patients.[35–37] It is a ubiquitous organism found in mammal and bird feces, particularly in pigeon droppings.[38,39] It represents the most common fungal CNS infection in AIDS, occurring in approximately 5% to 10% of patients.[37] The infection is acquired through inhalation and then disseminates hematogenously from the lung to the CNS, with pathogenesis similar to that of TBM.[37,40,41] CNS is the preferred site for cryptococcal infection because anticryptococcal factors present in serum are absent in CSF and the polysaccharide capsule of the fungus protects it from host inflammatory response.[35] Most patients with CNS cryptococcosis present with symptoms and signs of subacute meningitis or meningoencephalitis.[35,39] Immunocompetent patients tend to present with localized, indolent neurologic disease and more intense inflammatory responses, but have a better clinical outcome.[42]

CNS infection can be either meningeal or parenchymal.[43] Imaging findings are variable and frequently minimal. MR and CT abnormalities range from no abnormality to meningeal enhancement (Fig. 20), abscesses, intraventricular or intraparenchymal cryptococcomas, gelatinous pseudocysts, or hydrocephalus.[35,36,44] Hydrocephalus is the most common, although nonspecific, finding. Intraparenchymal and intraventricular mass lesions are less common,[44] because cryptococcus extends from the subarachnoid space along the perivascular (Virchow-Robin) spaces, which become dilated, resulting in pseudocyst formation without involvement of the brain parenchyma (Fig. 20). These widened perivascular spaces are visualized as hypodensities on CT and have CSF intensity on both T1WI and T2WI, which fail to enhance.[36,37] Evidence of clusters of these cysts in the basal ganglia and thalami strongly suggests cryptococcal infection.[43] Cerebral infarctions may occur in 4% of patients with cryptococcal meningitis in the acute stage and during the treatment and are usually observed in the basal ganglia, internal capsule, and thalamus.[45]

PARASITIC MENINGITIS

Parasitic diseases are common among tourists, immigrants from areas with highly endemic infection, and immunocompromised people.

CYSTICERCOSIS

Cysticercosis is the most common and most widely disseminated parasitic infection in the world, and is caused by ingestion of the ova of pork tapeworm (*Taenia solium*).[46] Humans become the intermediate host after ingestion of ova, usually on contaminated vegetables or water; however, the main intermediate host of *T solium* is pig. Humans can also become the definitive host when poorly cooked pork infected with cysticercosis is ingested. When the eggs mature, larvae

are released into the bloodstream, causing neurocysticercosis. The common locations include subarachnoid spaces, typically the basal cisterns and deep within the sulci, hemispheric parenchyma at the gray matter–white matter interface and in the ventricles (the fourth ventricle is most common) or combination of these sites.[15,21,37,47]

Three clinicopathologic forms may be identified: meningobasilar (55%), ventricular (15%), and parenchymal (30%).[48]

Cysticercal meningoencephalitis is caused by infiltration of the meninges and the parenchyma of the brain by many parasites, and inflammation in the surrounding tissue is responsible for meningitis and encephalitis.[49,50] Around 60% of cysticercal meningoencephalitis cases have been reported to have associated parenchymal lesions.[51] Most cases described are chronic in evolution,[52] and isolated acute meningitis is rare.[53] The diagnosis, suggested by epidemiologic and clinical findings, is confirmed by specific serologic tests,[54,55] and by imaging.[56–58] The presence of CSF eosinophilia and the coexistent inflammatory granuloma suggests the possibility of cysticercal meningitis. Cysticercosis is the commonest cause of CSF eosinophilia in endemic areas.[49] Other causes of eosinophilic meningitis are listed in Box 6.

Helminthic Eosinophilic Meningitis

Eosinophilic meningitis is a rare clinical entity and is defined by the presence of 10 or more eosinophils/L in the CSF or a CSF eosinophilia of at least 10%. The most common cause is invasion of the CNS by helminthic parasites, particularly *A cantonensis*, but other infections as well as noninfectious conditions may also be associated (see Box 6).[59,60]

A cantonensis, or rat lungworm, infection occurs by eating poorly cooked or raw fish, slugs, snails,

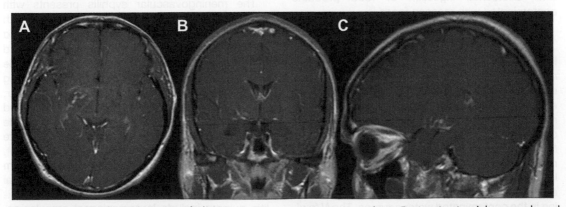

Fig. 20. Cryptococcal meningoencephalitis in an immunocompetent patient. Postcontrast axial, coronal, and sagittal images (*A–C*) show increased leptomeningeal enhancement. CSF showed India ink positive yeast, and culture confirmed it to be *Cryptococcus neoformans*.

Box 6
Causes of eosinophilic meningitis

- Coccidioidal meningitis
- *Angiostrongylus cantonensis*
- *Paragonimus westermani*
- *Gnathostoma spinigerum*
- Intrathecal injection of foreign proteins
- Insertion of rubber tubing into the CNS in the course of neurosurgery

---

or vegetables contaminated by infected rat, and humans are accidental hosts. Angiostrongyliasis is diagnosed by a history of exposure, CSF finding, and serology. CSF shows eosinophilia-increased protein with normal sugar level. A CT scan is usually normal. MR imaging may show prominence of Virchow-Robin spaces, periventricular hyperintense T2 signals, and enhancing subcortical lesions. Proton MRS may show decreased choline in the lesions. Diagnosis is confirmed by showing the larvae from CNS and by Western blot analysis to identify the presence of antibodies against *A cantonensis* in either the acute or convalescent phase of the illness. The prognosis is generally good and most symptoms resolve within weeks, and long-term sequelae are rare.[60,61]

G spinigerum, a gastrointestinal parasite of wild and domestic dogs and cats, may cause eosinophilic meningoencephalitis. This situation is common in Southeast Asia, China, and Japan but has been reported sporadically worldwide. Humans acquire the infection after ingestion of undercooked infected fish and poultry.[60]

B procyonis is an ascarid parasite that is prevalent in the raccoon populations in the United States and rarely causes human eosinophilic meningoencephalitis. Human infections occur after accidental ingestion of food products contaminated with raccoon feces.[60]

Amoebic Meningoencephalitis

Infection with free-living amoebas (eg, *Acanthamoeba*, *Balamuthia*, and *Naegleria*) is an infrequent but often life-threatening human illness, even in immunocompetent individuals, with nonspecific imaging findings.[62] *N fowleri* is the only recognized human pathogenic species of *Naegleria*, and it is the agent of primary amoebic meningoencephalitis. The parasite has been isolated in lakes, pools, ponds, rivers, tap water, and soil. Infection occurs when swimming or playing in the contaminated water sources. The *N fowleri* amoebas invade the CNS through the nasal mucosa and cribriform plate.[62]

Toxoplasmosis

Toxoplasmosis is caused by an obligate intracellular protozoan, *Toxoplasma gondii*. This is the most frequent opportunistic infection in patients with HIV. Toxoplasmosis is frequently multifocal, has a predilection for basal ganglia, does not show periventricular spread, and may occasionally hemorrhage. Infection may be acquired prenatally and may present with multiple small calcified lesions scattered in the parenchyma as well as in the periventricular region with hydrocephalus.[15,36,37] Although toxoplasmosis meningitis has been described, it is rare. In some series, the incidence of toxoplasmic meningoencephalitis has been reported from 3% to 50% in HIV-positive patients.[63] Because toxoplasmic meningitis is rare, purulent or TBM, lymphoma, and other infections should be considered in the differential diagnosis. The diagnosis is established with both serologic tests and histopathologic examinations.[64]

Neurosyphilis

Syphilis is usually a sexually transmitted disease caused by the spirochete *Treponema pallidum*. Three well-characterized clinical phases have been described; although CNS involvement can occur in any phase, it usually occurs in the tertiary stage. Neurosyphilis usually results from small vessel end arteritis of the meninges, brain, and spinal cord.[21,22] Acute syphilitic meningitis is a common manifestation in HIV-positive patients who are infected by *Treponema pallidum*.[22] Making the diagnosis is often difficult, because most patients are either asymptomatic or present with nonspecific symptoms, and there is a wide range of neuroimaging findings.[18,65,66] Neurosyphilis can be divided into (1) meningovascular syphilis and (2) syphilitic gumma.[22]

The meningovascular syphilis presents with widespread thickening of the meninges, with lymphocytic infiltration around the meninges and small vessels. This situation leads to cortical and subcortical infarcts in the basal ganglia and middle cerebral artery territories along with varying degrees of narrowing and ectasia of the basilar, proximal anterior cerebral, middle cerebral, and supraclinoid carotid arteries.[65] CT shows multiple low-density areas involving both gray and white matter with linear nonhomogenous enhancement. MR imaging is superior to CT and shows a gyriform pattern of enhancement along with meningeal enhancement.[37] The manifestations of syphilitic gumma include leptomeningeal granulomas, known as gummata in the meninges and blood vessels, which may also occur intra-axially into the brain parenchyma and be indistinguishable from primary brain tumors, meningiomas, or sarcoidosis.[65–67] Bilateral mesial temporal T2 hyperintensity has recently been reported in neurosyphilis, and represents an important although rare differential diagnostic consideration for characteristic herpes simplex encephalitis MR imaging findings.[37,68] Cranial nerve involvement has also been reported, with optic and vestibulocochlear nerves most commonly affected.[21] Later stages may show cerebral atrophy.[21,22]

Neuroborreliosis (Lyme Disease)

Lyme disease is caused by the spirochete *Borrelia burgdorferi*, transmitted most commonly by the deer tick (*Ixodes dammini*), and is endemic in 3 regions in the United States (the coastal northeast states [from Massachusetts to Maryland], the midwest [Minnesota and Wisconsin], and the west [California, Oregon, Utah, and Nevada]), certain parts of Europe, and Asia.[69–72] Approximately 10% to 15% of patients develop variable neurologic symptoms, ranging from meningitis, encephalopathy, cranial nerve palsies, and radiculoneuropathy.[73,74] The pathophysiology includes direct invasion of the parenchyma, or a vasculitic or immunologic process.[75] Diagnosis is based on clinical findings and serology and the most likely diagnosis in patients with moderate pleocytosis, high protein, and intrathecal immunoglobulin synthesis is neuroborreliosis in endemic areas.

On MR imaging, findings include (1) most commonly a normal scan; (2) high-signal abnormalities on T2 and FLAIR, which can vary in size from punctuate to large mass lesions; and (3) contrast-enhancing parenchymal lesions, meninges, labyrinth, and cranial nerves. Other abnormalities include hydrocephalus and high intensity in the pons, thalamus, or basal ganglia.[76–78]

Lymphocytic meningoradiculitis or Garin-Bujadoux-Bannwarth syndrome is a European variety of Lyme disease and is clinically characterized by severe radicular pains with sensory and motor impairment and cranial nerve palsies, especially unilateral or bilateral facial weakness. The disease is often self-limiting, and in some cases it may be difficult to distinguish Bannwarth syndrome from neurosyphilis.[79,80]

COMPLICATIONS OF MENINGITIS

Complications of bacterial meningitis include hydrocephalus, ventriculitis, extra-axial collections (sterile subdural effusion, subdural/epidural empyema), cerebritis, and abscess, edema with or without cerebral herniation, cranial nerve involvement, thrombosis/infarction, and vasculopathy.[1,15,21,81]

Hydrocephalus

A mild, transient communicating hydrocephalus is the most common complication in patients with meningitis.[82] It may develop either because of the blockage of CSF resorption in the Pachionian granulations by inflammatory debris (extraventricular or communicating hydrocephalus) or related to aqueductal obstruction (intraventricular or noncommunicating hydrocephalus).[1,12] It is easily detected by CT or MR imaging; however, in infants, cranial ultrasonography may be used for this purpose. The most useful indicators are dilatation of the third ventricle or temporal horns.[81] In some patients, the ventricular system remains dilated and never returns to normal, so-called arrested hydrocephalus, which requires no therapy (see **Fig. 6**). A CSF-shunting procedure may be required in some patients to avoid permanent CNS injury or death from brain herniation.[1,12]

Extra-axial Collections

Extra-axial fluid collections can be sterile (effusions) or infected/purulent (empyema).[83] Subdural effusion is a common complication and is seen in up to one-third of patients with meningitis. It is most commonly seen with pneumococcal infection.[81] These effusions are believed to be caused by irritation of the dura mater by infectious agents and their products, or secondary to inflammation of subdural veins.[83] It must be differentiated from the normal prominent subarachnoid spaces often seen in infants by the presence of veins coursing through the collection, which indicates that the fluid is located in the subarachnoid space. These collections usually occur along the frontal and temporal convexities, and tend to resolve spontaneously over weeks to months. Some may require drainage, mostly when they are large and result in mass effect.[12] On CT and MR imaging, these effusions are seen as crescentic extra-axial fluid collections and show the same density and signal intensity as CSF (see **Figs. 8**, **9** and **16**).[1,15] Some effusions develop a fibrin network and membranes and may show peripheral or central enhancement on contrast-enhanced MR imaging, which makes it difficult to distinguish them from empyema.[81] Empyema is an uncommon collection, which occurs secondary to meningitis, sinusitis, otitis media, osteomyelitis, and trauma.[83] Persistence of neurologic findings suggests the likelihood of an empyema. Empyema generally needs to be drained surgically.[12] Subdural empyema is the collection of pus between the dura and the leptomeninges and can be found over the convexities or interhemispherically. It occurs usually secondary to retrograde thrombophlebitis via the calvarial emissary veins from an adjacent infection.[1,83] Approximately up to 15% of all subdural fluid collections become or are empyema.[12] CT shows a hypodense or isodense, crescentric or lenticular extra-axial collection slightly denser than CSF. MR imaging is more sensitive than CT for delineating such collections. Compared with sterile collections, empyema may show slightly higher signal intensity on T1WI and especially FLAIR images. Contrast-enhanced CT and MR imaging show an intensely enhancing membrane surrounding the empyema.[12,83] High T2 signal intensity in the underlying cortex and presence of neighboring venous thrombosis, infarction, cerebritis, and abscess also support the diagnosis of subdural empyema. Similar to abscesses, empyemas are typically bright on DWI (see **Fig. 9**), consistent with restricted diffusion of pus, whereas sterile collections are similar to CSF.[84]

In epidural empyema, collection of pus occurs between the dura and calvaria. These patients have a more insidious and benign course because the dura acts as a barrier, protecting brain parenchyma from complications. This situation also explains the occasional presence of low or mixed signal intensity on DWI, because the pus becomes less viscous.[25,83] It shows similar signal characteristics on T1-weighted and T2-weighted images and the attenuation in CT, as for subdural empyema. Contrast administration shows a thick dural enhancement. Imaging studies may also show displacement of falx and dural sinuses away from the inner table, indicating epidural location of the collection.[1,15,83]

Cerebritis and Abscesses

Cerebritis and abscesses may have a variety of causes. In the context of the present discussion, spread by contiguous infection of the meninges by retrograde thrombophlebitis, or direct extension into the brain via the pia mater or along the perivascular spaces may occur in the later stages of the infectious process.[1] Initially, there is an area of focal cerebritis, characterized by vascular congestion, petechial hemorrhage, and edema.[12] CT shows an ill-defined area of low attenuation with subtle mass effect. It shows prolonged T1 and T2 signal intensity on MR images and little or no contrast enhancement (see **Figs. 17** and **18**; **Fig. 21**).[37,83] Because there is no purulent fluid, the key diagnostic sequence is DWI, with marked diffusion restriction, which might be attributed to hypercellularity from abundant infiltration of inflammatory cells, brain ischemia, or cytotoxic edema.[85] As the brain attempts to contain the infection, a capsule of collagen and granulation tissue is formed, the central portion undergoes liquefactive necrosis, and abscess develops.[1] These abscesses are commonly located at the gray matter–white matter junction, mostly in the frontal and temporal lobes.[12,86] Approximately 90% of abscesses are pyogenic, and despite the antibiotic treatment, the mortality remains as high as 14%.[12] Clinical diagnosis remains challenging, because the signs and symptoms often are nonspecific and usually overlap with the presence of a focal mass lesion.[67,86] In the initial stages of abscess formation, there is an incomplete rim of enhancement, which allows antibiotics to penetrate, and many lesions are arrested at this stage.[12] In due course, a mature abscess may form. Imaging at this stage shows a well-defined, smooth, complete capsular ring, which enhances

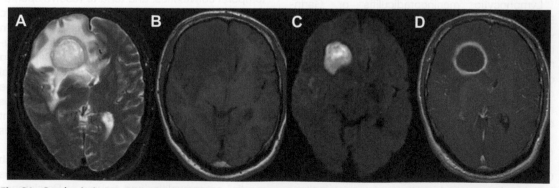

Fig. 21. Cerebral abscess in a 46-year-old man who presented with seizures and fever. Axial T2WI (*A*) at the level of ventricles showing a heterogeneous intensity lesion with surrounding edema in right frontal region. The lesion is hypointense on T1WI (*B*), with peripheral enhancement on postcontrast T1WI (*D*). On DWI (*C*), the lesion shows restricted diffusion. Pus culture grew *Staphylococcus aureus*.

strongly on contrast study. It is visualized as a thin, markedly hypointense ring on T2-weighted MR images, with prominent surrounding vasogenic edema.[12,87] The low T2-weighted signal intensity of the abscess rim is believed to be secondary to the presence of paramagnetic oxygen-free radicals inside macrophages.[12] The proteinaceous, necrotic fluid within the abscess cavity is hyperintense to CSF on T1 and FLAIR. Ring-enhancing brain lesions are nonspecific and need to be distinguished from other cystic lesions, primarily necrotic neoplasms.[37] In contrast to other ring-enhancing lesions, an abscess has a tendency to grow into the white matter, hence the abscess wall is usually thinner on the side that is closer to the ventricular system. The capsule is also generally smoother on the outside than on the inside.[12,25] On DWI, brain abscesses are seen as strong hyperintense foci with reduced ADC values (see Fig. 18). DWI is particularly useful in differentiating brain abscesses from necrotic or cystic tumor. Necrotic or cystic tumors generally have low to intermediate DWI signal and increased ADC values; however, cases of metastatic brain tumors with DWI hyperintensity and low ADC values have also been described.[88–90] In a recent study using DTI, it was shown that brain abscess cavity shows regions of increased FA values with restricted MD, compared with other cystic intracranial lesions. High FA in the brain abscess suggests inflammatory cell adhesion as a result of the presence of neuroinflammatory molecules, which suggests active inflammation. Hence DTI-derived FA could be used as potential surrogate marker of noninvasively assessing disease activity in patients with brain abscesses.[91] A perfusion MR study may also distinguish brain abscesses that show relative decrease in cerebral blood volume (CBV) from neoplasms, which show significantly increased CBV.[92] On MRS, spectra from brain abscesses reveal increased peaks of acetate (1.92 ppm), succinate (2.4 ppm), lactate (1.3 ppm), and other amino acids (0.9 ppm).[91] Main brain metabolites like N-acetylaspartate, creatine, and choline are usually not detectable. Although resonances of amino acids and lactate are seen in all bacterial abscesses, presence of acetate and succinate suggests anaerobic bacterial infection.[93]

Cranial Nerve Involvement

Cranial nerve dysfunction is likely related to direct inflammation or the result of direct stretching or pressure caused by shift of intracranial structures. The eighth nerve (vestibulocochlear) is most commonly affected and some degree of sensorineural hearing loss occurs in up to 30% of patients. It is most common after infection with Streptococcus pneumoniae. There is usually bilateral involvement, and once hearing loss occurs, it tends to be permanent. Hearing loss is probably the result of the spread of infection to the inner ear.[94] Other commonly affected nerves are the seventh (facial) and third (oculomotor) nerve. Second (optic) nerve involvement may occur, but is usually transient. Transient palsy of the sixth nerve can be seen as a sign of increased intracranial pressure or related to complication of lumbar puncture.

There are no specific imaging features for cranial nerve involvement in patients with pyogenic meningitis. In the chronic phase, CT may show sclerosis of the inner ear structures (labyrinthitis ossificans). However, thin-section T2-weighted MR imaging may show lack of normal high signal of the endolymph and perilymph in the labyrinth, before these changes become obvious on CT.[12] In addition, conductive-type hearing loss may be present in meningitis, secondary to middle ear infection or use of ototoxic antibiotics.[12]

Thrombosis and Infarct

Venous thrombosis results in cerebral infarctions in up to 30% of affected patients and is more commonly seen in children. It may arise as a direct consequence of meningitis or secondary to adjacent mastoiditis, which itself is a cause of meningitis.[12] It may affect the cortical venous sinuses or the cortical veins. The clinical manifestations of venous thrombosis are highly variable, ranging from no change in alertness, developing mild confusion, or progressing to coma. Focal neurologic deficits have also been described depending on the area of the involvement. Cranial nerve findings can also be present.[81] Venous infarcts involve nonarterial territories and are usually bilateral, show multiplicity, and tend to occur in the convexities. Areas of hemorrhage are seen in up to 25% of patients. On imaging, acute thrombosis of cortical veins or sinuses shows high attenuation on CT and is seen as high signal on T1-weighted MR images or as filling defects on MR or CT venography. Many venous infarcts are seen as nonspecific areas of high T2 signal intensity and are difficult to distinguish from areas of cerebritis. Because the identification of thrombosed cortical vein is difficult, many venous infarctions are only presumed diagnoses. DWI findings are also variable and are not predictive of infarction. Hemorrhages within these infarcts further affect ADC calculations.[95]

Vasculopathy

Cerebral infarcts associated with meningitis occur because of inflammatory-induced arterial spasms or because of direct inflammation of the walls of arteries/arterioles ending with an infectious arteritis and tend to affect the basal ganglia. However, occlusion of the large arterial branch can occur, resulting in cortical infarctions.[1] Narrowing and spasm of the larger-caliber arteries, irregularities of medium-size arteries, and occlusion of distal branches can be seen on catheter or MR angiography.[12]

VENTRICULITIS

Ventriculitis is a rare cerebral infection that has been variably referred to as ependymitis, intraventricular abscess, ventricular empyema, and pyocephalus.[96–100] With the increasing incidence of bacterial meningitis over the last 30 years because of nosocomial infections, the number of cases of ventriculitis is also likely to increase.[101] It is seen in 30% of all patients and is more common in the younger age group.[12,81] The 2 most common microorganisms causing ventriculitis are *Staphylococcus* and *Enterobacter*.[100]

There are multiple possible routes through which a pathogen might enter the intraventricular system, including direct implantation secondary to trauma or neurosurgical procedures, such as ventricular catheter placement; contiguous extension, such as rupture of a brain abscess; and extension into the ventricles and hematogenous spread to the subependyma or the choroid plexus.[1,97,101] Backflow of CSF from the extraventricular spaces into the intraventricular space might be considered as another possible route of infection leading to ventriculitis. This could be a potential explanation for the observation that ventriculitis is often associated with meningitis.[102]

Ventriculitis is important to recognize because its signs and symptoms may be subtle, its course can be indolent but lethal, and it is a potential source of persistent infection, even when meningitis is treated.[103–105] Early diagnosis is essential for the appropriate treatment of this life-threatening condition. Neuroimaging is one of the available diagnostic tools besides laboratory investigations that play an important role in diagnosing this condition.

Cranial sonography is a useful imaging modality in the evaluation of ventriculitis, especially in infants. The most common findings include an irregular and echogenic ependyma, the presence of intraventricular debris and stranding, often associated with ventricular dilatation. Intraventricular adhesions and septae are seen as chronic complications of meningitis in about 10% of patients and

their identification is important in planning for appropriate shunt placement. Sonography often shows them better than CT.[106–109]

On MR imaging, the ependyma is thick and enhances markedly (**Fig. 22**). The ventricular walls frequently show high T2 signal intensity, the ventricles themselves may be dilated, and debris are usually seen in their dependent portions.[100] Usually, these debris are of high signal on DWI, with reduced ADC value (see **Fig. 22**), and are seen as fluid levels of high signal intensity on FLAIR images.[100,110] However, higher ADC values might be observed when pus is diluted by nonpurulent CSF.[110] Presence of irregular ventricular debris is especially characteristic of ventriculitis. CT findings are similar to those of MR imaging. Intraventricular adhesions and septae may entrap portions of the ventricles and result in segmental dilation.[12,81] Choroid plexitis is another finding associated with ventriculitis. Imaging findings include a poorly defined margin of a swollen choroid plexus and enhancement on contrast study.[111] Unlike viral infections, pyogenic ventriculitis almost never results in periventricular calcifications.[12]

NONINFECTIOUS MENINGITIS

A diverse group of noninfectious processes can mimic CNS infections. Clinical manifestations primarily take the form of a chronic meningitic syndrome. They usually present with subacute onset, headache, fever, and stiff neck. Encephalitic signs also can occur, and seizures are not uncommon. CSF is marked by increased protein and decreased glucose levels, and usually lymphocytic pleocytosis.

Mild meningeal enhancement is present in most patients after neurosurgery, and should not be interpreted as meningitis. Leptomeningeal enhancement is rare after a lumbar puncture, and in the appropriate clinical setting, meningitis needs to be considered in such patients.[1]

Chemical Meningitis

The concept of chemical meningitis was first described by Cushing in 1920,[112] when he noted waves of fever after operating on cerebellar tumors. Chemical meningitis occurs in response to a nonbacterial irritant introduced into the subarachnoid space (eg, blood, dermoid cyst rupture and methotrexate instillation). Evaluation of CSF in these patients showed leukocytosis, increased protein low glucose levels, and negative cultures.[113]

Recurrent Meningitis

Recurrent meningitis is more common in adults and is said to have an incidence of 8%, and about

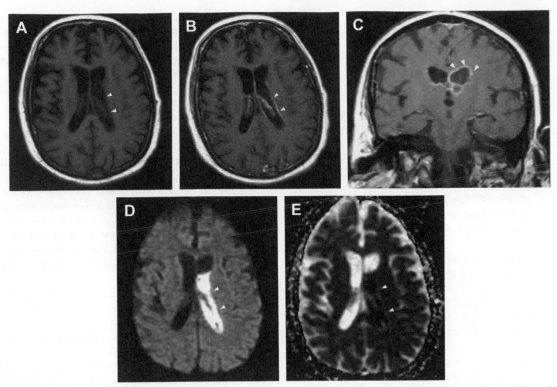

Fig. 22. Bacterial ventriculitis. (*A*) Axial T1WI shows subtle increased signal within the left lateral ventricle, indicating debris. (*B*, *C*) Axial and coronal T1WI after contrast shows increased ependymal enhancement along the left lateral ventricle consistent with ventriculitis. (*D*, *E*) DWI and corresponding ADC map show restricted diffusion within the left lateral ventricle, suggestive of abscess formation.

16% of all meningitis episodes are reported to be recurrent in nature. The interval between the bouts of meningitis may be months or even years. The most common underlying lesion (75%) is a bone defect, allowing for the intracranial compartment to communicate with the sinonasal or middle ear cavities, circumventing the usual immune defense mechanisms. The most common responsible microorganisms are streptococci and gram-negative bacilli.[1]

Mollaret Meningitis

Mollaret meningitis is a rare syndrome characterized by recurrent episodes of viral (aseptic) meningitis, most commonly seen in young females, with a possible link with herpes simplex virus. Each episode of Mollaret meningitis presents fulminantly with high fever, severe headache, and meningitic signs. Lumbar puncture reveals a neutrophilic and lymphocytic pleocytosis, with mildly increased protein and normal glucose levels. It can be diagnosed by polymerase chain reaction analysis of spinal fluid for the presence of viruses, in particular herpes simplex type 2. No specific imaging features have been described.[114]

SUMMARY

Many infectious and noninfectious inflammatory conditions can affect the cranial meninges. Knowledge of the normal anatomy of the meninges and the extra-axial spaces and its varied pathophysiologic states in meningitis aids in understanding the imaging appearances. Imaging studies can be normal in the early stages of the diseases, but MR imaging with its advanced techniques is a promising and sensitive technique in evaluation of patients suspected of having meningitis or its complications, or other processes affecting the subarachnoid space. One of the major roles of imaging is early identification of potentially serious complications, thus reducing morbidity and mortality.

ACKNOWLEDGMENTS

We are extremely grateful to Carolyn Nowak, B.A. and Michelle Kim, B.A., for their artistic skills rendered in creating the true-to-life medical illustrations that greatly enhanced the manuscript.

REFERENCES

1. Kanamalla US, Ibarra RA, Jinkins JR. Imaging of cranial meningitis and ventriculitis. Neuroimaging Clin North Am 2000;10:309–31.
2. Griffin DE. Approach to patient with infection of central nervous system. In: Gorbach SL, Barlett JG, Blacklow NR, editors. Infectious disease. 2nd edition. Philadelphia: WB Saunders; 1997. p. 1377.
3. Sze G, Soletsky S, Bronen R, et al. MR imaging of the cranial meninges with emphasis on contrast enhancement and meningeal carcinomatosis. Am J Neuroradiol 1989;10:965–75.
4. Meltzer CC, Fukui MB, Kanal E, et al. MR imaging of the meninges. Part I. Normal anatomic features and nonneoplastic disease. Radiology 1996;201:297–308.
5. Quint DJ, Eldevik OP, Cohen JK. Magnetic resonance imaging of normal meningeal enhancement at 1.5T. Acad Radiol 1996;6(3):463–8.
6. Smirniotopoulos JG, Murphy FM, Rushing EJ, et al. Patterns of contrast enhancement in the brain and meninges. Radiographics 2007;27(2):525–51.
7. Dietemann JL, Correia Bernardo R, Bogorin A, et al. Normal and abnormal meningeal enhancement: MRI features. J Radiol 2005;86(11):1659–83.
8. Sage MR, Wilson AJ, Scroop R. Contrast media and the brain: the basis of CT and MR imaging enhancement. Neuroimaging Clin N Am 1998;8:695–707.
9. Burke JW, Podrasky AE, Bradley WG Jr. Meninges: benign postoperative enhancement on MR images. Radiology 1990;174:99–102.
10. Mittl RL Jr, Yousem DM. Frequency of unexplained meningeal enhancement in the brain after lumbar puncture. Am J Neuroradiol 1994;15:633–8.
11. van de Beek D, de Gans J, Spanjaard L, et al. Clinical features and prognostic factors in adults with bacterial meningitis. N Engl J Med 2004;351(18):1849–59 [Erratum in: N Engl J Med. 2005 Mar 3; 352(9):950].
12. Castillo M. Imaging of meningitis. Semin Roentgenol 2004;39(4):458–64.
13. Becker LE. Infections of the developing brain. Am J Neuroradiol 1992;13(2):537–49.
14. Harris TM, Edwards MK. Meningitis. Neuroimaging Clin N Am 1991;1:39–56.
15. Wong J, Quint DJ. Imaging of central nervous system infections. Semin Roentgenol 1999;34(2):123–43.
16. Hasbun R, Abrahams J, Jekel J, et al. Computed tomography of the head before lumbar puncture in adults with suspected meningitis. N Engl J Med 2001;345:1727–33.
17. Kastrup O, Wanke I, Maschke M. Neuroimaging of infections of the central nervous system. Semin Neurol 2008;28(4):511–22.
18. Gee GT, Bazan C 3rd, Jinks JR. Miliary tuberculosis involving the brain: MR findings. AJR Am J Roentgenol 1992;159(5):1075–6.
19. Okagaki H. Fundamentals of neuropathology. 2nd edition. New York: Igaku-Shoin; 1989.
20. Jinkins JR. Computed tomography of intracranial tuberculosis. Neuroradiology 1991;33(2):126–35.
21. Osborn AG. Infections of the brain and its linings. In: Diagnostic neuroradiology. St Louis (MO): Mosby; 1994. p. 673–715.
22. Zee CS, Go JL, Kim P, et al. Cerebral infections and inflammation. In: Haaga JR, Lanzieri CF, Gilkeson RC, editors. CT and MR imaging of the whole body. 4th edition. St Louis (MO): Mosby; 2002. p. 207–10.
23. Parmar H, Sitoh YY, Anand P, et al. Contrast-enhanced FLAIR imaging in the evaluation of infectious leptomeningeal diseases. Eur J Radiol 2006;58(1):89–95.
24. Stuckey SL, Goh TD, Heffernan T, et al. Hyperintensity in the subarachnoid space on FLAIR MRI. AJR Am J Roentgenol 2007;189(4):913–21.
25. Karampekios S, Hesselink J. Cerebral infections. Eur Radiol 2005;15(3):485–93.
26. Kioumehr F, Dadsetan MR, Feldman N, et al. Postcontrast MRI of cranial meninges: leptomeningitis versus pachymeningitis. J Comput Assist Tomogr 1995;19(5):713–20.
27. Gupta RK, Kathuria MK, Pradhan S. Magnetization transfer MR imaging in CNS tuberculosis. Am J Neuroradiol 1999;20:867–75.
28. Kamra P, Azad R, Prasad KN, et al. Infectious meningitis: prospective evaluation with magnetization transfer MRI. Br J Radiol 2004;77(917):387–94.
29. Mishra AM, Gupta RK, Jaggi RS, et al. Role of diffusion-weighted imaging and in vivo proton magnetic resonance spectroscopy in the differential diagnosis of ring-enhancing intracranial cystic mass lesions. J Comput Assist Tomogr 2004;28(4):540–7.
30. Gupta RK. Tuberculosis and other non-tuberculous bacterial graunulomatous infections. In: Gupta RK, Lufkin RB, editors. MR imaging and spectroscopy of central nervous system infection. New York: Kluwer Academic/Plenum Publishers; 2001. p. 95–145.
31. Nath K, Husain M, Trivedi R, et al. Clinical implications of increased fractional anisotropy in meningitis associated with brain abscess. J Comput Assist Tomogr 2007;31:888–93.
32. Trivedi R, Malik GK, Gupta RK, et al. Increased anisotropy in neonatal meningitis: an indicator of meningeal inflammation. Neuroradiology 2007;49:767–75.
33. Yadav A, Malik GK, Trivedi R, et al. Correlation of CSF neuroinflammatory molecules with leptomeningeal cortical subcortical white matter fractional anisotropy in neonatal meningitis. Magn Reson Imaging 2009;27(2):214–21.

34. Malik GK, Trivedi R, Gupta A, et al. Quantitative DTI assessment of periventricular white matter changes in neonatal meningitis. Brain Dev 2008; 30:334–41.

35. Jain KK, Mittal SK, Kumar S, et al. Imaging features of central nervous system fungal infections. Neurol India 2007;55(3):241–50.

36. Kovoor JM, Mahadevan A, Narayan JP, et al. Cryptococcal choroid plexitis as a mass lesion: MR imaging and histopathologic correlation. Am J Neuroradiol 2002;23:273–6.

37. Rumboldt Z, Thurnher MM, Gupta RK. Central nervous system infections. Semin Roentgenol 2007;42(2):62–91.

38. Awasthi M, Patankar T, Shah P, et al. Cerebral cryptococcosis: atypical appearances on CT. Br J Radiol 2001;74:83–5.

39. Kathuria MK, Gupta RK. Fungal infections. In: Gupta RK, Lufkin RB, editors. MR imaging and spectroscopy of central nervous system infections. New York: Kluwer Press; 2001. p. 177–203.

40. Ruiz A, Post MJ, Bundschu CC. Dentate nuclei involvement in AIDS patients with CNS cryptococcosis: imaging findings with pathologic correlation. J Comput Assist Tomogr 1997;21:175–82.

41. Sibtain NA, Chinn RJ. Imaging of the central nervous system in HIV infection. Imaging 2002; 14:48–59.

42. Lui G, Lee N, Ip M, et al. Cryptococcosis in apparently immunocompetent patients. QJM 2006;99: 143–51.

43. Saigal G, Post MJD, Lolayekar S, et al. Unusual presentation of central nervous system cryptococcal infection in an immunocompetent patient. AJNR Am J Neuroradiol 2005;26:2522–6.

44. Vender JR, Miller DM, Roth T, et al. Intraventricular cryptococcal cysts. Am J Neuroradiol 1996;17: 110–3.

45. Aharon-Peretz J, Kliot D, Finkelstein R, et al. Cryptococcal meningitis mimicking vascular dementia. Neurology 2004;62:2135.

46. Pittella JE. Neurocysticercosis. Brain Pathol 1997; 7(1):681–93.

47. Salzman KL. Parasites, miscellaneous. In: Diagnostic imaging: brain. Salt Lake City (UT): Amirsys; 2004. p. 8–53.

48. La Mantia L, Costa A, Eoli M, et al. Racemose neurocysticercosis after chronic meningitis: effect of medical treatment. Clin Neurol Neurosurg 1995; 97(1):50–4.

49. Mishra D, Sharma S, Gupta S, et al. Acute cysticercal meningitis–missed diagnosis. Indian J Pediatr 2006;73(9):835–7.

50. Puri V, Sharma DK. Neurocysticercosis in children. Indian Pediatr 1991;28:1309–17.

51. Kalra V, Mittal R, Rana KS, et al. Neurocysticercosis: Indian experience. In: Perat MV, editor. New developments in neurology. Bologna (Italy): Monduzzi Editore S.P.A; 1998. p. 353–9.

52. Joubert J. Cysticercal meningitis–a pernicious form of neurocysticercosis which responds poorly to praziquantel. S Afr Med J 1990;77:528–30.

53. Visudhipan P, Chiemchanya S. Acute cysticercal meningitis in children: response to praziquantel. Ann Trop Paediatr 1997;17:9–13.

54. Jubelt B, Miller JR. Parasitic infections. In: Rowland LP, editor. Merritt's textbook of neurology. 8th edition. Philadelphia/London: Lea & Febiger; 1989. p. 164–76, chapter II.

55. Tsang VC, Brand JA, Boyer AE. An enzyme-linked immunoelectro-transfer blot assay and glycoprotein antigens for diagnosing human cysticercosis (Taenia solium). J Infect Dis 1989;159:50–9.

56. Zee CS, Segall HD, Apuzzo ML, et al. Intraventricular cysticercal cysts: further neuroradiological observations and neurosurgical implications. AJNR Am J Neuroradiol 1984;5:727–30.

57. Teitelbaum GP, Otto RJ, Lin M, et al. MR imaging of neurocysticercosis. Am J Radiol 1989;153:857–66.

58. Zee CS, Segall HD, Destian S, et al. MRI of intraventricular cysticercosis: surgical implications. J Comput Assist Tomogr 1993;17(6):932–9.

59. Ramirez-Avila L, Slome S, Schuster FL, et al. Eosinophilic meningitis due to Angiostrongylus and Gnathostoma species. Clin Infect Dis 2009;48(3):322–7.

60. Lo Re V 3rd, Gluckman SJ. Eosinophilic meningitis. Am J Med 2003;114(3):217–23.

61. Kanpittaya J, Jitpimolmard S, Tiamkao S, et al. MR findings of eosinophilic meningoencephalitis attributed to Angiostrongylus cantonensis. Am J Neuroradiol 2000;21(6):1090–4.

62. Singh P, Kochhar R, Vashishta RK, et al. Amebic meningoencephalitis: spectrum of imaging findings. Am J Neuroradiol 2006;27(6):1217–21.

63. Goto M, Takahashi T, Kanda T, et al. Detection of Toxoplasma gondii by polymerase chain reaction in cerebrospinal fluid from human immunodeficiency virus-1-infected Japanese patients with focal neurological signs. J Int Med Res 2004;32(6):665–70.

64. Okubo Y, Shinozaki M, Yoshizawa S, et al. Diagnosis of systemic toxoplasmosis with HIV infection using DNA extracted from paraffin-embedded tissue for polymerase chain reaction: a case report. J Med Case Reports 2010;4:265.

65. Brightbill TC, Ihmeidan IH, Post MJ, et al. Neurosyphilis in HIV-positive and HIV-negative patients: neuroimaging findings. Am J Neuroradiol 1995; 16:703–11.

66. Tien RD, Gean-Marton AD, Mark AS. Neurosyphilis in HIV carriers: MR findings in six patients. Am J Roentgenol 1992;158:1325–8.

67. Ances BM, Danish SF, Kolson DL, et al. Cerebral gumma mimicking glioblastoma multiforme. Neurocrit Care 2005;2(3):300–2.

68. Bash S, Hathout GM, Cohen S. Mesiotemporal T2-weighted hyperintensity: neurosyphilis mimicking herpes encephalitis. Am J Neuroradiol 2001;22: 314–6.

69. Agarwal R, Sze G. Neuro-lyme disease: MR imaging findings. Radiology 2009;253(1):167–73.

70. Finkel MF. Lyme disease and its neurologic complications. Arch Neurol 1988;45(1):99–104.

71. Falco RC, Fish D. Prevalence of Ixodes dammini near the homes of Lyme disease patients in Westchester County, New York. Am J Epidemiol 1988; 127(4):826–30.

72. Wright SW, Trott AT. North American tickborne diseases. Ann Emerg Med 1988;17(9):964–72.

73. Fernandez RE, Rothberg M, Ferencz G, et al. Lyme disease of the CNS: MR imaging findings in 14 cases. Am J Neuroradiol 1990;11(3):479–81.

74. Garcia-Monaco JC, Benach JL. Lyme neuroborreliosis. Ann Neurol 1995;37:691–702.

75. Ramesh G, Borda JT, Gill A, et al. Possible role of glial cells in the onset and progression of Lyme neuroborreliosis. J Neuroinflammation 2009;6:23.

76. Demaerel P, Wilms G, Van Lierde S, et al. Lyme disease in childhood presenting as primary leptomeningeal enhancement without parenchymal findings on MR. Am J Neuroradiol 1994;15(2): 302–4.

77. Kőchling J, Freitag HJ, Bollinger T, et al. Lyme disease with lymphocytic meningitis, trigeminal palsy and silent thalamic lesion. Eur J Paediatr Neurol 2008;12(6):501–4.

78. Huisman TA, Wohlrab G, Nadal D, et al. Unusual presentations of neuroborreliosis (Lyme disease) in childhood. J Comput Assist Tomogr 1999;23(1): 39–42.

79. Koudstaal PJ, Vermeulen M, Wokke JH. Argyll Robertson pupils in lymphocytic meningoradiculitis (Bannwarth's syndrome). J Neurol Neurosurg Psychiatry 1987;50(3):363–5.

80. Vianello M, Marchiori G, Giometto B. Multiple cranial nerve involvement in Bannwarth's syndrome. Neurol Sci 2008;29(2):109–12.

81. Hughes DC, Raghavan A, Mordekar SR, et al. Role of imaging in the diagnosis of acute bacterial meningitis and its complications. Postgrad Med J 2010;86(1018):478–85.

82. Cabral DA, Flodmark O, Farrell K, et al. Prospective study of computed tomography in acute bacterial meningitis. J Pediatr 1987;111:201–5.

83. Ferreira NP, Otta GM, do Amaral LL, et al. Imaging aspects of pyogenic infections of the central nervous system. Top Magn Reson Imaging 2005; 16(2):145–54.

84. Wong AM, Zimmerman RA, Simon EM, et al. Diffusion-weighted MR imaging of subdural empyema in children. Am J Neuroradiol 2004;25: 1016–21.

85. Tung GA, Rogg JM. Diffusion-weighted imaging of cerebritis. Am J Neuroradiol 2003;24:1110–3.

86. Rana S, Albayram S, Lin DD, et al. Diffusion-weighted imaging and apparent diffusion coefficient maps in a case of intracerebral abscess with ventricular extension. Am J Neuroradiol 2002; 23:109–12.

87. Falcone S, Post MJ. Encephalitis, cerebritis, and brain abscess: pathophysiology and imaging findings. Neuroimaging Clin N Am 2000;10:333–53.

88. Hartmann M, Jansen O, Heiland S, et al. Restricted diffusion within ring enhancement is not pathognomonic for brain abscess. Am J Neuroradiol 2001; 22:1738–42.

89. Holtas S, Geijer B, Stromblad LG, et al. A ring-enhancing metastasis with central high signal on diffusion-weighted imaging and low apparent diffusion coefficients. Neuroradiology 2000;42:824–7.

90. Guzman R, Barth A, Lovblad KO, et al. Use of diffusion-weighted magnetic resonance imaging in differentiating purulent brain processes from cystic brain tumors. J Neurosurg 2002;97:1101–7.

91. Gupta RK, Nath K, Prasad A, et al. In vivo demonstration of neuroinflammatory molecule expression in brain abscess with diffusion tensor imaging. Am J Neuroradiol 2008;29(2):326–32.

92. Erdogan C, Hakyemez B, Yildirim N, et al. Brain abscess and cystic brain tumor: discrimination with dynamic susceptibility contrast perfusion-weighted MRI. J Comput Assist Tomogr 2005;29:663–7.

93. Garg M, Gupta RK, Husain M, et al. Brain abscesses: etiologic categorization with in vivo proton MR spectroscopy. Radiology 2004;230:519–27.

94. Beijen J, Casselman J, Joosten F, et al. Magnetic resonance imaging in patients with meningitis induced hearing loss. Eur Arch Otorhinolaryngol 2009;266:1229–36.

95. Ducreux D, Oppenheim C, Vandamme X, et al. Diffusion-weighted imaging patterns of brain damage associated with cerebral venous thrombosis. Am J Neuroradiol 2001;22:261–8.

96. Bakshi R, Kinkel P, Mechtler L, et al. Cerebral ventricular empyema associated with severe adult pyogenic meningitis: computed tomography findings. Clin Neurol Neurosurg 1997;99:252–5.

97. Barloon TJ, Yuh WT, Knepper LE, et al. Cerebral ventriculitis: MR findings. J Comput Assist Tomogr 1990;14:272–5.

98. Bodino J, Lylyk P, Del Valle M, et al. Computed tomography in purulent meningitis. Am J Dis Child 1982;136:495–501.

99. Vachon L, Mikity V. Computed tomography and ultrasound in purulent ventriculitis. J Ultrasound Med 1987;6:269–71.

100. Fukui MB, Williams RL, Mudigonda S. CT and MR imaging features of pyogenic ventriculitis. Am J Neuroradiol 2001;22:1510–6.

101. Lambo A, Nchimi A, Khamis J, et al. Primary intra-ventricular brain abscess. Neuroradiology 2003;45: 908–10.

102. Fujikawa A, Tsuchiya K, Honya K, et al. Comparison of MRI sequences to detect ventriculitis. Am J Roentgenol 2006;187(4):1048–53.

103. Rahal JJ Jr, Hyams PJ, Simberkoff MS, et al. Combined intrathecal and intramuscular gentamicin for gram-negative meningitis: pharmacologic study of 21 patients. N Engl J Med 1974;290:1394–8.

104. Kaiser A, McGee Z. Aminoglycoside therapy of gram-negative bacillary meningitis. N Engl J Med 1975;293:1215–20.

105. Durand M, Calderwood S, Weber D, et al. Acute bacterial meningitis in adults: a review of 493 episodes. N Engl J Med 1993;328:21–8.

106. Yikilmaz A, Taylor GA. Sonographic findings in bacterial meningitis in neonates and young infants. Pediatr Radiol 2008;38(2):129–37.

107. Han BK, Babcock DS, McAdams L. Bacterial meningitis in infants: sonographic findings. Radiology 1985;154:645–50.

108. Tatsuno M, Hasegawa M, Okuyama K. Ventriculitis in infants: diagnosis by color Doppler flow imaging. Pediatr Neurol 1993;9:127–30.

109. Reeder JD, Sanders RC. Ventriculitis in the neonate: recognition by sonography. Am J Neuroradiol 1983;4:37–41.

110. Mathews VP, Smith RR. Choroid plexus infections: neuroimaging appearances of four cases. Am J Neuroradiol 1992;13:374–8.

111. Pezzullo JA, Tung GA, Mudigonda S, et al. Diffusion-weighted MR imaging of pyogenic ventriculitis. Am J Roentgenol 2003;180:71–5.

112. Cushing H. Experiences with the cerebellar astrocytomas: a critical review of seventy-six cases. Surg Gynecol Obstet 1931;52:129–91.

113. Sanchez GB, Kaylie DM, O'Malley MR, et al. Chemical meningitis following cerebellopontine angle tumor surgery. Otolaryngol Head Neck Surg 2008;138(3):368–73.

114. Prandota J. Mollaret meningitis may be caused by reactivation of latent cerebral toxoplasmosis. Int J Neurosci 2009;119(10):1655–92.

Imaging of Cerebritis, Encephalitis, and Brain Abscess

Tanya J. Rath, MD[a],*, Marion Hughes, MD[a],
Mohammad Arabi, MD, FRCR[b], Gaurang V. Shah, MD[b]

KEYWORDS

• Central nervous system • Infection • Magnetic resonance imaging

KEY POINTS

- The most common identified sources of brain abscess include: otomastoiditis, sinusitis, odontogenic abscess, hematogenous dissemination from a distant source and neurosurgical complication.
- MRI is sensitive for the detection of brain abscess. Restricted diffusion within a centrally T2 hyperintense ring enhancing mass is characteristic but not pathognomonic of pyogenic brain abscess.
- MRI can demonstrate the complications from brain abscess including intracranial herniation, hydrocephalus, meningitis, subdural or epidural empyema, venous sinus thrombosis and ventriculitis.
- Imaging is critical to the rapid diagnosis of brain abscess, provides guidance for stereotactic localization and is useful for monitoring response following treatment.
- Infectious encephalitis is usually viral in etiology and should be considered in patients complaining of fever and headache with altered level of consciousness or evidence of cerebral dysfunction.
- The MRI features of encephalitis are highly variable according to the offending organism and patient age.
- HSV encephalitis is associated with high mortality and in adults typically causes asymmetric bilateral FLAIR/T2WI hyperintensity in the medial temporal lobes, insular cortex and posterior-inferior frontal lobes with relative sparing of the basal ganglia.

INTRODUCTION

Cerebritis is an area of poorly defined acute inflammation in the brain with increased permeability of the local blood vessels, but without neovascularity or angiogenesis.[1] Cerebritis can result from a variety of etiological factors, including pyogenic infection, and if left untreated in this setting leads to pyogenic brain abscess formation. A pyogenic abscess is a focal area of parenchymal infection that contains a central collection of pus surrounded by a vascularized collagenous capsule.[1–3] Before the late 1800s brain abscess was typically fatal and only discovered on postmortem examination. In 1893, Sir William Macewen published the monograph *Pyogenic Infective Diseases of the Brain and Spinal Cord*, which described the successful surgical treatment of 18 of 25 reported intraparenchymal brain abscesses.[4] Macewen stressed the importance of aseptic surgery, cerebral localization, and early diagnosis as important factors essential to the successful surgical treatment of brain abscess.[4] After the addition of antibiotic treatment in the early 1940s, mortality from brain abscesses decreased over the next 2 decades but remained high. A multitude of imaging modalities including ventriculography, angiography, and thorotrast administration had a positive impact on the treatment of brain abscess by providing a means to sequentially image the

[a] Department of Radiology, University of Pittsburgh Medical Center, 200 Lothrop Street, Presby South Tower, 8th Floor North, Pittsburgh, PA 15213-2582, USA; [b] Department of Radiology, University of Michigan Health System, 1500 East Medical Center Drive, Ann Arbor, MI 48109, USA
* Corresponding author.
E-mail address: rathtj@upmc.edu

Neuroimag Clin N Am 22 (2012) 585–607
doi:10.1016/j.nic.2012.04.002
1052-5149/12/$ – see front matter © 2012 Elsevier Inc. All rights reserved.

abscess cavity.[5] Since the mid 1970s, mortality from brain abscess has decreased from 30% to 40% to 5% to 20%, with the higher rates reported in developing nations.[2,6–15] This reduction in mortality has largely been attributed to (1) the advent of commercially available computed tomography (CT) in 1974, and (2) improved targeted antibiotic therapy due to advances in bacteriologic techniques and new antimicrobial agents.[15–18] CT allows for rapid diagnosis and localization, stereotactic aspiration, and accurate serial postoperative evaluation.[19,20]

Encephalitis is a diffuse infection or inflammatory process of the brain itself with clinical evidence of brain dysfunction.[21,22] Infectious encephalitis is typically viral in origin. The diagnosis of viral encephalitis should be strongly considered in patients presenting with febrile disease accompanied by headache, altered level of consciousness, and evidence of cerebral dysfunction. Imaging plays a role in the diagnosis of encephalitis when combined with the medical history, physical examination, serologic studies, and cerebrospinal fluid (CSF) analysis. In addition, there are multiple nonviral causes of infectious encephalitis including bacterial, fungal, parasitic, and rickettsial origins.[21] The imaging appearances of several common and select uncommon infectious encephalitides along with causes of encephalitis in the pediatric patient population are reviewed in this article. Common causes of encephalitis in immunocompromised patients, and their imaging appearances, are also discussed in this article.

PYOGENIC INFECTION
Pathophysiology

Brain abscess is often categorized by the source of infection, which influences the location of the abscess and the offending organism. The most common identified causes of brain abscess include direct spread from local infections, hematogenous dissemination from a distant source, trauma, and neurosurgical complication. Up to 30% of brain abscesses are reported as cryptogenic.[2,3,12] Otomastoiditis, sinusitis, and odontogenic abscess are the primary sources of direct spread, which occurs through involvement of bone or via transmission of bacteria to the brain through the valveless emissary veins.[3] Otomastoiditis causes abscess formation in the adjacent temporal lobe and cerebellum (Figs. 1 and 2). Frontal and ethmoid sinusitis and odontogenic infection are frequently associated with formation of frontal lobe abscess.[23]

Abscesses secondary to hematogenous seeding from a distant source are more typically multiple, near the gray-white junction, and usually in the distribution of the middle cerebral artery.[23] Sources of hematogenous dissemination are variable. Identifying the source of infection is a crucial factor for adequate treatment to prevent recurrent disease. In children, there should be a high index of suspicion for congenital cyanotic heart disease.[2,24] Examples of other sources include pulmonary abscess, pulmonary arteriovenous malformation (AVM), bacterial endocarditis, and intra-abdominal infections. Dental abscess can result in bacteremia with hematogenous dissemination or local thrombophlebitis.

The epidemiologic trends of brain abscess are changing. Brain abscess is uniformly more common among males than females for unknown reasons, and most commonly occurs during the first 4 decades of life, although all age groups may be affected.[12] Aggressive medical and surgical management of otitis media has led to a decrease in otogenic-related brain abscess in developed countries, although it remains the principal source of brain abscess in developing countries such as India and China.[9,12] Similarly, there are reports of decreased incidence of brain abscess secondary to congenital cyanotic heart disease in developed countries, likely attributable to earlier and improved surgical repair.[9] Brain abscess secondary to trauma and neurosurgery has increased.[9,12,13,25–27] The rising incidence of postsurgical abscess has largely been attributed to the increased volume of neurosurgeries performed (Fig. 3). Additional predisposing factors include diabetes mellitus, alcoholism, intravenous drug abuse, pulmonary AVM, and immunosuppression.[9,13,14]

Clinical Presentation

Symptoms depend on the location of the abscess, degree of mass effect, and associated complications. Headache is the most frequent symptom. Additional symptoms include fever, focal neurologic deficit, nausea, vomiting, and seizure. Laboratory tests add little to the diagnosis. The white blood cell count is variably elevated and the absence of a leukocytosis does not exclude the diagnosis.[2,11,13,14] Lumbar puncture may be contraindicated because of mass effect and elevated intracranial pressure. CSF analysis can be normal, and when abnormal typically demonstrates a nonspecific elevation in protein and white blood cells that does not aid in diagnosis or treatment. In the absence of intraventricular rupture, CSF cultures are frequently sterile.[2,11,14] In cases of hematogenous dissemination blood cultures should be performed, as they may identify the causative organism.

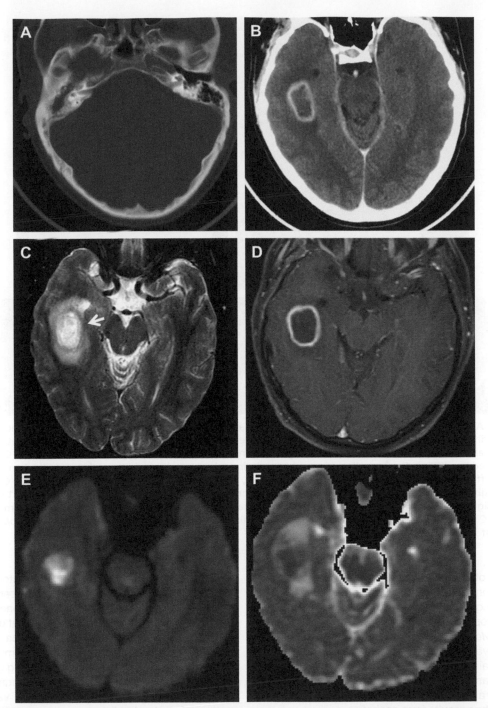

Fig. 1. A patient who presented with ear infection and headache. (*A*) CT bone window demonstrates complete opacification of the right middle ear cleft and poorly pneumatized right mastoid, consistent with chronic right otomastoiditis. (*B*) On contrast-enhanced CT there is an associated ovoid ring-enhancing mass in the right temporal lobe with surrounding vasogenic edema. (*C*) On axial T2-weighted sequence, it has central hyperintense signal corresponding to the pus cavity and the characteristic surrounding T2 hypointense signal of the abscess capsule (*white arrow*). Local mass effect results in entrapment of the adjacent mildly dilated right temporal horn. (*D*) Axial T1 postcontrast sequence demonstrates typical smooth ring enhancement of a mature abscess. (*E, F*) Corresponding diffusion-weighted sequence and apparent diffusion coefficient (ADC) maps confirm restricted diffusion within the abscess cavity.

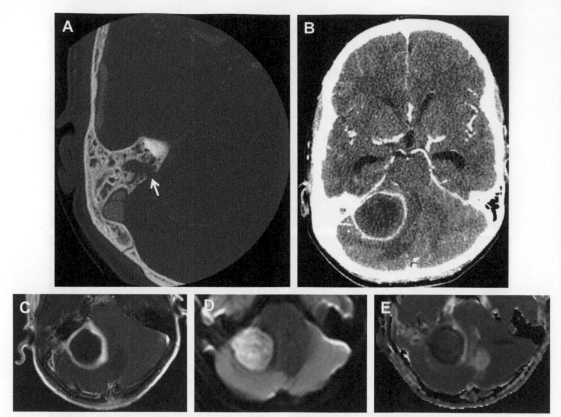

Fig. 2. A patient who presented with complaints of earache and fever. (*A*) Temporal bone CT demonstrates mastoiditis with opacification of the right mastoid air cells and bone dehiscence along the dorsal right petrous temporal bone (*white arrow*). An adjacent ring-enhancing mass is seen in the right posterior fossa. (*B*) Contrast-enhanced head CT confirms an adjacent round smooth rim-enhancing abscess in the right cerebellar hemisphere. Mass effect displaces the fourth ventricle to the left, and there is associated hydrocephalus. (*C*) On axial T1-weighted postcontrast MR imaging the abscess demonstrates a rind of enhancement with central T1 hypointense signal. (*D*) Diffusion-weighted sequence demonstrates central hyperintense signal. (*E*) On the corresponding ADC map there is central hypointense signal, confirming restricted diffusion in the abscess cavity. (*Courtesy of* Hemant Parmar, MD, University of Michigan.)

The offending microbes vary with the source of infection and frequently are polymicrobial. The most common implicated organisms include microaerophilic streptococci, anaerobic bacteria, *Staphylococcus aureus*, and facultative gram-negative bacteria.[2,3,9,11–14,26] In particular, nocardia brain abscess is reportedly difficult to treat and has been associated with high mortality.[28] Ideally antibiotic therapy should be targeted based on culture results from aspiration.

Radiologic Imaging

Progressing from cerebritis to abscess formation, the imaging characteristics change depending on the time of imaging. Britt and Enzmann[29] described the spectrum in 4 separate stages including early cerebritis, late cerebritis, early capsule formation, and late capsule formation,

based on observed gross surgical, histopathologic, and CT criteria. During the early cerebritis phase, bacteria arrive to the brain parenchyma, and there is an inflammatory response that grossly results in softening of the brain and histopathologically corresponds to perivascular inflammatory cuffing poorly delineated from surrounding normal brain. On noncontrast CT, this corresponds to an area of ill-defined low attenuation with a variable pattern of contrast enhancement ranging from no enhancement to nodular or ringlike enhancement. The enhancement pattern is unchanged or progresses on delayed images obtained at 30 to 60 minutes after contrast administration. During the late cerebritis phase, pathologically there is progression of central necrosis, and fibroblasts deposit an early reticulin matrix around the periphery. On noncontrast CT there is persistent poorly defined low-attenuation edema; however,

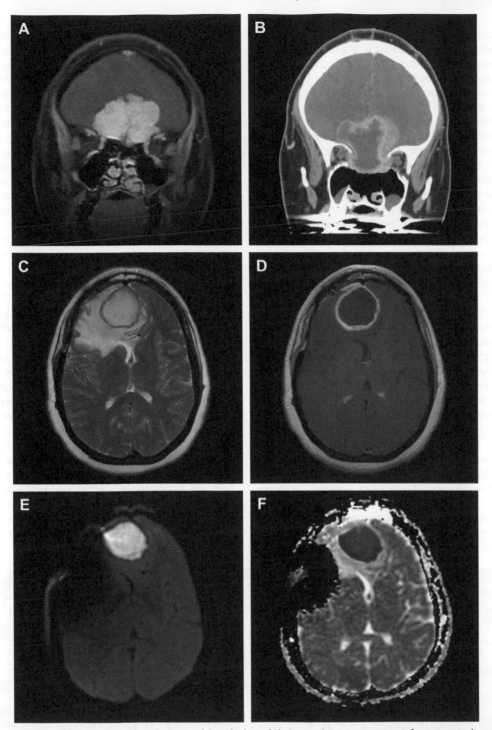

Fig. 3. A 36-year-old woman with a history of headaches. (*A*) Coronal T1 postcontrast fat-saturated sequence demonstrates an enhancing extra-axial mass along the floor of the anterior cranial fossa, characteristic of an olfactory groove meningioma. (*B*) Reconstructed coronal CT postcontrast image demonstrates partial resection of the mass that was done via a staged expanded endonasal and subfrontal approach. Postoperative course was complicated by recurrent frontal sinusitis and CSF leak requiring surgical repair. (*C, D*) Axial T2 and T1 post-contrast images demonstrate a large right frontal abscess with a characteristic T2 hypointense enhancing capsule. There is extensive surrounding vasogenic edema and mass effect displacing the anterior falx cerebri toward the left. There is associated opacification of the frontal sinus related to chronic sinusitis. (*E, F*) Hyperintense signal on the diffusion-weighted image and hypointense signal on the ADC map within the mass are consistent with restricted diffusion and typical of pyogenic abscess. Cultures from the abscess grew *Streptococcus milleri*. Suscep-tibility artifact in the right frontal region is from surgical hardware.

on postcontrast images there is thick ringlike or nodular enhancement that is stable or increases on delayed images. During the early and late capsule stage, there is a central core containing pus that may be round, oval, or multiloculated, with a surrounding capsule. The capsule consists of a reticulin network with scant collagen during the early stage, and progresses to a mature collagen capsule with a zone of surrounding gliosis during the late stage. On noncontrast CT during both the early and late capsule stages, the pus-containing core appears as a round or ovoid area of low attenuation with a sometimes faintly visible surrounding capsule ring. Following contrast administration, there is ring enhancement that decays on delayed images corresponding to the granulation tissue of the capsule. The medial or ventricular wall of the abscess cavity may be thinner than the lateral wall, attributed to differences in capsule blood supply. It is more prone to rupture and can lead to daughter abscess formation.

Magnetic resonance (MR) imaging is more sensitive than CT in the detection of brain abscess because it has greater sensitivity to changes in tissue water content, resulting in greater contrast between edematous brain and normal brain during the early stages of cerebritis and abscess formation.[30] During the early cerebritis stage, there is nonspecific poorly defined hyperintensity on T2-weighted sequence that is isointense to mildly hypointense on T1-weighted images, with ill-defined enhancement (**Fig. 4**).[31] The characteristic MR imaging features of the necrotic center of a mature brain abscess include fluid hyperintense relative to CSF and hypointense relative to white matter on the T1-weighted sequence. On T2-weighted sequences, the fluid in the abscess cavity is iso- to hyperintense to CSF and gray matter. This characteristic pattern of T2 prolongation relative to normal brain and T1 shortening relative to CSF reflects the proteinaceous nature of the abscess fluid.[30] Vasogenic edema surrounding the abscess cavity is characterized by surrounding hypointensity on the T1-weighted sequence and hyperintensity on the T2-weighted sequence. Interposed between the abscess cavity and the surrounding vasogenic edema is the abscess capsule, which is a smooth, circumferential ring that is iso- to hyperintense to white matter on the T1 sequence, iso- to hypointense on the T2-weighted sequence, and enhances on postcontrast images. The unique hypointensity of the capsule relative to white matter on T2-weighted sequences has been attributed to T1 and T2 shortening, occurring as a result of free radicals generated by phagocytic macrophages entering the capsule wall.[30]

The pathologic and imaging features of pyogenic abscess formation reflects the attempt by the host's immune system at containing the infection in immunocompetent patients. Experimental brain abscess models in immunocompetent mice indicate that microglia and astrocytes release chemokines and cytokines that result in an inflammatory response aimed at containing and eradicating the infection.[31] In immunocompromised patients with an impaired inflammatory response, there may be a lack of ring enhancement and less vasogenic edema in comparison with immunocompetent patients, features considered to be a poor prognostic finding.[32,33]

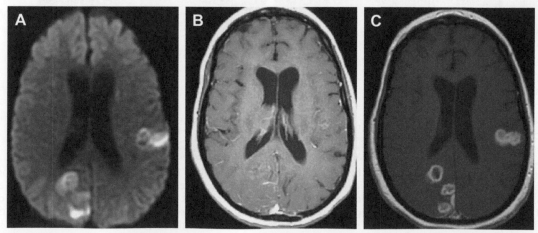

Fig. 4. Progression from cerebritis to abscess. (*A, B*) Axial diffusion-weighted sequence and T1 postcontrast image demonstrate areas of restricted diffusion in the left temporal lobe and the posterior right cerebral hemisphere that demonstrate some poorly defined enhancement. (*C*) Follow-up axial T1 postcontrast sequence 7 days later demonstrates progression to rim enhancement typical of abscess formation. (*Courtesy of* Hemant Parmar, MD, University of Michigan.)

Complicating factors that may be present on imaging include local mass effect with intracranial herniation, hydrocephalus, meningitis, and extra-axial fluid collection (**Figs. 5** and **6**). Local thrombophlebitis can result in venous sinus thrombosis. Intraventricular rupture with ventriculitis is a devastating complication associated with high mortality, and appears as ventricular debris and abnormal ependymal enhancement (**Figs. 7** and **8**).[34]

The classic ring-enhancing appearance of a capsule stage abscess on CT and conventional MR imaging is, however, nonspecific, and the differential diagnosis includes nonpyogenic abscess, high-grade primary central nervous system (CNS) neoplasm, metastasis, infarct, hematoma, thrombosed giant aneurysm, radiation necrosis, and demyelinating disease. Immunocompromised patients deserve special consideration because they are uniquely susceptible to a variety of opportunistic infections and neoplastic processes. *Toxoplasmosis gondii* infection, primary CNS lymphoma, and nonpyogenic abscesses should also be considered in these patients. Clinical data may be helpful in narrowing the differential of a ring-enhancing intraparenchymal brain mass, but is frequently of limited value in differentiating abscess from metastases or high-grade glioma because of the unreliable presence of infectious signs in the setting of abscess. Imaging features favoring abscess include (1) 2- to 7-mm continuous smooth, thin rim of enhancement, (2) T2 hypointense rim, and (3) thinning along the medial wall. However, these features are not consistently present and none are 100% specific.[1,30,35] Consequently, attempts have been made to differentiate ring-enhancing neoplasm from brain abscess using additional noninvasive imaging techniques.

Nuclear medicine has a limited role in the evaluation of brain abscess. Brain abscesses are usually localized by MR imaging or CT because patients present with headache or other neurologic signs. Some investigators report that the use of the oncotropic tracer thallium-201 chloride in conjunction with MR imaging or CT improves diagnostic confidence in distinguishing abscess from neoplasm.[36] However, this application has not been reliable and there are reports of false-positive thallium-201 chloride uptake in brain abscesses.[37] Its main application has been in distinguishing CNS lymphoma from *T gondii* infection in human immunodeficiency virus (HIV)-positive patients, with sensitivity of 92% and specificity of 89% for the diagnosis of CNS lymphoma.[38]

Diffusion-weighted imaging is helpful in distinguishing ring-enhancing neoplasm from pyogenic abscess. The central nonenhancing portion of a ring-enhancing neoplasm usually demonstrates facilitated diffusion while restricted diffusion within a ring-enhancing mass is characteristic, but not pathognomonic, of a brain abscess.[35,39–42] It appears as a central bright signal on the diffusion-weighted sequence and reduced apparent diffusion coefficient (ADC) values on the ADC map. Whereas some investigators attribute the restriction of water proton mobility within the abscess cavity to necrotic debris, macromolecules, and viscosity of pus, in vivo and ex vivo studies by Mishra and colleagues[35,39,43] suggest viable bacteria and inflammatory cells in the abscess cavity primarily account for the restricted diffusion. Furthermore, there are reports of higher ADCs in treated abscesses, as well as some data to suggest that persistent low ADC or recurrent low ADC in an abscess cavity following treatment indicates reactivation of infection or failed therapy.[44,45] Infrequently there is overlap of the diffusion-weighted imaging features of neoplasm and abscess, with some aseptic ring-enhancing neoplasms demonstrating restricted diffusion and some reports of facilitated diffusion within pyogenic abscess cavities, typically when empiric antibiotic therapy has preceded imaging.[46–51] The reported sensitivity and specificity of diffusion-weighted imaging in differentiating abscess from other pathology ranges from 72% to 95% and from 96% to 100%, respectively.[43,48]

Advanced Imaging

In vivo ^{1}H nuclear MR (^{1}H-NMR) spectroscopy complements diffusion-weighted imaging and conventional MR imaging. ^{1}H-NMR can improve diagnostic confidence in distinguishing cystic or necrotic tumor from abscess.[48] In the late capsule stage, bacterial abscesses have necrotic centers that lack the normal brain metabolites of N-acetylaspartate (NAA), choline, and creatine. Elevated levels of cytosolic amino acids (0.9 ppm) and lactate (1.3 ppm) with or without acetate (1.9 ppm) and succinate (2.4 ppm) are the characteristic resonances within the cavity of untreated pyogenic abscess.[52–54] While lactate and lipid signal can be found in the in vivo ^{1}H-NMR spectra of both brain tumor and abscess, cytosolic amino acids (valine, leucine, and isoleucine) are a key marker of pyogenic abscess which, when present, suggest its diagnosis (**Fig. 9**). These amino acids are not detectable on in vivo ^{1}H-NMR spectra from cystic or necrotic brain tumors.[55] The increased levels of lactate, acetate, and succinate are the by-product of glycolysis and fermentation by the causative bacteria. The amino acids are a result of proteolysis by polymorphonucleocytes in pus.[51,53] Acetate, with or without succinate, is not typically present

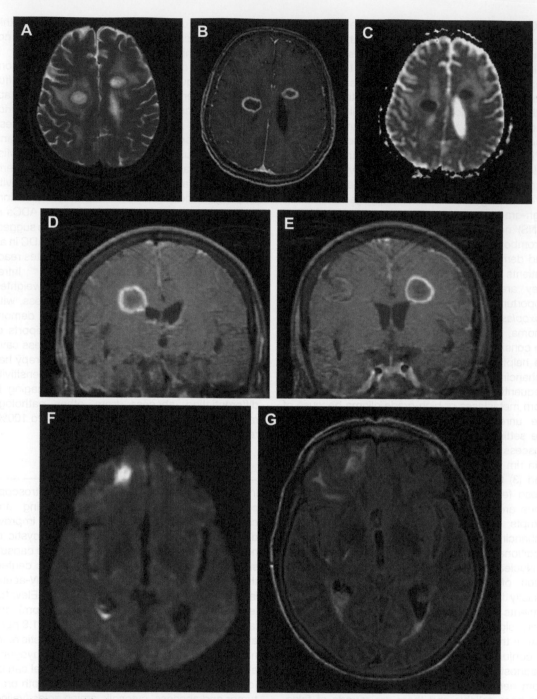

Fig. 5. A 68-year-old who woman presented with altered mental status. (*A–C*) T2, T1 postcontrast, and ADC maps demonstrate multiple bilateral abscesses with central T2 hyperintense signal and surrounding T2 hypointense signal, peripheral smooth rim enhancement, and reduced ADC values. There is characteristic thinning of the capsules along the ventricular margins. (*D, E*) Coronal T1 postcontrast images redemonstrate thinning along the medial margin of the abscess capsules where they communicate with the ventricular system. There is associated abnormal ependymal enhancement (*white arrow*). (*F, G*) Diffusion-weighted sequence and fluid-attenuated inversion recovery (FLAIR) sequence confirm intraventricular rupture and ventriculitis, with debris layering dependently in the ventricular system. (*Courtesy of* William Delfyett, MD, University of Pittsburgh.)

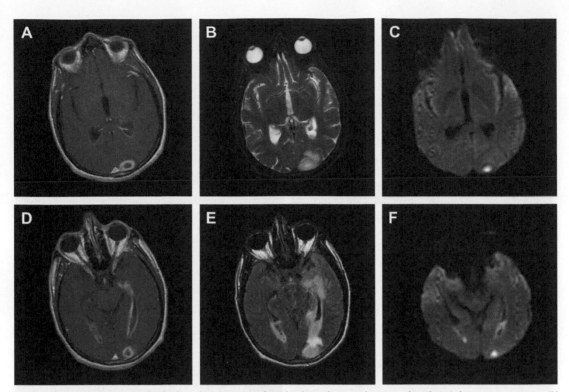

Fig. 6. A 57-year-old male alcoholic who presented with altered mental status. (*A–C*) Axial T1 postcontrast, T2, and diffusion-weighted sequences demonstrate a characteristic left occipital abscess with rim enhancement, central T2 hyperintensity, and bright signal on the diffusion-weighted sequence, which was confirmed to represent true restricted diffusion by ADC maps. There is surrounding mild vasogenic edema. (*D–F*) Axial T1 postcontrast, FLAIR, and diffusion-weighted sequences demonstrate associated intraventricular rupture with ventriculitis as demonstrated by abnormal ependymal enhancement, and layering debris in the ventricular system that restricts diffusion. (*Courtesy of* William Delfyett, MD, University of Pittsburgh.)

in brain abscesses caused by aerobic infection, but has been reported in abscesses caused by anaerobic and facultative anaerobic microorganisms.[54,56] Following treatment, the resonances of amino acids have been reported to disappear.[41,48,51,57] The reported sensitivity and specificity of MR spectroscopy in distinguishing abscess from other pathology is 72% to 96% and 30% to 100%, respectively.[48,50,54–56]

There are few published articles on the role of perfusion imaging in distinguishing brain abscess from necrotic or cystic ring-enhancing neoplasms. In a recent prospective study, Chiang and colleagues found that the mean relative cerebral blood volume of brain tumor walls was statistically significantly higher than that of cerebral abscesses. This difference was attributed to a greater degree of vascularity and blood-brain barrier breakdown in the wall of neoplasm versus the collagenous wall of a mature abscess.[58,59]

Recent research has focused on the microstructure of the abscess cavity using diffusion tensor imaging (DTI). Elevated DTI-derived fractional anisotropy within brain abscess cavities has been demonstrated, and has a positive correlation with neuroinflammatory molecules in pus.[60,61] Similarly, a positive correlation between fractional anisotropy in heat-killed *S aureus*–treated cell lines has been demonstrated.[61] These findings support the hypothesis that increased fractional anisotropy is due to upregulation of neuroinflammatory adhesion molecules, causing a structured orientation of inflammatory cells in the abscess cavity. In a small study, Nath and colleagues[51] found that increased fractional anisotropy and reduced mean diffusivity had 100% and 75% sensitivity, respectively, in predicting pyogenic abscess. Furthermore, fractional anisotropy in abscess cavities has been shown to decrease following treatment while mean diffusivity did not significantly change, suggesting that in the future, surveillance of fractional anisotropy may serve as a marker of inflammation and could help to guide therapy, although additional research is required.[62]

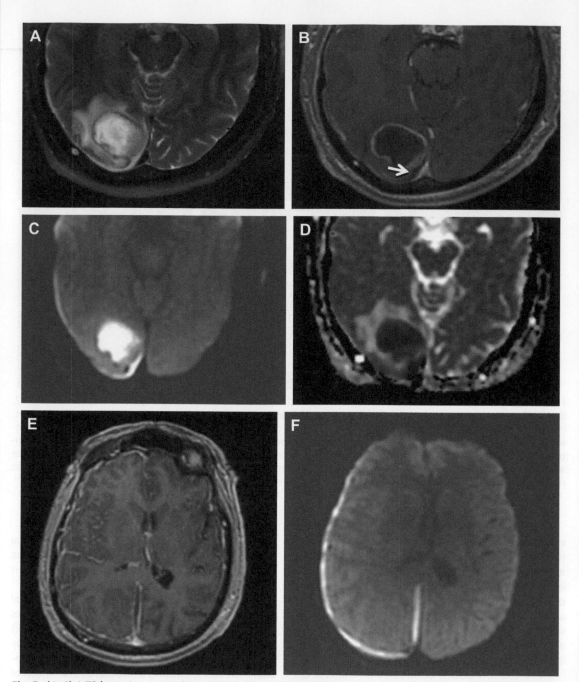

Fig. 7. (*A, B*) A T2 hyperintense right occipital abscess demonstrates central T2 hyperintense signal in the abscess cavity, T2 hypointense signal in the capsule, and capsule rim enhancement. There is surrounding vasogenic edema. There is an adjacent small subdural empyema medial to the abscess (*white arrow*). (*C, D*) Axial diffusion-weighted sequence and ADC map confirm restricted diffusion in the abscess cavity and within the small right tentorium subdural empyema. (*E*) On axial T1 postcontrast sequence there is a rim-enhancing subdural fluid collection extending over the right cerebral convexity and along the right posterior falx cerebri. There is associated mild local mass effect and meningitis with leptomeningeal enhancement over the right cerebral hemisphere (*F*). On the diffusion-weighted sequence the subdural fluid collection demonstrates restricted diffusion, consistent with an associated subdural empyema.

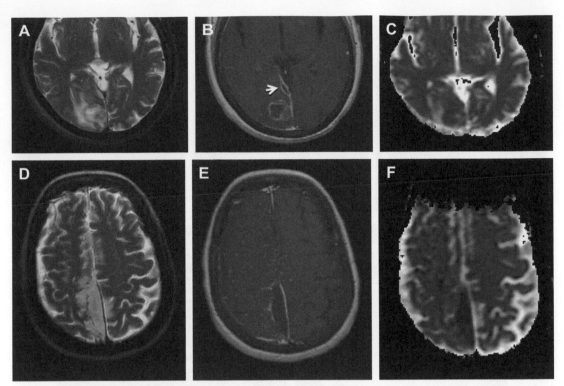

Fig. 8. (*A–C*) Axial T2-weighted sequence, T1 postcontrast sequence, and ADC maps demonstrate a typical brain abscess in the right occipital lobe with central T2 hyperintense signal, surrounding rim enhancement, and hypointense signal on ADC, consistent with restricted diffusion. There is daughter abscess formation beginning along its medial margin. There is a rim-enhancing small subdural empyema along the right tentorium (*white arrow*). (*D–F*) There is an associated right posterior parafalcine T2 hyperintense rim-enhancing subdural fluid collection with reduced ADC, consistent with a subdural empyema. In addition, there is evidence of meningitis with leptomeningeal enhancement noted in the right cerebral hemisphere. (*Courtesy of* Barton F. Branstetter IV, MD, University of Pittsburgh.)

Treatment

Cerebritis is typically treated with high-dose intravenous antibiotics alone and serial imaging to ensure response to therapy.[63] Brain abscesses larger than 2.5 cm or associated with mass effect are usually treated with stereotactic aspiration or excision combined with intravenous antibiotics. Antibiotic therapy is continued for 6 to 8 weeks with serial imaging weekly or biweekly, depending on the patient's clinical condition.[2,63] Patients who are poor surgical candidates, have numerous small abscesses or have surgically inaccessible disease may be treated with intravenous antibiotics alone. However, diagnostic aspiration should be performed when possible to optimize targeted antibiotic therapy. Unfavorable outcomes have been associated with the presence of an underlying medical condition, sepsis, nocardia abscess, poor neurologic status at presentation, and intraventricular rupture.[9,12,14,25,28,64,65]

ENCEPHALITIDES
Herpes Simplex Encephalitis

Herpes simplex encephalitis (HSE) is the most common cause of sporadic fatal encephalitis in the United States, with approximately 2000 cases per year.[21,66] HSE results in necrotizing encephalitis.[67] About 90% of the cases of HSE are caused by herpes simplex virus type 1 (HSV-1) with approximately 10% of cases being caused by HSV-2; the latter typically is seen in neonates, and is discussed in the pediatrics article by Parmar and colleagues elsewhere in this issue.[21] Patients with HSE typically present with headache, fever, seizures, viral prodrome, and mental status changes. The classic imaging findings are bilateral asymmetric involvement of the temporal and inferior frontal lobes with less common involvement of the insula and cingulate gyri.[68] The involved brain typically demonstrates high signal on T2-weighted images and gyral expansion. Fluid-attenuated

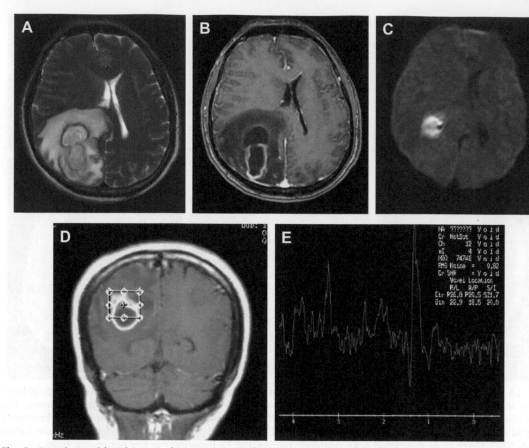

Fig. 9. A patient with a history of intravenous drug abuse who complained of drowsiness, headache, and left hemiparesis. (*A–C*) Axial T2, T1 postcontrast, and diffusion-weighted images demonstrate a bilobed cystic mass in the right parietal lobe with some surrounding T2 hypointense signal, rim enhancement, and restricted diffusion typical of an abscess in the anterior cystic portion. (*D, E*) Single-voxel, 144 millisecond echo time, proton MR spectroscopy supports the diagnosis of brain abscess, showing a prominent lipid and smaller inverted lactate peak at 1.3 ppm, amino acids at 0.9 ppm, acetate at 1.9 ppm, and presence of succinate at 2.4 ppm. Mildly elevated choline is also noted at 3.2 ppm. (*Courtesy of* Suyash Mohan, MD, Penn State University.)

inversion recovery (FLAIR)/T2-weighted sequences demonstrate increased signal in both the swollen cortex and subcortical white matter. Restricted diffusion and petechial hemorrhages may be seen. Gyriform enhancement may be noted, but is typically a later finding.[68,69] The basal ganglia are rarely involved in HSE, which helps to distinguish this disease process from other encephalitides.[68] Thus when insular and subinsular involvement is noted but the signal abnormality abruptly stops at the lateral putamen, HSE should be considered (**Fig. 10**). Corresponding CT findings include areas of hypoattenuation and gray-white differentiation loss. Metabolic alterations have been demonstrated by MR spectroscopy in cases of HSE with reduced NAA, elevated choline compounds, and sometimes elevated lactate.[70–72] However, the role of MR spectroscopy in the diagnosis of HSE is limited, as treatment is typically initiated when there is clinical

suspicion and corresponding imaging findings are consistent with HSE. Acyclovir is the treatment of choice for HSE (Class IA evidence).[22] Furthermore, treatment with acyclovir for HSE should be immediately begun when there is clinical suspicion of HSE, as mortality rates in untreated HSE are approximately 70%; early initiation of acyclovir decreases mortality to 20% to 30%.[22]

HSV-2, the genital strain, causes infections typically in the neonatal period, and is thought to be transmitted to the fetus transplacentally or to the neonate during delivery from a mother with genital herpes. HSV-2 is covered in the pediatrics article in this issue.

Varicella Zoster Virus

Primary varicella zoster virus (VZV) infection typically occurs in children and is known as

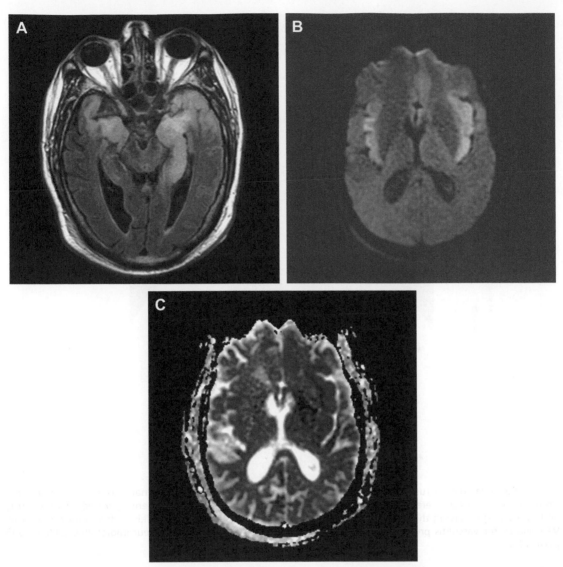

Fig. 10. Herpes simplex encephalitis. Axial FLAIR (A) image demonstrates bilateral, asymmetric temporal lobe signal abnormalities. Diffusion-weighted image (B) and the corresponding ADC map (C) demonstrate areas of restricted diffusion. Postcontrast T1 images (not shown) demonstrated minimal associated enhancement.

chickenpox or varicella. Subsequently the virus becomes latent in ganglionic neurons along the neuroaxis.[73] VZV can reactivate in patients, typically in elderly individuals whose cell-mediated immunity to VZV has declined or in immunosuppressed patients. When VZV reactivates the result is zoster or shingles, a painful rash that is caused when the virus travels along the sensory nerve from the dorsal root ganglion to the skin. Zoster is frequently followed by chronic pain known as post-herpetic neuralgia.[73] However, other sequela of VZV infection include vasculopathy, myelopathy, retinal necrosis, and cerebellitis. Of note, the CNS complications of VZV reactivation can occur in the absence of a rash.[73] VZV infection

has frequently been described as a meningoencephalitis and vasculopathy, but the vasculopathy is thought to be the dominant component.[73] Typically both large-vessel and small-vessel arteries are involved, although involvement of either small or large arteries alone can be seen (Fig. 11).[73,74] The infection is primarily in the media of the arteries.[73] Patients often present with an acute stroke or transient ischemic attacks; additional common clinical presentations include headache, cranial neuropathies, changes in mental status, aphasia, ataxia, hemisensory loss, and vision loss. The imaging appearance is of multiple areas of high signal on the T2-weighted image, classically involving the gray-white junction, with purely

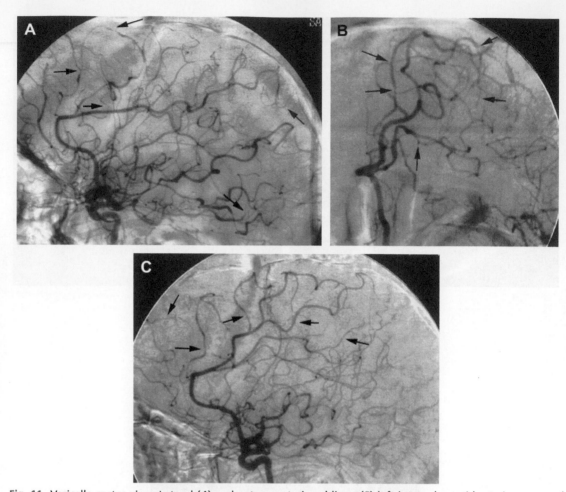

Fig. 11. Varicella zoster virus. Lateral (*A*) and anteroposterior oblique (*B*) left internal carotid arteriograms and right internal carotid lateral (*C*) arteriograms, showing multiple scattered segments (*arrows*) of irregularity and narrowing involving the small and medium-sized vessels. (*From* Jain R, Deveikis J, Hickenbottom S, et al. Varicella-zoster vasculitis presenting with intracranial hemorrhage. AJNR Am J Neuroradiol 2003;24:972; with permission.)

gray and white matter lesions also seen. Deep and superficial infarcts, some with associated hemorrhage, are seen. Less frequently, VZV vasculopathy results in aneurysm formation, subarachnoid or parenchymal hemorrhage, vascular ectasia, or dissection.[73] The treatment for VZV infection is acyclovir.[22]

Cytomegalovirus

Cytomegalovirus (CMV) is a ubiquitous herpes virus, which is present in its latent form in the majority of the population. In normal hosts, CMV infection presents with nonspecific clinical manifestations such as a febrile illnesses, and the course is usually self limited.[75] However, reactivation of CMV in an immunocompromised patient can result in disseminated infections, typically of the respiratory system, gastrointestinal system, and occasionally

the CNS. Meningoencephalitis and ventriculitis are the intracranial manifestations (see later discussion). Other neurologic manifestations include retinitis, polyradiculitis, and myelitis, which are not discussed further in this article. Because of the HIV epidemic, CMV encephalitis has emerged as an important clinical entity in adults.[75] With the introduction of highly active antiretroviral therapy (HAART), there has been a decrease in the prevalence of CMV infection, but familiarity with the entity remains critical.

Imaging findings of CNS infection with CMV include ependymal and subependymal enhancement, which when present is very suspicious for CMV ventriculitis in a patient with AIDS.[75] Other imaging findings include atrophy and periventricular white matter hyperintensities on T2-weighted/FLAIR imaging. Generalized atrophy is the most commonly reported CT abnormality, but is a nonspecific finding seen frequently in patients who have AIDS.[66] Of note, imaging studies may be unremarkable in patients with CMV encephalitis.[75,76] Rarely CNS infection with CMV may manifest as a ring-enhancing or space-occupying lesion.[66,76] CMV encephalitis is an important opportunistic infection in HIV-infected and, less frequently, in other immunocompromised individuals.[75] For CMV encephalitis, combination therapy with intravenous ganciclovir and foscarnet is advocated.[21,22] However, response of CMV encephalitis and ventriculitis to antiviral drugs is poor.[21,22,76]

Japanese Encephalitis

Japanese encephalitis (JE) is a flaviviral encephalitis that is a major health problem in Asia, where it is a leading cause of viral encephalitis with 30,000 to 50,000 cases reported annually.[66] Case fatality rates are reported as up to 60%.[77] Lesions are typically T2 hyperintense and T1 hypointense on MR imaging, and are seen involving the thalami and brainstem, in particular the substantia nigra, basal ganglia, cerebral cortex, corpus striatum, and cerebellum (**Fig. 12**).[77] The most consistent finding in JE is bilateral thalamic lesions with or without hemorrhagic changes on MR imaging.[66] Handique and colleagues[77] reported that temporal lobe involvement is present in 17% of patients with JE, but involves the body and tail of the hippocampus and spares the anterior temporal lobe and insula, in contradistinction to HSV-1 encephalitis.

West Nile Virus

West Nile virus (WNV) is a member of the Flaviviridae family that can cause a meningoencephalitis. The WNV appeared in the Western hemisphere in 1999 with an outbreak of encephalitis in the greater New York area.[78,79] Mosquitoes are the vectors of transmission. Roughly 1 in 150 individuals infected with WNV will develop significant CNS disease, defined as encephalitis, meningitis, or a combination of the two.[78] Positive MR imaging studies in patients with WNV meningoencephalitis are common though nonspecific. WNV infection should be included in the differential of signal abnormalities involving the deep gray matter, brainstem, or mesial temporal lobes, where it is typically cortical (**Fig. 13**). Infarcts have also been reported.[78] Of note, MR studies may be normal in patients with WNV encephalitis. Flaccid paralysis has been reported in multiple cases of WNV, and spine MR findings include anterior horn signal abnormalities and enhancement of the cauda equina.[78]

Rabies

Rabies encephalitis is a rare acute infection of the CNS by caused by an RNA virus of the rhabdovirus family. The mode of transmission to humans is primarily via the bites of rabid animals. After inoculation the virus reaches the CNS through retrograde axoplasmic flow.[80] Human rabies presents in two forms: encephalitic and paralytic. In the CNS there is an initial proclivity toward infection

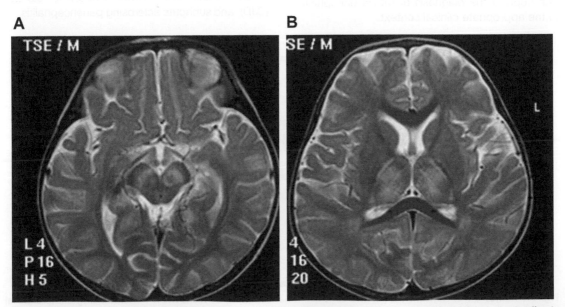

Fig. 12. Japanese encephalitis. (*A, B*) T2-weighted image demonstrates abnormal signal involving the midbrain (*A*) and bilateral thalami (*B*). (*Courtesy of* Hemant Parmar, MD, University of Michigan.)

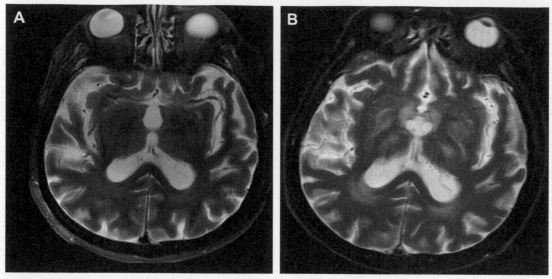

Fig. 13. West Nile virus. (*A*) T2-weighted images are initially unremarkable other than for age-related volume loss. (*B*) T2-weighted image acquired 2 months later demonstrates abnormal T2 signal involving the thalami and imaged portions of the inferior basal ganglia bilaterally.

of the gray matter. Reports of imaging findings in patients infected with the rabies virus are sparse. Reported imaging findings include areas of hypo-attenuation on CT and hyperintensity on T2-weighted imaging involving the brainstem, basal ganglia, and thalamus (**Fig. 14**).[80,81] An abnormal signal on the T2-weighted image involving the hippocampi, cerebral white matter, and central gray matter of the cord can also be seen.[66] Associated mild to moderate enhancement of these lesions is a late feature.[80] The imaging findings can support the diagnosis of rabies encephalitis in the appropriate clinical context.

Subacute Encephalitis

Subacute encephalitis refers to cases in which the onset of symptoms is insidious when compared with the clinical course of acute encephalitis, examples of which are discussed earlier in this article. Many infections fall into this category. Some disease processes that radiologists should be aware of include HIV encephalitis (HIVE), progressive multifocal leukoencephalopathy (PML), cytomegalovirus encephalitis, which can result in either acute or chronic encephalitis, Creutzfeldt-Jakob disease (CJD), and subacute sclerosing panencephalitis.

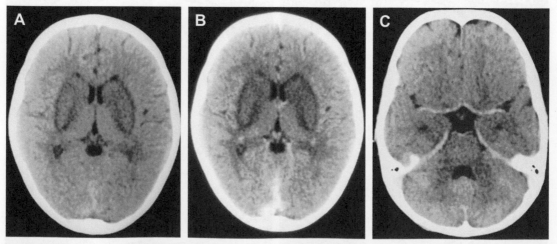

Fig. 14. Rabies. (*A–C*) Noncontrast (*A*) and contrast-enhanced (*B, C*) CT scans show nonenhancing bilateral basal ganglia hypodensities. (*From* Awasthi M, Parmar H, Patankar T, et al. Imaging findings in rabies encephalitis. AJNR Am J Neuroradiol 2001;22:678; with permission.)

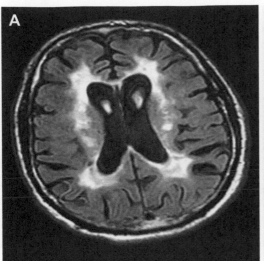
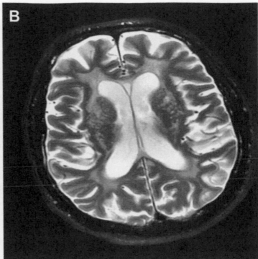

Fig. 15. Human immunodeficiency virus encephalitis. FLAIR (A) and T2-weighted (B) MR images demonstrate volume loss and periventricular and deep white matter signal abnormality without mass effect.

HIV Encephalitis

AIDS dementia complex is a syndrome of cognitive, behavioral, and motor abnormalities attributed to direct HIV infection of the brain. The imaging findings of AIDS dementia complex are frequently referred to as HIVE.[76] The typical imaging appearance is the combination of atrophy and periventricular, relatively symmetric areas of T2 signal abnormality. HIVE does not result in mass effect or enhancement. If either of these findings is present, another diagnosis must be considered (Fig. 15). Proton ^{1}H-NMR spectroscopy reveals decreased NAA and elevated peaks of choline and myo-inositol.[82] Magnetization transfer ratios (MTR) are reported to help differentiate HIVE from PML. There is a marked decrease in MTR with PML lesions, thought to be secondary to demyelination.[83] DTI has been reported to depict abnormalities in mean diffusivity and fractional anisotropy in the subcortical white matter, even when the brain appears normal on conventional MR images in HIV-positive patients. Of note, the patients in whom statistically significant differences were noted were those not receiving HAART and with detectable viral loads.[84] Other investigators have found DTI to be not fully helpful in identifying patients with early HIV infection.[85] The clinical role of imaging with DTI in HIV patients seems to be relatively limited at this point. Nonetheless, imaging plays a crucial role in the management and evaluation for infections in HIV patients.

Progressive Multifocal Leukoencephalopathy

PML results from infection of the oligodendrocytes with a papovavirus, JC virus, named after the index patient.[86] PML is most commonly seen in patients with AIDS, but can occur in a spectrum of immuno-compromised patients. PML results in progressive neurologic decline. The JC virus directly infects the oligodendrocytes, which are thus unable to maintain myelin. The resultant white matter lesions are typically multiple, bilateral, asymmetric, and confluent.[86] Any region of the brain may be infected, but there is some increased prevalence of lesions seen in the parietal lobe, and overall supratentorial lesions predominate over infratentorial lesions.[86] The lesions demonstrate increased T2 and decreased T1 signal, and corresponding low attenuation on CT images (Figs. 16 and 17).

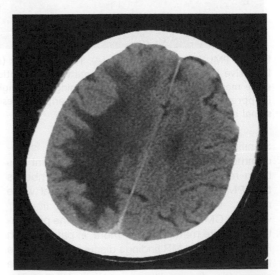

Fig. 16. Progressive multifocal leukoencephalopathy (PML). Noncontrast head CT demonstrates extensive abnormal low attenuation within the right frontal and parietal lobes.

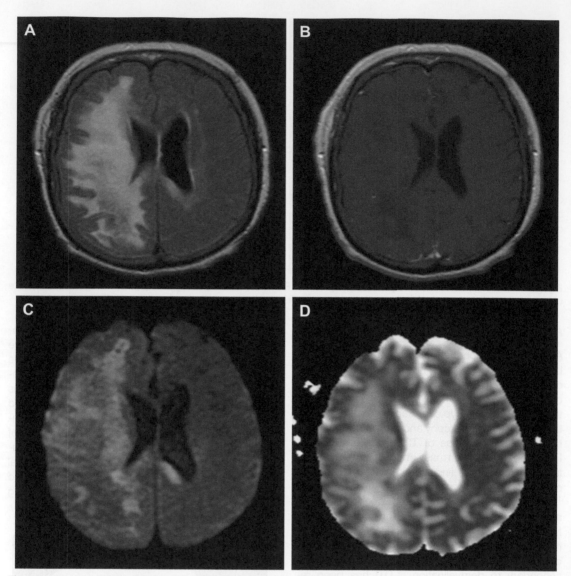

Fig. 17. PML. MR imaging FLAIR (*A*), T1 postcontrast (*B*), diffusion-weighted, (*C*), and ADC map (*D*) images. (*A*) Extensive right hemispheric white matter and subtle left periventricular signal abnormality is noted, with some mass effect in the form of flattening of the right lateral ventricle. (*B*) Minimal associated enhancement is appreciated. (*C*, *D*) Scattered areas of peripheral restricted diffusion are noted with corresponding decreased signal on the ADC maps.

Significant mass effect or enhancement is uncommon; although peripheral enhancement has been reported.[76,86] A key point to remember is that PML typically involves the peripheral white matter, involving the subcortical U fibers,[87] whereas CMV and HIV tend to involve the periventricular white matter. Furthermore, in patients with PML the CT and MR findings discussed earlier are typically asymmetric compared with the more symmetric abnormalities noted with HIVE.[76] The degree of brain atrophy is significantly milder in PML than that seen in HIVE,[86] although considerable overlap of these disease processes exists.[76]

PML lesions can demonstrate patchy restricted diffusion that is frequently peripheral and is thought to correlate with areas of lesion expansion.[87,88]

There is some evidence that diffusion-weighted images can evaluate for response of PML to HAART. Specifically, Usiskin and colleagues[89] described PML lesions demonstrating marked reduction in lesional ADC and reconstitution of anisotropy in the affected areas that correlated with treatment response, although this was a case report (see **Fig. 17**). Some early research also suggests that patients with rapid clinical progression following initiation of HAART have lesions with higher ADC values and are at risk of developing immune reconstitution inflammatory syndrome.[88] MR spectroscopic analysis of the affected white matter may demonstrate decreased NAA, elevated choline, presence of lactate, increased lipids, and potential elevation in *myo*-inositol levels.[90] Again, MTR are reported to help differentiate HIVE and PML. There is a marked decrease in MTR with PML lesions, thought to be secondary to demyelination.[83]

Creutzfeldt-Jakob Disease

CJD is a spongiform encephalopathy characterized by progressive dementia. The infecting organism is a prion. CJD is classified into sporadic CJD, familial CJD, and acquired forms. The so-called acquired forms include new variant CJD, kuru, and iatrogenic CJD. New variant CJD has similarities to bovine spongiform encephalopathy, which is thought to be transmitted from infected cattle to humans. Kuru was first described in brain-eating cannibals in New Guinea.[91] Iatrogenic CJD has been described in patients following corneal transplants, ingestion of prior contaminated human growth hormone, and following transplantation of cadaveric dural matter.[91] Approximately 85% of the cases are classified as sporadic CJD with an unknown source of infection.[66] Hereditary CJD accounts for approximately 10% of cases. Rapidly progressive dementia, periodic synchronous discharges on the electroencephalogram, and myoclonus are classic

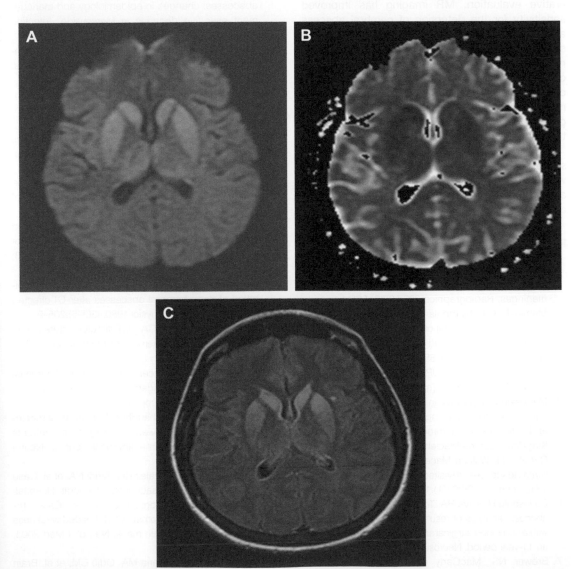

Fig. 18. Creutzfeldt-Jakob disease. MR diffusion-weighted (*A*), ADC map (*B*), and FLAIR (*C*) images. True restricted diffusion involving the basal ganglia and thalamus (pulvinar) are noted.

features of sporadic CJD. Typical MR imaging findings in sporadic CJD are areas of restricted diffusion along the cortex and involving the deep gray matter structures; corresponding hyperintensity on the T2-weighted and FLAIR sequences can be seen.[74] The characteristic MR imaging abnormality in new variant CJD is restricted diffusion and hyperintensity on T2-weighted imaging involving the pulvinar nuclei (**Fig. 18**).[92]

SUMMARY

CT and MR imaging have had a great impact on the diagnosis and management of brain abscess. CT provides a rapid means of localization, guidance for stereotactic aspiration, and serial postoperative evaluation. MR imaging has improved sensitivity for the detection of cerebral abscess and its associated complications. Restricted diffusion within a ring-enhancing mass is typical but not pathognomonic of a brain abscess. In cases of uncertainty, MR spectroscopy complements diffusion-weighted imaging and can improve diagnostic confidence. Abscess drainage with targeted antimicrobial therapy remains the standard treatment.

The cause of encephalitis can be suggested in some cases based on imaging findings, particularly when combined with CSF and serologic studies and patient history including age, immune status, and geographic and seasonal information.

REFERENCES

1. Smirniotopoulos JG, Murphy FM, Rushing EJ, et al. Patterns of contrast enhancement in the brain and meninges. Radiographics 2007;27(2):525–51.
2. Mamelak AN, Mampalam TJ, Obana WG, et al. Improved management of multiple brain abscesses: a combined surgical and medical approach. Neurosurgery 1995;36(1):76–85 [discussion: 6].
3. Mathisen GE, Johnson JP. Brain abscess. Clin Infect Dis 1997;25(4):763–79 [quiz: 80–1].
4. Macewen W. Pyogenic infective disease of the brain and spinal cord. Meningitis, abscess of the brain and infective sinus thrombosis. Glasgow (United Kingdom): James Maclehose and Sons; 1893.
5. Canale DJ. William Macewen and the treatment of brain abscesses: revisited after one hundred years. J Neurosurg 1996;84(1):133–42.
6. Cavusoglu H, Kaya RA, Turkmenoglu ON, et al. Brain abscess: analysis of results in a series of 51 patients with a combined surgical and medical approach during an 11-year period. Neurosurg Focus 2008;24(6):E9.
7. Brewer NS, MacCarty CS, Wellman WE. Brain abscess: a review of recent experience. Ann Intern Med 1975;82(4):571–6.
8. Carey ME, Chou SN, French LA. Experience with brain abscesses. J Neurosurg 1972;36(1):1–9.
9. Carpenter J, Stapleton S, Holliman R. Retrospective analysis of 49 cases of brain abscess and review of the literature. Eur J Clin Microbiol Infect Dis 2007; 26(1):1–11.
10. Garfield J. Management of supratentorial intracranial abscess: a review of 200 cases. Br Med J 1969;2(5648):7–11.
11. Hakan T, Ceran N, Erdem I, et al. Bacterial brain abscesses: an evaluation of 96 cases. J Infect 2006;52(5):359–66.
12. Menon S, Bharadwaj R, Chowdhary A, et al. Current epidemiology of intracranial abscesses: a prospective 5 year study. J Med Microbiol 2008;57(Pt 10):1259–68.
13. Sharma R, Mohandas K, Cooke RP. Intracranial abscesses: changes in epidemiology and management over five decades in Merseyside. Infection 2009;37(1):39–43.
14. Xiao F, Tseng MY, Teng LJ, et al. Brain abscess: clinical experience and analysis of prognostic factors. Surg Neurol 2005;63(5):442–9 [discussion: 9–50].
15. Alderson D, Strong AJ, Ingham HR, et al. Fifteen-year review of the mortality of brain abscess. Neurosurgery 1981;8(1):1–6.
16. de Louvois J. Bacteriological examination of pus from abscesses of the central nervous system. J Clin Pathol 1980;33(1):66–71.
17. Miller ES, Dias PS, Uttley D. CT scanning in the management of intracranial abscess: a review of 100 cases. Br J Neurosurg 1988;2(4):439–46.
18. Rosenblum ML, Hoff JT, Norman D, et al. Decreased mortality from brain abscesses since advent of computerized tomography. J Neurosurg 1978; 49(5):658–68.
19. Walsh PR, Larson SJ, Rytel MW, et al. Stereotactic aspiration of deep cerebral abscesses after CT-directed labeling. Appl Neurophysiol 1980;43(3–5):205–9.
20. Wise BL, Gleason CA. CT-directed stereotactic surgery in the management of brain abscess. Ann Neurol 1979;6(5):457.
21. Kennedy PG. Viral encephalitis: causes, differential diagnosis, and management. J Neurol Neurosurg Psychiatry 2004;75(Suppl 1):i10–5.
22. Steiner I, Budka H, Chaudhuri A, et al. Viral meningoencephalitis: a review of diagnostic methods and guidelines for management. Eur J Neurol 2010;17(8):999. e57.
23. Friedlander RM, Gonzalez RG, Afridi NA, et al. Case records of the Massachusetts General Hospital. Weekly clinicopathological exercises. Case 16-2003. A 58-year-old woman with left-sided weakness and a right frontal brain mass. N Engl J Med 2003; 348(21):2125–32.
24. Saez-Llorens XJ, Umana MA, Odio CM, et al. Brain abscess in infants and children. Pediatr Infect Dis J 1989;8(7):449–58.

25. Lu CH, Chang WN, Lin YC, et al. Bacterial brain abscess: microbiological features, epidemiological trends and therapeutic outcomes. QJM 2002;95(8): 501–9.

26. Prasad KN, Mishra AM, Gupta D, et al. Analysis of microbial etiology and mortality in patients with brain abscess. J Infect 2006;53(4):221–7.

27. Yang KY, Chang WN, Ho JT, et al. Postneurosurgical nosocomial bacterial brain abscess in adults. Infection 2006;34(5):247–51.

28. Mamelak AN, Obana WG, Flaherty JF, et al. Nocardial brain abscess: treatment strategies and factors influencing outcome. Neurosurgery 1994;35(4):622–31.

29. Britt RH, Enzmann DR. Clinical stages of human brain abscesses on serial CT scans after contrast infusion. Computerized tomographic, neuropathological, and clinical correlations. J Neurosurg 1983;59(6):972–89.

30. Haimes AB, Zimmerman RD, Morgello S, et al. MR imaging of brain abscesses. AJR Am J Roentgenol 1989;152(5):1073–85.

31. Baldwin AC, Kielian T. Persistent immune activation associated with a mouse model of Staphylococcus aureus-induced experimental brain abscess. J Neuroimmunol 2004;151(1–2):24–32.

32. Enzmann DR, Britt RH, Yeager AS. Experimental brain abscess evolution: computed tomographic and neuropathologic correlation. Radiology 1979; 133(1):113–22.

33. Yuh WT, Nguyen HD, Gao F, et al. Brain parenchymal infection in bone marrow transplantation patients: CT and MR findings. AJR Am J Roentgenol 1994;162(2):425–30.

34. Seydoux C, Francioli P. Bacterial brain abscesses: factors influencing mortality and sequelae. Clin Infect Dis 1992;15(3):394–401.

35. Desprechins B, Stadnik T, Koerts G, et al. Use of diffusion-weighted MR imaging in differential diagnosis between intracerebral necrotic tumors and cerebral abscesses. AJNR Am J Neuroradiol 1999; 20(7):1252–7.

36. Kita T, Hayashi K, Yamamoto M, et al. Does supplementation of contrast MR imaging with thallium-201 brain SPECT improve differentiation between benign and malignant ring-like contrast-enhanced cerebral lesions? Ann Nucl Med 2007;21(5):251–6.

37. Martinez del Valle MD, Gomez-Rio M, Horcajadas A, et al. False positive thallium-201 SPECT imaging in brain abscess. Br J Radiol 2000;73(866):160–4.

38. Skiest DJ. Focal neurological disease in patients with acquired immunodeficiency syndrome. Clin Infect Dis 2002;34(1):103–15.

39. Ebisu T, Tanaka C, Umeda M, et al. Discrimination of brain abscess from necrotic or cystic tumors by diffusion-weighted echo planar imaging. Magn Reson Imaging 1996;14(9):1113–6.

40. Kim YJ, Chang KH, Song IC, et al. Brain abscess and necrotic or cystic brain tumor: discrimination with signal intensity on diffusion-weighted MR imaging. AJR Am J Roentgenol 1998;171(6):1487–90.

41. Lai PH, Ho JT, Chen WL, et al. Brain abscess and necrotic brain tumor: discrimination with proton MR spectroscopy and diffusion-weighted imaging. AJNR Am J Neuroradiol 2002;23(8):1369–77.

42. Noguchi K, Watanabe N, Nagayoshi T, et al. Role of diffusion-weighted echo-planar MRI in distinguishing between brain abscess and tumour: a preliminary report. Neuroradiology 1999;41(3):171–4.

43. Mishra AM, Gupta RK, Saksena S, et al. Biological correlates of diffusivity in brain abscess. Magn Reson Med 2005;54(4):878–85.

44. Cartes-Zumelzu FW, Stavrou I, Castillo M, et al. Diffusion-weighted imaging in the assessment of brain abscesses therapy. AJNR Am J Neuroradiol 2004;25(8):1310–7.

45. Fanning NF, Laffan EE, Shroff MM. Serial diffusion-weighted MRI correlates with clinical course and treatment response in children with intracranial pus collections. Pediatr Radiol 2006;36(1):26–37.

46. Park SH, Chang KH, Song IC, et al. Diffusion-weighted MRI in cystic or necrotic intracranial lesions. Neuroradiology 2000;42(10):716–21.

47. Holtas S, Geijer B, Stromblad LG, et al. A ring-enhancing metastasis with central high signal on diffusion-weighted imaging and low apparent diffusion coefficients. Neuroradiology 2000;42(11):824–7.

48. Lai PH, Hsu SS, Ding SW, et al. Proton magnetic resonance spectroscopy and diffusion-weighted imaging in intracranial cystic mass lesions. Surg Neurol 2007;68(Suppl 1):S25–36.

49. Tung GA, Evangelista P, Rogg JM, et al. Diffusion-weighted MR imaging of rim-enhancing brain masses: is markedly decreased water diffusion specific for brain abscess? AJR Am J Roentgenol 2001;177(3):709–12.

50. Mishra AM, Gupta RK, Jaggi RS, et al. Role of diffusion-weighted imaging and in vivo proton magnetic resonance spectroscopy in the differential diagnosis of ring-enhancing intracranial cystic mass lesions. J Comput Assist Tomogr 2004; 28(4):540–7.

51. Nath K, Agarwal M, Ramola M, et al. Role of diffusion tensor imaging metrics and in vivo proton magnetic resonance spectroscopy in the differential diagnosis of cystic intracranial mass lesions. Magn Reson Imaging 2009;27(2):198–206.

52. Kim SH, Chang KH, Song IC, et al. Brain abscess and brain tumor: discrimination with in vivo H-1 MR spectroscopy. Radiology 1997;204(1):239–45.

53. Lai PH, Li KT, Hsu SS, et al. Pyogenic brain abscess: findings from in vivo 1.5-T and 11.7-T in vitro proton MR spectroscopy. AJNR Am J Neuroradiol 2005; 26(2):279–88.

54. Pal D, Bhattacharyya A, Husain M, et al. In vivo proton MR spectroscopy evaluation of pyogenic

brain abscesses: a report of 194 cases. AJNR Am J Neuroradiol 2010;31(2):360–6.

55. Grand S, Passaro G, Ziegler A, et al. Necrotic tumor versus brain abscess: importance of amino acids detected at 1H MR spectroscopy–initial results. Radiology 1999;213(3):785–93.

56. Garg M, Gupta RK, Husain M, et al. Brain abscesses: etiologic categorization with in vivo proton MR spectroscopy. Radiology 2004;230(2): 519–27.

57. Burtscher IM, Holtas S. In vivo proton MR spectroscopy of untreated and treated brain abscesses. AJNR Am J Neuroradiol 1999;20(6):1049–53.

58. Chiang IC, Hsieh TJ, Chiu ML, et al. Distinction between pyogenic brain abscess and necrotic brain tumour using 3-tesla MR spectroscopy, diffusion and perfusion imaging. Br J Radiol 2009;82(982): 813–20.

59. Chan JH, Tsui EY, Chau LF, et al. Discrimination of an infected brain tumor from a cerebral abscess by combined MR perfusion and diffusion imaging. Comput Med Imaging Graph 2002;26(1):19–23.

60. Gupta RK, Hasan KM, Mishra AM, et al. High fractional anisotropy in brain abscesses versus other cystic intracranial lesions. AJNR Am J Neuroradiol 2005;26(5):1107–14.

61. Gupta RK, Nath K, Prasad A, et al. In vivo demonstration of neuroinflammatory molecule expression in brain abscess with diffusion tensor imaging. AJNR Am J Neuroradiol 2008;29(2):326–32.

62. Nath K, Ramola M, Husain M, et al. Assessment of therapeutic response in patients with brain abscess using diffusion tensor imaging. World Neurosurg 2010;73(1):63–8 [discussion: e6].

63. Mampalam TJ, Rosenblum ML. Trends in the management of bacterial brain abscesses: a review of 102 cases over 17 years. Neurosurgery 1988;23(4):451–8.

64. Tattevin P, Bruneel F, Clair B, et al. Bacterial brain abscesses: a retrospective study of 94 patients admitted to an intensive care unit (1980 to 1999). Am J Med 2003;115(2):143–6.

65. Zeidman SM, Geisler FH, Olivi A. Intraventricular rupture of a purulent brain abscess: case report. Neurosurgery 1995;36(1):189–93 [discussion: 93].

66. Tali ET. Viruses and prion in the CNS. Preface. Neuroimaging Clin N Am 2008;18(1):xiii–xxiv.

67. Baringer JR. Herpes simplex infections of the nervous system. Neurol Clin 2008;26(3):657–74, viii.

68. Falcone S, Post MJ. Encephalitis, cerebritis, and brain abscess: pathophysiology and imaging findings. Neuroimaging Clin N Am 2000;10(2): 333–53.

69. Noguchi T, Yoshiura T, Hiwatashi A, et al. CT and MRI findings of human herpesvirus 6-associated encephalopathy: comparison with findings of herpes simplex virus encephalitis. AJR Am J Roentgenol 2010; 194(3):754–60.

70. Foerster BR, Thurnher MM, Malani PN, et al. Intracranial infections: clinical and imaging characteristics. Acta Radiol 2007;48(8):875–93.

71. Menon DK, Sargentoni J, Peden CJ, et al. Proton MR spectroscopy in herpes simplex encephalitis: assessment of neuronal loss. J Comput Assist Tomogr 1990;14(3):449–52.

72. Samann PG, Schlegel J, Muller G, et al. Serial proton MR spectroscopy and diffusion imaging findings in HIV-related herpes simplex encephalitis. AJNR Am J Neuroradiol 2003;24(10):2015–9.

73. Gilden D, Cohrs RJ, Mahalingam R, et al. Varicella zoster virus vasculopathies: diverse clinical manifestations, laboratory features, pathogenesis, and treatment. Lancet Neurol 2009;8(8):731–40.

74. Katchanov J, Siebert E, Klingebiel R, et al. Infectious vasculopathy of intracranial large- and medium-sized vessels in neurological intensive care unit: a clinico-radiological study. Neurocrit Care 2010; 12(3):369–74.

75. Arribas JR, Storch GA, Clifford DB, et al. Cytomegalovirus encephalitis. Ann Intern Med 1996;125(7): 577–87.

76. Smith AB, Smirniotopoulos JG, Rushing EJ. From the archives of the AFIP: central nervous system infections associated with human immunodeficiency virus infection: radiologic-pathologic correlation. Radiographics 2008;28(7):2033–58.

77. Handique SK, Das RR, Barman K, et al. Temporal lobe involvement in Japanese encephalitis: problems in differential diagnosis. AJNR Am J Neuroradiol 2006;27(5):1027–31.

78. Petropoulou KA, Gordon SM, Prayson RA, et al. West Nile virus meningoencephalitis: MR imaging findings. AJNR Am J Neuroradiol 2005; 26(8):1986–95.

79. Asnis DS, Conetta R, Teixeira AA, et al. The West Nile Virus outbreak of 1999 in New York: the Flushing Hospital experience. Clin Infect Dis 2000; 30(3):413–8.

80. Laothamatas J, Hemachudha T, Mitrabhakdi E, et al. MR imaging in human rabies. AJNR Am J Neuroradiol 2003;24(6):1102–9.

81. Awasthi M, Parmar H, Patankar T, et al. Imaging findings in rabies encephalitis. AJNR Am J Neuroradiol 2001;22(4):677–80.

82. Laubenberger J, Haussinger D, Bayer S, et al. HIV-related metabolic abnormalities in the brain: depiction with proton MR spectroscopy with short echo times. Radiology 1996;199(3):805–10.

83. Ernst T, Chang L, Witt M, et al. Progressive multifocal leukoencephalopathy and human immunodeficiency virus-associated white matter lesions in AIDS: magnetization transfer MR imaging. Radiology 1999;210(2):539–43.

84. Filippi CG, Ulug AM, Ryan E, et al. Diffusion tensor imaging of patients with HIV and normal-appearing white matter on MR images of the brain. AJNR Am J Neuroradiol 2001;22(2):277–83.

85. Thurnher MM, Castillo M, Stadler A, et al. Diffusion-tensor MR imaging of the brain in human immunodeficiency virus-positive patients. AJNR Am J Neuroradiol 2005;26(9):2275–81.

86. Post MJ, Yiannoutsos C, Simpson D, et al. Progressive multifocal leukoencephalopathy in AIDS: are there any MR findings useful to patient management and predictive of patient survival? AIDS Clinical Trials Group, 243 Team. AJNR Am J Neuroradiol 1999;20(10):1896–906.

87. Kuker W, Mader I, Nagele T, et al. Progressive multifocal leukoencephalopathy: value of diffusion-weighted and contrast-enhanced magnetic resonance imaging for diagnosis and treatment control. Eur J Neurol 2006;13(8):819–26.

88. Buckle C, Castillo M. Use of diffusion-weighted imaging to evaluate the initial response of progressive multifocal leukoencephalopathy to highly active antiretroviral therapy: early experience. AJNR Am J Neuroradiol 2010;31(6):1031–5.

89. Usiskin SI, Bainbridge A, Miller RF, et al. Progressive multifocal leukoencephalopathy: serial high-b-value diffusion-weighted MR imaging and apparent diffusion coefficient measurements to assess response to highly active antiretroviral therapy. AJNR Am J Neuroradiol 2007;28(2):285–6.

90. Chang L, Ernst T, Tornatore C, et al. Metabolite abnormalities in progressive multifocal leukoencephalopathy by proton magnetic resonance spectroscopy. Neurology 1997;48(4):836–45.

91. Ukisu R, Kushihashi T, Tanaka E, et al. Diffusion-weighted MR imaging of early-stage Creutzfeldt-Jakob disease: typical and atypical manifestations. Radiographics 2006;26(Suppl 1):S191–204.

92. Zeidler M, Sellar RJ, Collie DA, et al. The pulvinar sign on magnetic resonance imaging in variant Creutzfeldt-Jakob disease. Lancet 2000;355(9213):1412–8.

Fungal Infections of the Central Nervous System

Mahan Mathur, MD[a],*, Carl E. Johnson, MD[b],
Gordon Sze, MD[a]

KEYWORDS

- Fungal infection • Abscess • Central nervous system • Meningitis • Cerebritis

KEY POINTS

- The increasing incidence of central nervous system (CNS) fungal infections is thought to be related to the AIDS epidemic, an increase in transplants, and resistance to antifungal agents.
- MRI, given its superior contrast resolution relative to CT imaging, remains the preferred imaging modality in the evaluation of CNS infection.
- Imaging findings of fungal disease are nonspecific but may be organized as parenchymal (granulomas, cerebritis, and abscess), extra-axial (meningitis, sinusitis), and vascular (vasculitis, mycotic aneurysm).
- In general, morphology may predict imaging manifestations: large, hyphal organisms (Aspergillus) commonly involve the brain parenchyma, whereas small unicellular organisms (Candida, Cryptococcus) commonly cause meningitis.
- Advanced imaging techniques, including diffusion-weighted imaging, MR perfusion, and MR spectroscopy, may aid in differentiating fungal from pyogenic or neoplastic disease.

INTRODUCTION

Fungi are a ubiquitous and distinct set of organisms that are often nonpathogenic or result in a self-limited illness in otherwise healthy humans.[1] Fungal spores typically travel through the upper airways to the lung parenchyma where they are most often removed by an immunocompetent immune system.[1,2] Fungemia may occasionally occur related to indwelling catheters, fungal disease in other organs, or trauma, with the infection subsequently being eliminated by a combination of the host's reticuloendothelial, cellular, and humoral defense system.[1,3] Infection of the bloodstream may rarely penetrate the blood-brain barrier in immunocompetent hosts, resulting in meningitis or infection of the brain parenchyma. Infection of the central nervous system (CNS) may also occur secondary to direct penetration of the blood-brain barrier, as can be seen in the setting of neurosurgical procedures or secondary to adjacent sinus disease.[4,5]

The incidence of fungal CNS infection has been increasing over the past 3 decades.[6] Data from 8124 autopsies performed by Groll and colleagues[7] at a university hospital in Germany from 1978 to 1992 showed a rise in the number of invasive fungal infections, ranging from 2.2% and 3.2% in 1978 to 1982 and 1983 to 1987, respectively, to 5.1% from 1987 to 1992. A follow-up study over the next decade showed a continuous increase in the number of invasive fungal infections, with the incidence increasing from 6.6% from 1993 to 1996 to 10.4% in 2001 to 2005.[8]

The increase in the incidence of invasive fungal infections is thought to be related to the AIDS

The authors have no disclosures to make.
[a] Department of Radiology, Yale University Medical Center, 333 Cedar Street, New Haven, CT 06510, USA;
[b] Department of Radiology, New York-Presbyterian Hospital, 525 East 68th Street, New York, NY 10065, USA
* Corresponding author.
E-mail address: mahan.mathur@gmail.com

epidemic, an increase in both solid organ and hematopoietic stems cell transplants and resistance to antifungal agents.[9] A study of 1048 patients with invasive fungal disease in the San Francisco Bay Area from 1992 to 1993 showed that more than 80% of patients were immunocompromised in some manner, with HIV infection being the most prevalent cause (47.4%).[10] Although the advent of highly active antiretroviral therapy (HAART) has led to a decrease in the incidence of AIDS-related opportunistic fungal infection in the developed world, invasive fungal disease remains a significant cause of morbidity and mortality in the developing world.[11] The incidence of invasive fungal disease in the transplant population has continued to rise, with Marr and colleagues[12] showing an increase in invasive aspergillosis from 7.3% in 1992 to 16.9% in 1998 in patients who underwent hematopoietic stem cell transplantation. Patterns of antimicrobial prophylaxis practices have further contributed to the rise of invasive fungal infections, as shown by an increase of mycelial infections from 18% in patients without fluconazole prophylaxis to 29% in patients who received the prophylactic antifungal.[13]

The following discussion includes the general imaging manifestations of fungal CNS disease, highlighting salient differences that may allow radiologists to differentiate fungal disease from bacterial or tuberculous infections and neoplastic disease. Some of the more commonly encountered fungal pathogens are considered in greater detail, emphasizing both the typical and atypical imaging findings that individual fungi may exhibit in the CNS.

RADIOGRAPHIC MANIFESTATIONS

Although the radiologic differentiation of fungal infections is nonspecific, grouping fungal pathogens by the immune status of the infected host may aid in generating a differential diagnosis. Fungal infections that affect immunocompetent hosts include Cryptococcus neoformans, Coccidioides immitis, Histoplasma capsulatum, and Blastomyces dermatitidis, whereas Aspergillus and Candida are most often seen in immunocompromised hosts.[14] The past 4 decades have shown a shift in the epidemiologic data regarding the most common organisms involved in fungal CNS disease. Although a study by Parker and colleagues[15] of 39 patients over a 13-year period (1964–1976) found that Candida was the most common fungal infection of the brain, more recent data by Dubey and colleagues[16] in 40 patients over a 23-year period (1980–2003) not only found that Aspergillus is more common but also noted the increased incidence of other fungal organisms, such as the Zygomycetes.[15,16]

Certain fungal organisms have a geographic predilection that may further help provide a differential diagnosis in otherwise equivocal imaging findings. Histoplasma capsulatum is often seen in the greater Mississippi valley, along the United States/Mexico border, and in scattered regions in Central and South America.[2] Coccidioides immitis may be a consideration in the southwest United States, central California, northern Mexico, and in regions of Argentina. Blastomyces dermatitidis may be seen in the Midwest, the St. Lawrence Seaway, and some Mideastern states, although it has also been found outside the United States in Africa, the Middle East, and India. Most fungal organisms, including Cryptococcus neoformans, Aspergillus, and Candida, are widespread in their distribution and can occur in countries across the world.[1]

Knowledge of fungal morphology may help in understanding the imaging findings, because the pathophysiology often follows from this.[17] Morphologically, fungi may be divided into three major categories: yeast (small, unicellular organisms), hyphae (growth in branchlike colonies), or dimorphic (unicellular organisms or branchlike, depending on the ambient temperature).[18] The vegetative form of fungus consisting of a mass of branching hyphae is a mycelium. Examples of fungi that grow as yeast include Candida and Cryptococcus, whereas Aspergillus and Mucormycoses grow with branching hyphae. Coccidiomycosis is an example of a dimorphic fungus. Fungi that grow as yeasts spread hematogenously, entering the meningeal microcirculation owing to their small size, resulting in seeding of the subarachnoid space and meningitis.[19] Although parenchymal disease is less common with yeast organisms, both Candida and Cryptococcus may manifest as primarily parenchymal abnormalities with the formation of granulomas or abscesses.[20] The hyphal forms of fungal pathogens often cause parenchymal disease, because the larger morphology precludes access to the meningeal microcirculation.[21] The larger cerebral vessels may also become involved, resulting in vasculitis with thrombosis and mycotic aneurysm formation.[22]

Parenchymal Disease

Parenchymal involvement of CNS fungal disease may result in granuloma formation, cerebritis, and/or abscess formation. Although radiographic differentiation of the cause of the intracranial abnormality is difficult and often nonspecific, certain clues may help differentiate fungal infection from other infectious origins, such as bacteria and tuberculosis.

Fungal granulomatous masses are an uncommon presentation of invasive CNS infection. Granulomas form as a response to the hematogenous or direct dissemination of fungal disease to the brain parenchyma. A 22-year retrospective review of 40 patients with intracranial fungal granulomas by Dubey and colleagues[16] demonstrated that the most common organisms were *Aspergillus* (63%) followed by *Mucormycosis* (18%). The study found that the most common locations of disease were in the frontal lobes (25%) and anterior cranial fossa without frontal lobe involvement (20%). CT findings in these patients were nonspecific, showing irregular hypoattenuating lesions with heterogeneous, faint contrast enhancement and perilesional edema. Although MRI findings of granulomas are often nonspecific, certain features may suggest a specific origin. Aspergillomas, for example, may demonstrate intermediate T2 signal within the granuloma, with surrounding high T2 signal representing edema.[23] This finding is supported by Gupta and colleagues,[24] who reported an intracranial aspergilloma that simulated a meningioma by demonstrating isointense T1 signal to the brain parenchyma and isointense T2 signal to the white matter.

Imaging findings of cerebritis are nonspecific but typically include increased T2/FLAIR (fluid attenuated inversion recovery) signal abnormality associated with a variable amount of enhancement (**Fig. 1**). Diffusion weighted imaging (DWI) may demonstrate restricted diffusion, although these findings can be variable (**Fig. 2**). In a study by Gaviani and colleagues,[25] two of eight patients with fungal CNS infection had histopathologic evidence of cerebritis. Imaging findings in these patients included one to several lesions that demonstrated minimal to no enhancement, as opposed to ring enhancement in fungal abscesses, and heterogeneously hyperintense DWI signal in distinction to the predominantly central hyperintense restricted diffusion in fungal abscesses. The lesions had increased surrounding T2 signal corresponding to vasogenic edema. The lack of enhancement was likely related to the rapid clinical deterioration in both of these patients, which precluded the time progression needed for abscess formation.

The imaging appearance of an intracranial fungal abscess is similar to a pyogenic abscess typically demonstrating a ring-enhancing lesion with a hypointense T2 rim,[26] which may show restricted diffusion. Immunocompromised patients may have a variable imaging appearance, as shown by Enzmann and colleagues,[27] who studied 15 immunocompromised patients with CNS infections and concluded that six of eight patients afflicted with *Aspergillus* had minimal to no enhancement on imaging with intravenous contrast. These findings are likely reflective of the host's failing immune system, which is unable to isolate and/or encapsulate the offending agent (**Fig. 3**). Other

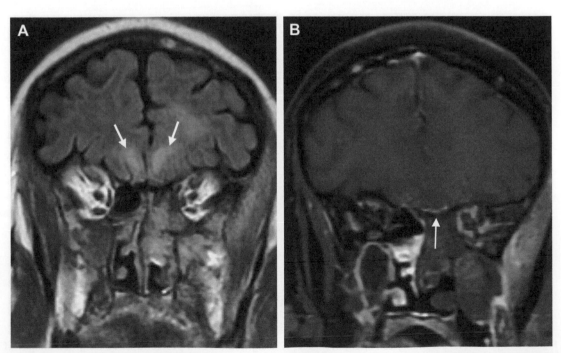

Fig. 1. Cerebritis related to aspergillosis. Coronal FLAIR (*A*) and coronal postcontrast T1-weighted images (*B*) of the brain show high signal intensity bilaterally in the frontal lobes (*arrows*). Minimal dural enhancement is noted after administration of contrast (*arrow* in *B*).

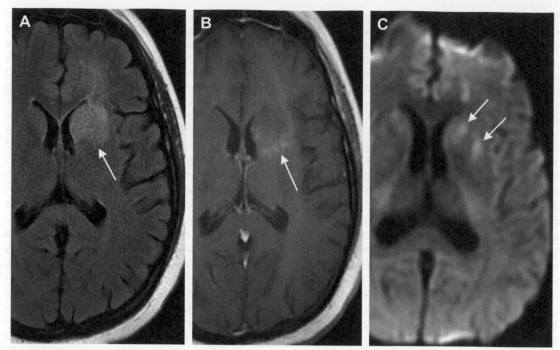

Fig. 2. Cerebritis in a patient with aspergillosis. Axial FLAIR (*A*) and T1-weighted postcontrast images (*B*) at the level of the lateral ventricles show nonspecific increased FLAIR signal intensity involving the head of the left caudate and left basal ganglia, which minimally enhances after the administration of intravenous gadolinium contrast (*arrows* in *A, B*). Diffusion-weighted images (*C*) show two foci of restricted diffusion in the region reflecting early ischemic changes related to the underlying infection (*arrows* in *C*).

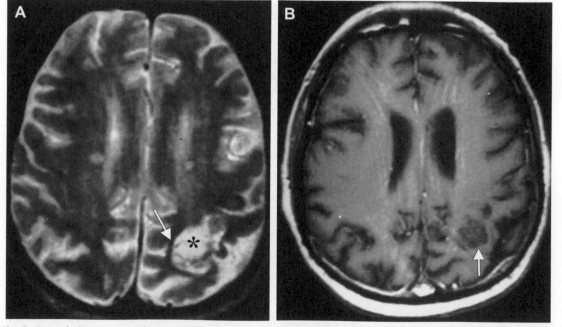

Fig. 3. Fungal abscess secondary to *Aspergillus*. Axial T2-weighted (*A*) and postcontrast T1-weighted images of the brain (*B*) show a mass in the left occipital lobe which is predominantly of high T2 signal intensity centrally (*asterisk* in *A*) and is delineated by a hypointense rim (*arrow* in *A*). Minimal ring enhancement is seen after the administration of intravenous contrast (*arrow* in *B*).

features that may help distinguish fungal from pyogenic abscess include number and location, with fungal abscesses often multiple and near the gray-white matter junction related to the hematologic distribution of fungal organisms.[28] Fungal abscesses may also involve the deep gray matter nuclei involvement of the deep gray-matter nuclei (Fig. 4). Bacterial abscesses are more often single and spare the basal ganglia.[28,29]

Recent data suggest that the morphology of an intracranial abscess may help differentiate fungal from bacterial and tuberculous origins. In a study by Luthra and colleagues[30] that examined 110 surgically proven brain abscesses (91 bacterial, 11 tubercular, and 8 fungal), 4 of 8 fungal lesions demonstrated a lobulated outer contour, whereas the remaining 4 had a crenated border. This differed from pyogenic and tubercular abscesses, most of which demonstrated smooth or lobulated borders (60.4% and 54.5%, respectively). Only 1 tuberculous abscess had a crenated border. In addition, 8 of 8 fungal lesions demonstrated nonenhancing intracavitary projections from the wall of the abscess, which were isointense to hypointense on T1-weighted images and hypointense on the T2-weighted images. These findings were distinct for fungal disease and thought to be related to fungal hyphae projecting into the abscess lumen (Fig. 5). On DWI, the wall and intracavitary projections of 8 of 8 fungal abscesses demonstrated restricted diffusion, with the core of the lesion showing no restricted diffusion (see Fig. 5; Fig. 6). The cavity of bacterial and tuberculous abscesses, however, demonstrated the typical restricted diffusion associated with an intracranial abscess. Therefore, intracranial fungal abscesses may be distinguished by their crenated border and nonenhancing intracavitary projections, which demonstrate restricted diffusion.

Magnetic resonance spectroscopy (MRS) demonstrated similar findings in fungal and bacterial abscesses, with peaks corresponding to amino acids, lipid, and lactate.[30] A distinct feature in five of eight fungal abscesses, however, was the presence of multiple signals between 3.6 and 3.8 ppm (parts per million), which were attributed to trehalose, a disaccharide found in the fungal wall (Fig. 7). Identification of multiple signals between 3.6 and 3.6 ppm may confer further specificity to the diagnosis.

Fungal abscesses may be difficult to distinguish from intracranial cystic neoplasms, although some general guidelines may aid in this differentiation. In a study of 53 rim-enhancing intracranial lesions, Fertikh and colleagues[31] showed that

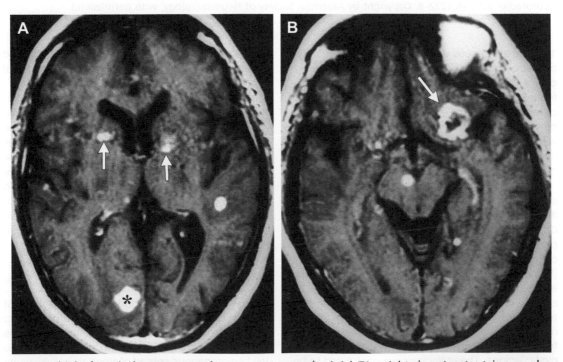

Fig. 4. Multiple fungal abscesses secondary to cryptococcosis. Axial T1-weighted postcontrast images show multiple homogenously (asterisk in A) and ring-enhancing (arrows in B) lesions scattered throughout the parenchyma, compatible with abscesses. Note the bilateral involvement of the basal ganglia, a finding that is more commonly seen with fungal abscesses (arrows in A).

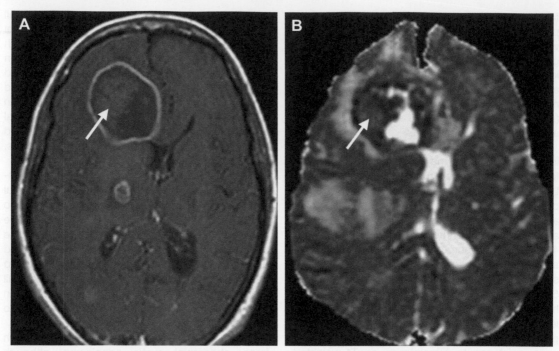

Fig. 5. Fungal abscess. Axial T1-weighted postcontrast image (*A*) shows a ring-enhancing abscess in the right frontal lobe in a patient with aspergillosis. Note the hyperintense intracavitary projections, which are thought to represent fungal hyphae (*arrow*). Axial apparent diffusion coefficient (*B*) map of the same lesion shows dark signal corresponding to the projections, indicative of restricted diffusion. Culture from pus grew *Aspergillus flavus*. (*Reprinted from* Luthra G, Parihar A, Nath K, et al. Comparative evaluation of fungal, tubercular and pyogenic abscesses with conventional and diffusion MR imaging and proton MR spectroscopy. AJNR Am J Neuroradiol 2007;28:1332–8. Copyright by American Society of Neuroradiology; with permission.)

19 of 26 abscesses demonstrated a complete hypointense rim on T2-weighted images, whereas only 4 of 27 neoplasms demonstrated this same feature, with most lesions (23/27) showing a partial or lack of a definable rim. Furthermore, apparent diffusion coefficient (ADC) ratios in neoplasm were significantly higher than in abscesses, thus conferring a high degree of accuracy in their differentiation.

Newer imaging techniques may help further differentiate an intracranial fungal abscess from a necrotic tumor, although more work needs to be done. Both diffusion tensor imaging (DTI) and MR perfusion may prove of benefit. Gupta and colleagues[32] compared the fractional anisotropy (FA) and mean diffusivity in 12 cystic intracranial lesions (5 pyogenic abscesses, 2 cysticercus cysts, and 5 low-grade astrocytomas) demonstrating regions of relative increased FA with restricted mean diffusivity in 5 of 5 abscesses, as opposed to low FA and high mean diffusivity in the remaining cystic lesions. These findings are postulated to be secondary to an upregulation of adhesive molecules in the presence of bacteria that aggregate leukocytes into organized clumps with high diffusion anisotropy. No data have been published regarding the distinguishing characteristics of fungal abscesses using DTI. Chan and colleagues[33] studied 16 patients with cystic or necrotic intracranial lesions using MR perfusion demonstrating significantly lower regional cerebral blood volume (rCBV) within the walls of pyogenic abscesses compared with rCBV values in cystic or necrotic neoplasms. Although specific data are lacking for fungal abscesses, perfusion imaging may help differentiate a fungal abscess from a neoplastic origin, because the relative angiogenesis of tumors maintains blood flow at the tumor periphery that can be demonstrated on MR perfusion.[33]

Extra-Axial

Fungal disease is an uncommon but important source for meningitis in the immunocompromised population. Although any of the fungal pathogens may cause meningitis, it is typically secondary to the hematogenous spread of small, unicellular yeast organisms (such as *Candida* and *Cryptococcus*) to the meningeal microcirculation, resulting in inflammation of the meninges.[19] This assertion is supported

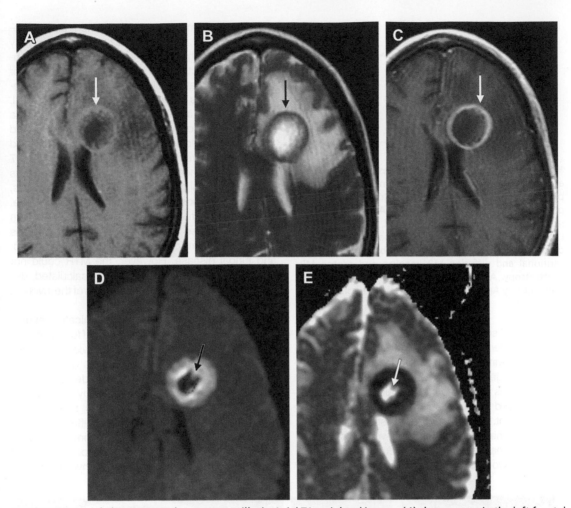

Fig. 6. Intracranial abscess secondary to aspergillosis. Axial T1-weighted images (*A*) show a mass in the left frontal lobe with a hypointense center. Axial T2-weighted (*B*) images show a hypointense periphery delineating a mass that has a hyperintense center. Adjacent regions of high T2 signal are compatible with vasogenic edema. Axial T1-weighted postcontrast images (*C*) show ring enhancement of the left frontal lobe abscess. Axial DWI image (*D*) with apparent diffusion coefficient map (*E*) shows restricted diffusion in most of the abscess, except for the central portion, a finding that has been attributed to coagulative necrosis.

in a study by Safdieh and colleagues,[34] who retrospectively reviewed 77 patients with cancer and positive cerebrospinal fluid (CSF) cultures. Although most cultures were of bacterial origin, of the 8% caused by fungal disease, 7% were *Cryptococcus* and 1% was *Candida*. The incidence of fungal meningitis in the AIDS population within the Western hemisphere has slowly declined over the past 2 decades owing to the introduction of azoles and HAART.[35] An 8-year review of patients with cryptococcal meningitis in patients with AIDS in Atlanta demonstrated a decrease in incidence from 6.6% in 1992 to 0.7% in 2000.[36] Fungal meningitis in patients with HIV, however, remains an important source of morbidity and mortality in developing nations, with the incidence in Africa ranging from 26.5% in Malawi to 45% in Zimbabwe.[37,38]

Although meningitis is largely a clinical diagnosis, certain radiographic findings, such as nodular leptomeningeal enhancement, particularly at the base of the skull, may be appreciated on gadolinium-enhanced T1-weighted images (**Fig. 8**).[39] FLAIR imaging may occasionally demonstrate increased leptomeningeal signal abnormality in the setting of meningitis, although contrast-enhanced T1-weighed images remain the more sensitive study.[40] These findings were substantiated by Kamran and colleagues,[41] who studied 28 patients diagnosed with meningitis showing sensitivities of 57% and 82% on FLAIR and postcontrast T1-weighted images, respectively, with 18% demonstrating no imaging abnormalities. Newer imaging techniques, such as DTI, have shown increased sensitivity for detecting meningitis compared with contrast-enhanced

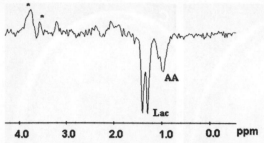

Fig. 7. MRS findings in a fungal abscess. Multiple peaks at 3.6 and 3.8 ppm are shown corresponding to trehalose present within the fungal wall (*asterisk*). Additional peaks corresponding to amino acid (AA, 0.9 ppm) and lactate (Lac, 1.3 ppm) are also noted. (*Reprinted from Luthra G, Parihar A, Nath K, et al. Comparative evaluation of fungal, tubercular and pyogenic abscesses with conventional and diffusion MR imaging and proton MR spectroscopy. AJNR Am J Neuroradiol 2007;28:1332–8. Copyright by American Society of Neuroradiology; with permission.*)

T1-weighted sequences. A study of 10 patients with pyogenic meningitis versus 10 controls showed increased FA in enhancing and nonenhancing cortical regions, suggesting the presence of early inflammation in regions where the blood-brain barrier was not compromised enough for detectable meningeal enhancement.[42] No current published data have compared the sensitivity of DTI versus contrast-enhanced images for detecting fungal meningitis, and further work remains to be done.

Overall, leptomeningeal enhancement is a nonspecific finding that, in addition to fungal disease, may also be seen with other entities, such as leptomeningeal tumor, bacterial or tuberculous meningitis, or other granulomatous disease. Other imaging techniques, such as magnetization transfer (MT) MRI, may play a role in this differentiation, although data are currently conflicted. A study by Gupta and colleagues[40] calculated the MT ratios of thickened meninges relative to normal brain parenchyma in 27 patients with meningitis, finding that tuberculous meningitis had higher MT ratios than viral meningitis, but lower than those for pyogenic and fungal disease. A subsequent study by Kamra and colleagues,[43] in contrast, showed higher MT ratios in tuberculous meningitis when compared with viral, pyogenic, and fungal disease. However, the MTR could not always be reliably and reproducibly calculated, depending on the location and thickness of the involved meninges.

As with all meningitides, communicating hydrocephalus is a possible complication of fungal meningitis apparent at imaging (Fig. 9). A review by Cornell and Jacoby[44] found 7 of 12 patients with intracranial cryptococcosis showing some degree of ventricular dilatation. In a larger series by Rozenbaum and Gonçalves,[45] who studied 130 patients with *Cryptococcus* meningitis in three different patient populations (immunocompetent, immunocompromised secondary to AIDS, and immunocompromised from another cause), 15 developed hydrocephalus,

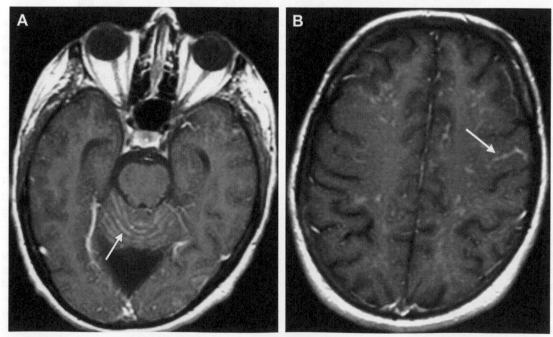

Fig. 8. Cryptococcal meningitis. Axial T1-weighted images (*A, B*) show diffuse leptomeningeal enhancement throughout the meninges. Note the diffuse enhancement of the cerebellar folia (*arrows in A and B*).

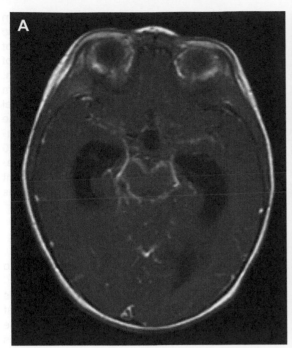 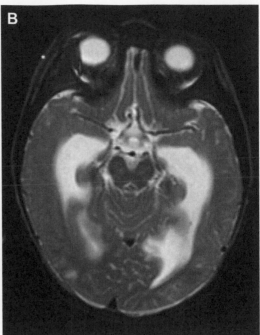

Fig. 9. Cryptococcal meningitis with hydrocephalus. Axial T1-weighted postcontrast (*A*) image shows diffuse basilar leptomeningeal enhancement. Axial T2-weighted image (*B*) shows dilatation of the temporal horns of the lateral ventricles, compatible with hydrocephalus, a sometimes fatal complication of meningitis.

with the distributions across the patient populations found to be not statistically significant.

Intracranial fungal infection can arise from extension of adjacent fungal sinus disease. At imaging, fungal sinusitis may have a characteristic appearance. Regions of increased attenuation on noncontrast CT images were demonstrated in 19 of 25 patients with documented fungal sinusitis in a review by Zinreich and colleagues.[46] This finding is postulated to be secondary to a combination of increased metal ions in mycetomas and calcium salts within necrotic regions of the hyphae, although these imaging features are nonspecific and may also be seen with thick pus, thrombus, or hemorrhage. MRI features are more specific, demonstrating decreased signal intensity on both T1- and T2-weighted images, in contrast to bacterial sinusitis or neoplasm, which often demonstrate hyperintense T2 signal. The decreased T2 signal with fungal sinusitis is thought to be related to the presence of ferromagnetic material (iron, magnesium, and manganese) within the hyphae. Fungal sinus disease is often seen with *Mucormycosis* and *Aspergillus* species. A large series by Klossek and colleagues[47] showed the presence of *Aspergillus* in 33 of 109 patients, with the remaining majority showing no growth on cell culture. Immunocompromised patients have an increased risk for invasive fungal sinusitis,

which may rapidly progress to osteomyelitis with subsequent vascular and parenchymal involvement of the adjacent CNS structures.[48] Clinically, these patients may present with chronic sinusitis not resolved with antibiotics or sinus disease in the setting of a depressed immune system.[46]

Vascular

Vascular complications of fungal CNS infection include vasculitis and mycotic aneurysms. Fungal organisms can gain access to the blood stream through hematogenous spread from the lungs or other primary locations, and through direct invasion, as can be seen with sinus disease. Certain hyphal fungal organisms, such as *Aspergillus* and *Mucormycosis*, have a predilection for angioinvasion through the production of the enzyme elastase, which compromises the elastin component present in the walls of blood vessels.[49] In vitro studies of 198 strains of *Aspergillus* obtained from patients with invasive disease, noninvasive fungal balls, and simple colonization have shown a correlation between the elastase activity and pathogenicity, with higher values found in invasive disease.[50] Digestion of elastin subsequently elicits an inflammatory reaction, resulting in vasculitis, in situ thrombosis, or embolization of the hyphal lesions. Given the tendency to involve large and medium-sized vessels at the base of the brain, fungal cerebral arteritis may be further complicated by infarction.[51] These findings are reflected as regions of hypodensity on noncontrast CT and hyperintensity with restricted diffusion on T2-weighted FLAIR and DWI MR sequences, respectively.[39,52] Superimposed hemorrhage, manifest as hyperdensity on CT and increased T1 with decreased T2 signal on MR images, is typically associated with underlying *Aspergillus* infection.[39,53]

The incidence of infectious CNS aneurysms is rare, compromising 1% to 3% of all causes of intracranial aneurysms.[54] Infectious origins are most often bacterial in origin, with fungal causes being very uncommon.[49] Between 1990 and 2005, 33 patients with intracranial fungal aneurysms have been reported in the literature, with most cases related to surgery or primary infection elsewhere in the body.[55] Data from prior case reports spanning 40 years (1950–1990) show that *Aspergillus* is the most common cause (7/8 reports) and that the most common site involves the internal carotid artery at the base of the brain.[56]

Several pathogenic mechanisms for aneurysm formation have been proposed, including embolic occlusion of the vasa vasorum, direct invasion of the arterial from within the lumen, invasion of the arterial wall from adjacent structures (sinus, bone, and meninges), and vascular injury from the deposition of immune complexes.[55,56] Fungal hyphae may compromise long segments of the vessel wall, resulting in fusiform aneurysmal dilatation of the proximal cerebral vasculature (**Figs. 10** and **11**).[57] These findings are in contrast to bacterial infectious aneurysms, which typically present as multiple, small (2–5 mm), spherical lesions arising in the distal cerebral vasculature.

ASPERGILLOSIS

Aspergillus is a commonly encountered mold found in soil, water, and decaying vegetation.[58] Although more than 350 individual species of this fungus exist, *Aspergillus fumigatus* is the most common pathogen involved in invasive tissue disease.[59] Inhalation of *Aspergillus* spores incites a granulomatous response in the lungs of an

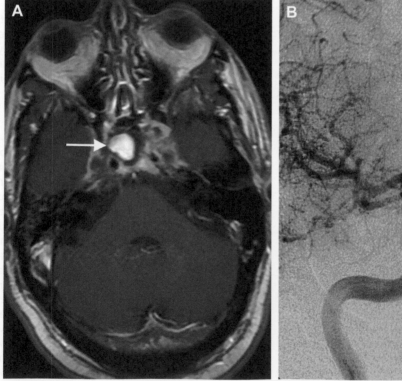
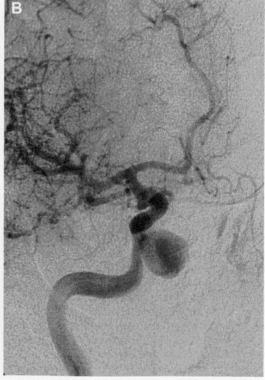

Fig. 10. Mycotic aneurysm related to aspergillosis. Axial T1-weighted postcontrast image shows an aneurysm involving the cavernous portion of the right carotid artery (*arrow* in *A*). This finding was confirmed on cerebral angiography (*B*), which shows an outpouching off the cavernous left internal carotid artery compatible with a mycotic aneurysm.

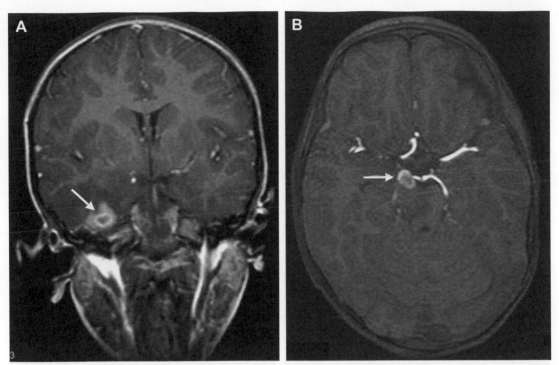

Fig. 11. Aspergillosis with posterior cerebral artery aneurysm. Coronal contrast enhanced T1-weighted image of the brain (*A*) shows a ring-enhancing lesion within the right temporal lobe (*arrow*) in this 3-year-old patient with chronic granulomatous disease. Multiple similar lesions were noted throughout the brain parenchyma. Axial image from a time-of-flight sequence through the Circle of Willis (*B*) shows a focal aneurysm of the right posterior cerebral artery (*arrow*).

immunocompetent host, typically resulting in a chronic infection.[58] Disseminated disease may occur in the setting of immunodeficiency or immunosuppression, with the fungi having a tendency to cause CNS infection. In a study of 98 patients with aspergillosis, Young and colleagues[60] found that 34 patients had evidence of disseminated disease at autopsy, with 44% showing involvement of the brain. In addition to spread from the lung, *Aspergillus* may also enter the CNS from paranasal sinus infection or through direct inoculation in the setting of head trauma.[59]

Although the imaging findings of aspergillosis are nonspecific, certain imaging characteristics may help in narrowing a differential diagnosis. Given that *Aspergillus* grows as branching hyphae at physiologic body temperatures, brain parenchymal involvement is more commonly found than the meningeal infection typically associated with unicellular yeast organisms.[59] Invasive aspergillosis can result in granuloma formation and/or encephalitis, with or without abscess formation (**Fig. 12**). In a retrospective analysis of 53 patients treated for fungal infection, Nadkarni and Goel[61] found that 18 had a diagnosis of intracranial aspergillosis. Autopsy data on 10 of 14 described findings of *Aspergillus* granuloma and/or abscesses. *Aspergillus* is among the most commonly isolated organism from fungal brain abscesses. In a study of 17 posttransplant patients with a documented fungal abscess, *Aspergillus* was isolated in 11 (65%).[28] *Aspergillus* abscesses may be surrounded by a low signal intensity on T2-weighted and gradient-echo images. The hypointense T2 signal rim has been attributed to small amount of hemorrhage with hemosiderin-laden macrophages and a dense population of hyphae at the abscess rim.[62] Peripherally restricted diffusion may be present (**Fig. 13**).

Another striking feature of *Aspergillus* is the tendency for the organism to invade blood vessels. In the retrospective analysis by Nadkarni and Goel,[61] 3 of 10 patients were found to have autopsy-proven evidence of intracranial vascular invasion with secondary thrombosis. Vascular invasion is thought to be facilitated by the release of the enzyme elastase, which facilitates intramural vascular invasion. Secondary complications of vascular invasion include vasculitis, infarction, rarely mycotic aneurysms, and intracranial hemorrhage.[49,51,55] Imaging findings of hemorrhage are common in association with *Aspergillus* infection. *Aspergillus* is also commonly encountered in the setting of fungal sinus disease, with distinct MR imaging findings as previously described.

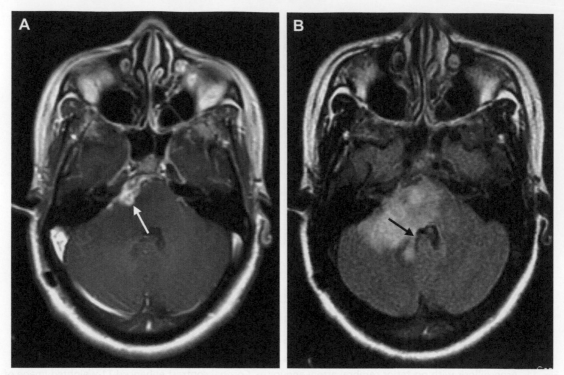

Fig. 12. Aspergillosis. Axial postcontrast image of the brain (*A*) shows abnormal enhancement in the prepontine cistern extending into the right cerebellopontine angle (*white arrow*). Note the adjacent regions of high FLAIR signal resulting in mass effect on the fourth ventricle (*B, black arrow*).

MUCORMYCOSIS

Mucormycosis, which has been used interchangeably with *phycomycosis* and *zygomycosis*, generally refers to infection from any fungi within the family Mucoraceae.[59] It is characteristically found in patients with diabetes, although other debilitating conditions, such as chronic renal failure, cirrhosis, and chronic diarrhea, are associated with the development of invasive disease.[63] The Mucoraceae are ubiquitous in their distribution, but are most commonly found in decaying organic material.[61,64] Spores of these organisms can be found in the nasal mucosa, oropharynx, or respiratory airways, from which they can directly invade the brain parenchyma through paranasal sinus and orbital extension (rhinocerebral mucormycosis) or, less commonly, hematogenously disseminate to the CNS, typically via a primary infection in the lung.[59] Rhinocerebral mucormycosis has such a high correlation with diabetes that this entity should be considered in any patients with diabetes who have sinusitis, facial, or eye pain, regardless of their glycemic control.[65] Isolated cerebral mucormycosis, however, has a high correlation with intravenous drug use, as shown by Stave and colleagues,[66] who found that 11 of

22 individuals with isolated cerebral involvement had some history of intravenous drug abuse.

Imaging findings of cerebral mucormycosis are similar to aspergillosis, with the most characteristic features including a propensity for sino-orbital disease and vascular invasion. Sinus disease manifests as nonspecific nodular mucosal thickening, typically without the presence of air-fluid levels.[67] The ethmoid sinus is most commonly involved, with disease subsequently spreading via the valveless veins to the orbit, nose, cavernous sinuses, or brain parenchyma.[68] Extension to the orbit results in thickening and lateral displacement of the adjacent medial rectus muscle, preseptal edema, proptosis, and fat infiltration, particularly at the orbital apex. Parenchymal involvement from sino-orbital disease portends a bad prognosis, with one series finding a 100% mortality rate in 11 patients with rhinocerebral mucormycosis (**Fig. 14**).[68] Like aspergillosis, vascular invasion in mucormycosis is thought to occur through the presence of an elastase that compromises the vessel wall.[49] Vascular thromboses and pseudoaneurysm formation are uncommon but associated findings. Bergstrom and colleagues[69] found cavernous sinus involvement in 14 patients in their series of 48 patients with intracranial mucormycosis (**Fig. 15**).

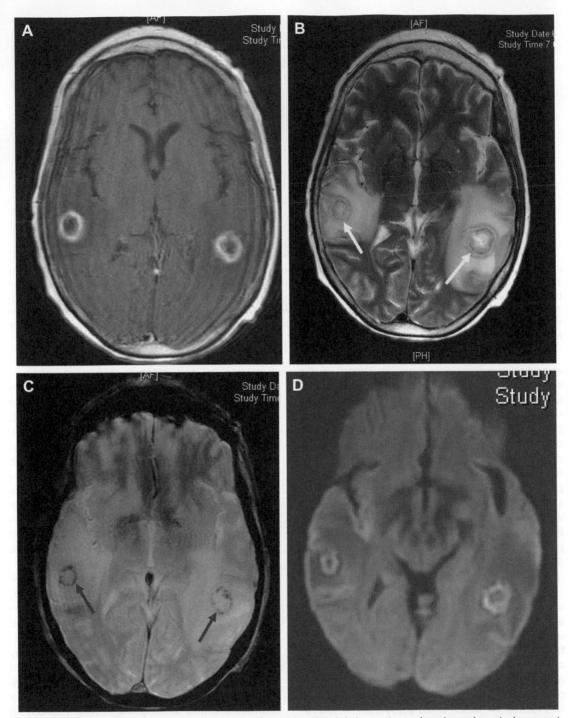

Fig. 13. Aspergillus abscesses. Axial T1 contrast-enhanced image (*A*) shows ring-enhancing subcortical masses in the posterior temporal lobes. The T2-weighted image (*B*) shows a hypointense rim (*yellow arrows*) and associated edema. On the gradient echo image (*C*) a hypointense rim is present, consistent with susceptibility effect related to hemorrhage (*red arrows*.) The diffusion-weighted image (*D*) shows restricted diffusion at the periphery.

HISTOPLASMOSIS

Histoplasmosis is the sequelae of infection with the unicellular yeast, *Histoplasma capsulatum*.[59] In the United States the organism is most commonly found in the Ohio, Mississippi, and St. Lawrence River valleys, with spores often present in bat caves, bird droppings, and chicken coops.[63] In

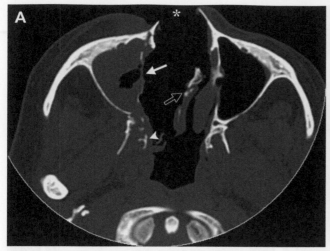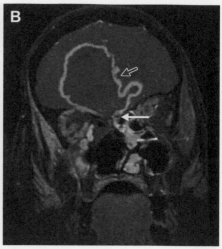

Fig. 14. Mucormycosis of the right orbit with intraparenchymal extension. Axial noncontrast CT scan of the orbits on bone windows (*A*) shows destruction of the nasal bone (*asterisk*), nasal septum (*black arrow*), medial wall of the right maxillary sinus (*white arrow*), and right pterygoid plate (*arrowhead*). Coronal contrast-enhanced T1-weighted image of the brain (*B*) shows abnormal enhancement of the nasal cavity with superior extension of the infectious process through the cribriform plate (*white arrow*) resulting in a bilobed abscess spanning the frontal lobes (*block arrow*).

immunocompetent individuals, inhalation of the spores may result in a mildly symptomatic respiratory illness, with a subsequent granulomatous response to the offending pathogen. Studies have shown that immunocompetent patients at risk for disseminated disease include infants and young children, and adults older than 40, the latter being attributed to greater occupational exposure in this population.[70] Disseminated disease is seen with impaired immune function, particularly in patients with AIDS in endemic areas.[71,72] Although CNS involvement is clinically evident in 5% to 10% of patients with disseminated histoplasmosis, autopsy studies have found CNS histoplasmosis in approximately 25% of patients.[73]

Imaging findings are nonspecific, but unlike aspergillosis and mucormycosis, a relatively higher tendency for isolated meningeal involvement exists in CNS histoplasmosis. Other CNS manifestations include granuloma and abscess formation and cerebritis, although the latter is uncommon. A review by Wheat and colleagues[74] found the presence of cerebritis in only 2 of 77 patients. Granuloma formation is more common, with a reported incidence as high as 25%, although the imaging findings are nonspecific, with low signal rims on T1- and T2-weighted images, thought to be secondary to paramagnetic substances.[74,75]

CANDIDIASIS

Candida albicans is responsible for most cases of human candidiasis.[59] *Candida* is part of the normal human flora and is most commonly seen in the gastrointestinal tract and mucocutaneous membranes.[63] Disseminated disease can occur through imbalances in the equilibrium of this pathogen relative to other normal flora found in humans. One of the most common factors that contribute to this imbalance is treatment with antibiotics, steroids, or chemotherapy.[11] Other factors that may result in disseminated disease include the presence of indwelling catheters or intravenous drug use with resulting Candida endocarditis.[76] Although CNS involvement may be seen in 18% to 52% of patients, the most common site for disseminated candidiasis is the kidneys.[77]

Four main clinicopathologic disease groups have been identified: cerebral microabscesses, meningitis, cerebral macroabscesses, and vascular complications.[78] Patients with cerebral microabscesses have evidence of systemic disease and show signs of diffuse encephalopathy on neurologic examination. The incidence of cerebral microabscesses (<3 mm) varies between 0.2% and 0.5%, as corroborated by Pendlebury and colleagues,[79] who found that 35 of 92 patients with documented CNS candidiasis showed these abscesses on postmortem examination. On contrast-enhanced CT images, these lesions demonstrate punctate nodular enhancement and are isodense to hypodense on the noncontrast images, although most often these lesions are too small to be confidently detected in the antemortem state.[39,78] Unenhanced MR may show hypointense T2 lesions secondary

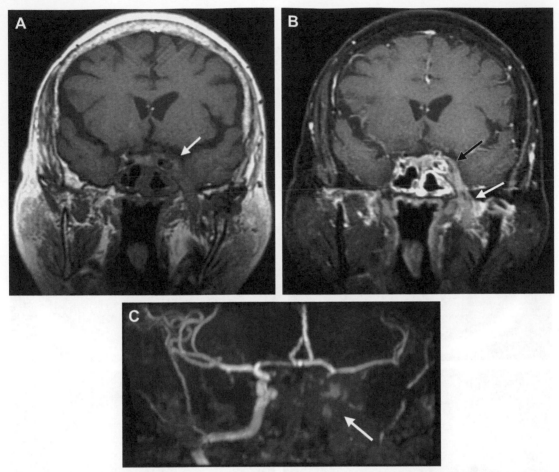

Fig. 15. Mucormycosis with occlusion of the cavernous left internal carotid artery. Coronal precontrast (*A*) and postcontrast (*B*) T1-weighted images of the brain shows abnormal enhancement of the left cavernous sinus (*white arrow* in *A, block arrow* in *B*) from extension from left maxillary/orbital mucormycosis infection for which the patient was status postenucleation. Note the extension of infection through the left foramen ovale (*white arrow* in *B*) with abnormal enhancement of the left masticator space. Three-dimensional reconstructed time-of-flight image of the Circle of Willis (*C*) shows complete occlusion of the left internal carotid artery, a result of extensive mucormycosis infection (*white arrow*).

to hemorrhage, or nonspecific hyperintense white matter lesions.[80] Small enhancing lesions are seen, which may have restricted diffusion (**Fig. 16**). Candida meningitis has been found to occur in fewer than 15% of patients. Meningeal infection is likely facilitated by the small size of the spores, which allows easier access to the meningeal microcirculation.[78] Cerebral macroabscesses are uncommon, but have been reported in both immunocompetent and immunocompromised individuals.[79–81] Abscesses can be single or multiple. They are usually found in the parietooccipital region, although cases of cerebellar involvement have been reported.[82] Cerebral vascular involvement has been demonstrated in up to 23%

of autopsy studies.[80] Like other fungal disease, Candida vascular involvement may lead to infarctions, particularly in the basal ganglia, and mycotic aneurysm with subarachnoid hemorrhage.[77] Cerebral atrophy has been a reported finding with CNS candidiasis, although this is usually attributed to the underlying medical condition (HIV infection, radiotherapy) rather than the fungus itself.[83]

COCCIDIOIDOMYCOSIS

Coccidioides immitis is a dimorphic fungus endemic to the southwestern United States, particularly southern California and Arizona, and

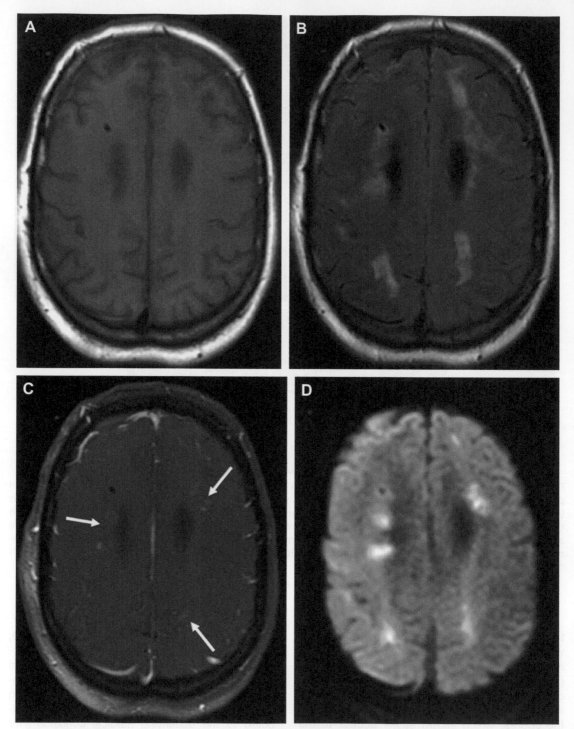

Fig. 16. Candida micoabscesses. No lesions are apparent on the unenhanced T1 weighted image (*A*). Axial T2 weighted FLAIR images (*B*) show nonspecific white matter increased signal intensity. Following contrast injection multiple small deep frontoparietal enhancing lesions are seen (*arrows*) (*C*). Restricted diffusion is seen associated with the enhancing lesions (*D*). (*Images courtesy of* John Go, MD, Los Angeles, California.)

parts of Central and South America.[59] Inhalation of the fungal spores usually results in a self-limited mild respiratory illness with fever, cough, and chest pain.[63] Dissemination occurs in fewer than 1% of patients, with the incidence increasing up to 30% in patients with HIV.[84]

Extrapulmonary sites of infection include osteomyelitis, cutaneous lesions, and CNS involvement, with the meninges involved in one-third to one-half of all patients with disseminated disease.[85] Erly and colleagues[86] described MR imaging findings of meningitis, including enhancement of the basal

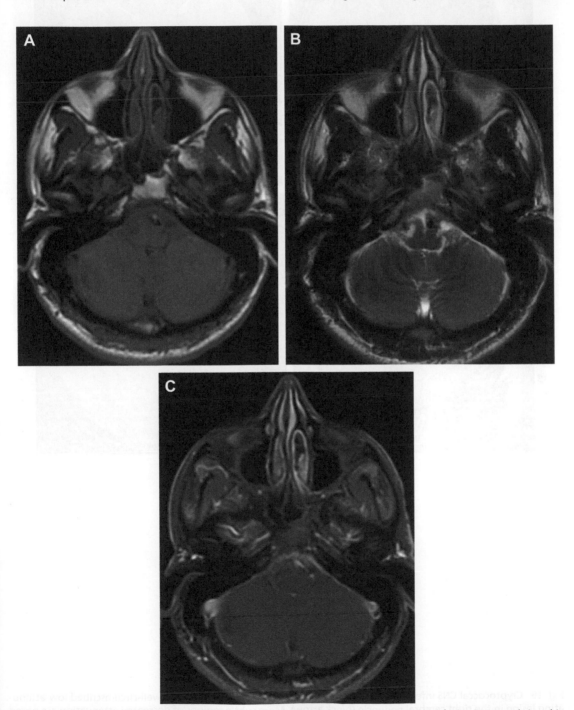

Fig. 17. Coccidiomycosis basilar meningitis. Axial T1-weighted image (A) shows subtle relative increased signal in the basilar cisterns with (B) increased T2 signal intensity similar to CSF. After contrast injection, diffuse enhancement of the basilar cisterns is seen (C). (Courtesy of John Go, MD.)

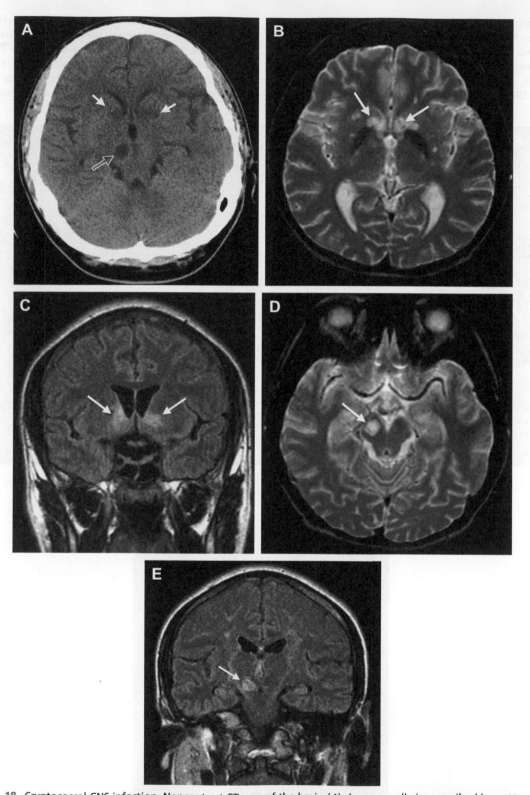

Fig. 18. Cryptococcal CNS infection. Noncontrast CT scan of the brain (*A*) shows a well-circumscribed low-attenu-ating lesion in the right cerebral peduncle (*block arrow*). More subtle regions of decreased attenuation are noted in the basal ganglia bilaterally (*white arrows*). Axial T2 (*B, D*) and coronal FLAIR (*C, E*) images show high signal intensity lesions in the basal ganglia and right cerebral peduncle corresponding to cryptococcomas in this patient with HIV and positive CSF cryptococcal antigen.

cisterns, sylvian fissures, and pericallosal regions in 10 of 14 patients who presented with acute CNS coccidioidomycosis (**Fig. 17**). The resulting dense meningeal exudates have been related to the development of hydrocephalus in 68% to 93% of patients.[21,87]

Vascular involvement has been reported in up to 40% of patients, with ischemia occurring in 58%.[88,89] Erly and colleagues,[86] also found ischemic changes in 4 of 14 patients (29%), with the ischemic regions noted in areas of perforating vessels that had evidence of meningitis involving the parent vessel. The ischemic changes were attributed to vasospasm or direct invasion of the vessel itself.

Intracerebral coccidioidomycosis including granuloma and abscess is uncommon, with Bañuelos and colleagues[90] reporting a total of 39 cases in their review spanning 1905 through 1996. When present, lesions were single or multiple, and their distribution suggested hematogenous dissemination from the lung or infected meningeal sources, rather than direct invasion from the meninges itself. In fact, 11 of 32 patients with intraparenchymal abscesses in whom data were available showed no evidence of underlying meningitis.[90,91] No distinct imaging findings were reported. Abscesses typically showed ring enhancement on contrast-infused images.

CRYPTOCOCCOSIS

Cryptococcus neoformans thrives in soil contaminated with bird feces, particularly pigeon droppings, which contain the organic nitrogen that allows the pathogen to grow.[59] Although cryptococcosis is most often seen in patients with some degree of immune dysfunction, up to 30% of patients may demonstrate no underlying predisposing condition.[91] Cryptococcosis is the most common fungal pathogen to infect the CNS and is the most frequently identified fungal CNS infection in patients with AIDS.[92,93] The disease is more commonly identified in men (80%), which may be related to a greater occupational exposure to the fungal spores.[70] Inhalation of spores seldom results in clinical pulmonary disease, with subsequent dissemination occurring in the context of impaired immunity.[59] *Cryptococcus neoformans* has a tendency to spread to the CNS, with one study showing autopsy findings of CNS involvement in 90% of patients with cryptococcal infection.[70] The propensity for CNS dissemination is postulated to occur because the soluble anticryptococcal factors present in serum are absent in CSF.[94] Furthermore, the polysaccharide capsule of the fungal pathogen confers protection against the host inflammatory response.

Cryptococcosis often causes meningeal disease, as shown in a study of 145 individuals with AIDS, among whom meningitis was present in 9 of 10 patients with underlying cryptococcosis.[95] Although meningeal enhancement is most prominent at the base of the brain (see **Fig. 9**), imaging findings are often lacking, especially in immunocompromised patients. In these cases, the diagnosis is more definitively obtained through detecting the presence of the fungal antigen in the CSF and blood.[39,96]

Invasion of the adjacent brain parenchyma in cases of cryptococcal meningitis may give rise to cryptococcomas, which represent chronic granulomas composed of lymphocytes, macrophages, and giant cells.[39] Cryptococcomas have been previously reported to demonstrate intermediate to low signal on T1-weighted images and high signal on T2-weighted images. Most of these lesions are usually found in the basal ganglia. In immunocompromised patients, these lesions rarely demonstrate enhancement after the administration of intravenous contrast (**Figs. 18** and **19**). In a study by Miszkiel and colleagues,[97] 9 of 25 patients with AIDS developed cryptococcomas, most of which were in the basal ganglia (7/9) and none of which showed contrast enhancement. Granulomas have also been reported to form along the ependyma of the choroid plexus, a finding that has been reported to be a specific

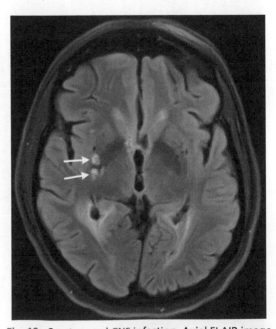

Fig. 19. Cryptococcal CNS infection. Axial FLAIR image of the brain shows two FLAIR hyperintense foci (*arrows*) within the right basal ganglia compatible with cryptococcomas in this patient with known cryptococcal meningitis.

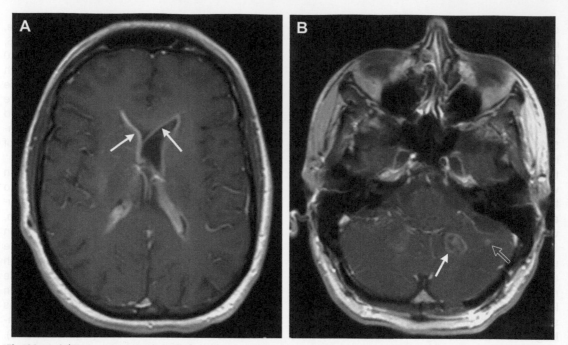

Fig. 20. Axial T1 postcontrast image showing cryptococcal CNS infection. (*A*) Abnormal ependymal enhancement is compatible with ventriculitis (*arrows*). (*B*) A ring-enhancing lesion in the left cerebellar hemisphere (*white arrow*) and a smaller adjacent enhancing focus compatible with multiple abscesses (*block arrow*) are seen.

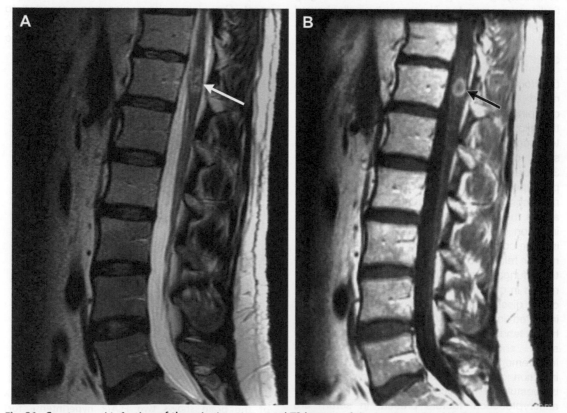

Fig. 21. Cryptococcal infection of the spinal cord. Sagittal T2 images of the lumbar spine (*A*) show a hyperintense focus within the conus medullaris (*white arrow*). The lesion shows ring enhancement on the sagittal T1 postcontrast image (*B, black arrow*). These findings are compatible with cryptococcus infection of the spinal cord in this HIV-positive patient with positive CSF cryptococcal antigen.

feature of cryptococcosis (**Fig. 20**).[98] Involvement of the spinal cord is an uncommon but reported finding, with the imaging features showing nonspecific increased T2 signal within the cord, with or without contrast enhancement (**Fig. 21**).

Cryptococcal meningeal infection may spread along the perivascular (Virchow-Robin) spaces penetrating the brain parenchyma, resulting in the formation of gelatinous pseudocysts.[39] MR imaging demonstrates nonenhancing lesions, which are usually isointense to CSF on T1- and T2-weighted images, although occasionally they may be slightly hyperintense on T1-weighted images.[48] Post-mortem studies reviewed by Tien and colleagues[99] correlated these lesions to perivascular spaces filled with fungi and mucoid gelatinous material produced by the capsule of the organism. The pseudocysts are often bilateral and symmetric, and have a predilection for the midbrain and basal ganglia. They seldom demonstrate significant mass effect, although findings may vary, depending on the size of the lesions. Pseudocysts may demonstrate restricted diffusion, which is attributed to decreased molecular diffusibility within the thick gelatinous content of the lesion.[100]

SUMMARY

Although the imaging features of fungal CNS infection are often nonspecific, various fungal infections of the CNS have some characteristic imaging and associated clinical findings. CNS fungal infection more often occurs in the immunocompromised or debilitated host. CNS fungal infection manifestations may be organized into extra-axial, parenchymal, and vascular categories. Small unicellular organisms such as *Candida* or *Cryptococcus* more commonly cause meningitis. *Mucormycosis* and *Aspergillus* have a predilection for sinus disease with secondary CNS involvement. Larger, hyphal organisms such as *Aspergillus* tend to involve the brain parenchyma and the cerebral vascular structures, giving rise to cerebritis, abscess, vasculitis, and mycotic aneurysm formation. Dimorphic organisms such ss *Coccidiomycosis* may cause meningeal or parenchymal infection. Imaging features of fungal infection, such as the lower T2 signal intensity of intracavitary projections in fungal abscesses or hemorrhage associated with *Aspergillus*, may aid in differentiating fungal from pyogenic or tuberculous infections. DWI in addition to other imaging techniques, including MR perfusion and MR spectroscopy, may help differentiate abscess from other mimickers, such as a cystic metastases, and help differentiate a fungal from a pyogenic origin. Fungal infectious aneurysms are rare, although certain clues, such as the morphology and location, may

suggest the diagnosis in the appropriate clinical setting.

REFERENCES

1. Davis LE. Fungal infections of the central nervous system. Neurol Clin 1999;17(4):761–81.
2. Medoff G, Kobayashi GS. Systemic fungal infections: an overview. Hosp Pract 1991;26:41.
3. Parker JC Jr, McCloskey JJ, Lee RS. Human cerebral candidosis—a postmortem evaluation of 19 patients. Hum Pathol 1981;12:23.
4. Lucas S, Bell J, Chimelli L. Parasitic and fungal infections. In: Love S, Louis DN, Ellison DW, editors. Greenfield's neuropathology. 8th edition. London: Edward Arnold; 2008. p. 1488–511.
5. Chakrabarti A. Epidemiology of central nervous system mycoses. Neurol India 2007;55(3):191–7.
6. Pfaller MA, Pappas PG, Wingard JR. Invasive fungal pathogens: current epidemiological trends. Clin Infect Dis 2006;43(Suppl 1):S3–14.
7. Groll AH, Shah PM, Mentzel C, et al. Trends in the postmortem epidemiology of invasive fungal infections at a university hospital. J Infect 1996;33(1):23–32.
8. Lehrnbecher T, Frank C, Engels K, et al. Trends in the postmortem epidemiology of invasive fungal infections at a university hospital. J Infect 2010; 61(3):259–65.
9. Richardson M, Lass-Florl C. Changing epidemiology of systemic fungal infections. Clin Microbiol Infect 2008;14(Suppl 4):5–24.
10. Rees JR, Pinner RW, Hajjeh RA, et al. The epidemiological features of invasive mycotic infections in the San Francisco Bay area, 1992-1993: results of population-based laboratory active surveillance. Clin Infect Dis 1998;27(5):1138–47.
11. Richardson MD. Changing patterns and trends in systemic fungal infections. J Antimicrob Chemother 2005;56(Suppl 1):i5–11.
12. Marr KA, Carter RA, Crippa F, et al. Epidemiology and outcome of mould infections in hematopoietic stem cell transplant recipients. Clin Infect Dis 2002;34(7):909–17.
13. van Burik JH, Leisenring W, Myerson D, et al. The effect of prophylactic fluconazole on the clinical spectrum of fungal diseases in bone marrow transplant recipients with special attention to hepatic candidiasis. An autopsy study of 355 patients. Medicine (Baltimore) 1998;77(4):246–54.
14. Lyons RW, Andriole VT. Fungal infections of the CNS. Neurol Clin 1986;4:159–70.
15. Parker JC Jr, McCloskey JJ, Solanki KV, et al. Candidosis: the most common postmortem cerebral mycosis in an endemic fungal area. Surg Neurol 1976;6:123–8.
16. Dubey A, Patwardhan RV, Sampath S, et al. Intracranial fungal granuloma: analysis of 40 patients

and review of the literature. Surg Neurol 2005;63:
254–60.

17. Kobayashi GS. Fungi. In: Davis BD, Dulbecco R, Eisen HN, et al, editors. Microbiology. New York: Harper and Row; 1980. p. 817–50.

18. Black KE, Baden LR. Fungal infections of the CNS: treatment strategies for the immunocompromised patient. CNS Drugs 2007;21(4):293–318.

19. Murthy JM. Fungal infections of the central nervous system: the clinical syndromes. Neurol India 2007; 55(3):221–5.

20. Sundaram C, Umabala P, Laxmi V, et al. Histopathology of fungal infections of central nervous system: a seventeen years experience from south India. Histopathology 2006;49:396–405.

21. Parker JC Jr, Dyer MC. Neurologic infections due to bacteria fungi, and parasites. In: Doris RL, Robertson DM, editors. Textbook of neuropathology. Baltimore (MD): Williams & Wilkins; 1985. p. 632–703.

22. Somer T, Finegold SM. Vasculitides associated with infections, immunization and antimicrobial drugs. Clin Infect Dis 1993;20:1010–46.

23. Mikhael MA, Rushovich AM, Ciric I. Magnetic resonance imaging of cerebral aspergillosis. Comput Radiol 1985;9(2):85–9.

24. Gupta R, Singh AK, Bishnu P, et al. Intracranial aspergillus granuloma simulating meningioma on MR imaging. J Comput Assist Tomogr 1990;14:467–9.

25. Gaviani P, Schwartz RB, Hedley-Whyte ET, et al. Diffusion-weighted imaging of fungal cerebral infection. AJNR Am J Neuroradiol 2005;26(5):1115–21.

26. Haimes AB, Zimmerman RD, Morgello S, et al. MR imaging of brain abscesses. AJR Am J Roentgenol 1989;152:1073–85.

27. Enzmann DR, Brant-Zawadzki M, Britt RH. CT of central nervous system infections in immunocompromised patients. AJR Am J Roentgenol 1980; 135(2):263–7.

28. Ashdown BC, Tien RD, Felsberg GJ. Aspergillosis of the brain and paranasal sinuses in immunocompromised patients: CT and MR imaging findings. AJR Am J Roentgenol 1994;162(1):155–9.

29. Baddley JW, Salzman D, Pappas PG. Fungal brain abscess in transplant recipients: epidemiologic, microbiologic, and clinical features. Clin Transplant 2002;16(6):419–24.

30. Luthra G, Parihar A, Nath K, et al. Comparative evaluation of fungal, tubercular, and pyogenic brain abscesses with conventional and diffusion MR imaging and proton MR spectroscopy. AJNR Am J Neuroradiol 2007;28(7):1332–8.

31. Fertikh D, Krejza J, Cunqueiro A, et al. Discrimination of capsular stage brain abscesses from necrotic or cystic neoplasms using diffusion-weighted magnetic resonance imaging. J Neurosurg 2007; 106(1):76–81.

32. Gupta RK, Hasan KM, Mishra AM, et al. High fractional anisotropy in brain abscesses versus other cystic intracranial lesions. AJNR Am J Neuroradiol 2005;26(5):1107–14.

33. Chan JH, Tsui EY, Chau LF, et al. Discrimination of an infected brain tumor from a cerebral abscess by combined MR perfusion and diffusion imaging. Comput Med Imaging Graph 2002;26(1):19–23.

34. Safdieh JE, Mead PA, Sepkowitz KA, et al. Bacterial and fungal meningitis in patients with cancer. Neurology 2008;70(12):943–7.

35. Jarvis JN, Harrison TS. HIV-associated cryptococcal meningitis. AIDS 2007;21(16):2119–29.

36. Mirza SA, Phelan M, Rimland D, et al. The changing epidemiology of cryptococcosis: an update from population-based active surveillance in 2 large metropolitan areas, 1992–2000. Clin Infect Dis 2003;36:789–94.

37. Gordon SB, Walsh AL, Chaponda M, et al. Bacterial meningitis in Malawian adults: pneumococcal disease is common, severe, and seasonal. Clin Infect Dis 2000;31:53–7.

38. Hakim JG, Gangaidzo IT, Heyderman RS, et al. Impact of HIV infection on meningitis in Harare, Zimbabwe: a prospective study of 406 predominantly adult patients. AIDS 2000;14:1401–7.

39. Jain KK, Mittal SK, Kumar S, et al. Imaging features of central nervous system fungal infections. Neurol India 2007;55(3):241–50.

40. Gupta RK, Kathuria MK, Pradhan S. Magnetization transfer MR imaging in CNS tuberculosis. AJNR Am J Neuroradiol 1999;20(5):867–75.

41. Kamran S, Bener AB, Alper D, et al. Role of fluid-attenuated inversion recovery in the diagnosis of meningitis: comparison with contrast-enhanced magnetic resonance imaging. J Comput Assist Tomogr 2004;28(1):68–72.

42. Nath K, Husain M, Trivedi R, et al. Clinical implications of increased fractional anisotropy in meningitis associated with brain abscess. J Comput Assist Tomogr 2007;31(6):888–93.

43. Kamra P, Azad R, Prasad KN, et al. Infectious meningitis: prospective evaluation with magnetization transfer MRI. Br J Radiol 2004;77(917):387–94.

44. Cornell SH, Jacoby CG. The varied computed tomographic appearance of intracranial cryptococcosis. Radiology 1982;143:703–7.

45. Rozenbaum R, Gonçalves AJ. Clinical epidemiological study of 171 cases of cryptococcosis. Clin Infect Dis 1994;18(3):369–80.

46. Zinreich SJ, Kennedy DW, Malat J, et al. Fungal sinusitis: diagnosis with CT and MR imaging. Radiology 1988;169(2):439–44.

47. Klossek M, Serrano E, Peloquin L, et al. Functional endoscopic sinus surgery and 109 mycetomas of paranasal sinuses. Laryngoscope 1997;107: 112–7.

48. Ferguson BJ. Fungus balls of the paranasal sinuses. Otolaryngol Clin North Am 2000;33(2):389–98.

49. Hurst RW, Judkins A, Bolger W, et al. Mycotic aneurysm and cerebral infarction resulting from fungal sinusitis: imaging and pathologic correlation. AJNR Am J Neuroradiol 2001;22(5):858–63.

50. Blanco JL, Hontecillas R, Bouza E, et al. Correlation between the elastase activity index and invasiveness of clinical isolates of Aspergillus fumigatus. J Clin Microbiol 2002;40(5):1811–3.

51. Kalita J, Bansal R, Ayagiri A, et al. Midbrain infarction: a rare presentation of cryptococcal meningitis. Clin Neurol Neurosurg 1999;101:23–5.

52. Keyik B, Edgüer T, Hekimoglu B. Conventional and diffusion-weighted MR imaging of cerebral aspergillosis. Diagn Interv Radiol 2005;11:199–201.

53. McKee EE. Mycotic infection of the brain with arteritis and sub-arachnoid hemorrhage: report of case. Am J Clin Pathol 1950;20:381–4.

54. Frazee J. Inflammatory aneurysms. In: Wilkins R, Rengachary S, editors. Neurosurgery. New York: McGraw Hill; 1996. p. 2378–82.

55. Sundaram C, Goel D, Uppin SG, et al. Intracranial mycotic aneurysm due to Aspergillus species. J Clin Neurosci 2007;14(9):882–6.

56. Horten BC, Abbott GF, Porro RS. Fungal aneurysms of intracranial vessels. Arch Neurol 1976; 33:577–9.

57. Lau A, Takeshita M, Ishii N. Mycotic (aspergillus) arteritis resulting in fatal subarachnoid hemorrhage: a case report. Angiology 1991;42:251–5.

58. Kleinschmidt-DeMasters BK. Central nervous system aspergillosis: a 20-year retrospective series. Hum Pathol 2002;33(1):116–24.

59. Ostrow TD, Hudgins PA. Magnetic resonance imaging of intracranial fungal infections. Magn Reson Imaging 1994;6(1):22–31.

60. Young RC, Bennett JE, Vogel CL, et al. Aspergillosis. The spectrum of disease in 98 patients. Medicine 1970;49:147–73.

61. Nadkarni T, Goel A. Aspergilloma of the brain: an overview. J Postgrad Med 2005;51(Suppl 1):S37–41.

62. Cox J, Murtagh FR, Wilfrong A, et al. Cerebral aspergillosis: MR imaging and histopathologic correlation. AJNR Am J Neuroradiol 1992;5:1489–92.

63. Verma A, Brozman B, Petito CK. Isolated cerebral mucormycosis: report of a case and review of the literature. J Neurol Sci 2006;240(1–2):65–9.

64. Sugar AM. Mucormycosis. Clin Infect Dis 1992; 14(Suppl 1):S126–9.

65. Terk MR, Underwood DJ, Zee CS, et al. MR imaging in rhinocerebral and intracranial mucormycosis with CT and pathologic correlation. Magn Reson Imaging 1992;10(1):81–7.

66. Stave GM, Heimberger T, Kerkering TM. Zygomycosis of the basal ganglia in intravenous drug users. Am J Med 1989;86:115–7.

67. Yousem DM, Galetta SL, Gusnard DA, et al. MR findings in rhinocerebral mucormycosis. J Comput Assist Tomogr 1989;13(5):878–82.

68. Straatsma MR, Zimmerman LE, Gass JD. Phycomycosis: a clinicopathologic study of 51 cases. Lab Invest 1962;11:963–85.

69. Bergstrom L, Hemenway WG, Barnhart RA. Rhinocerebral mucormycosis. Ann Otol Rhinol Laryngol 1970;79:70–81.

70. Corez KJ, Walsh TJ. Space-occupying fungal lesions of the central nervous system. In: Scheld WM, Whitley RJ, Marra CM, editors. Infections of the central nervous system. 3rd edition. Philadelphia: Lippincott-Raven Publishers; 2004. p. 729.

71. Wheat J. Endemic mycoses in AIDS: a clinical review. Clin Microbiol Rev 1995;8:146–59.

72. Wheat LJ, Musial CE, Jenny-Avital E. Diagnosis and management of central nervous system histoplasmosis. Clin Infect Dis 2005;40:844–52.

73. Mawhorter SD, Curley GV, Kursh ED, et al. Prostatic and central nervous system histoplasmosis in an immunocompetent host: case report and review of the prostatic histoplasmosis literature. Clin Infect Dis 2000;30:595–8.

74. Wheat LJ, Batteiger BE, Sathapatayavongs B. Histoplasma capsulatum infections of the central nervous system. A clinical review. Medicine (Baltimore) 1990;69(4):244–60.

75. Dion FM, Venger BH, Landon G, et al. Thalamic histoplasmoma: CT and MR imaging. J Comput Assist Tomogr 1987;11(1):193–5.

76. Kay JH, Bernstein S, Feinstein D, et al. Surgical cure of Candida albicans endocarditis with open-heart surgery. N Engl J Med 1961;264:907–10.

77. Lipton SA, Hickey WF, Morris JH, et al. Candidal infection in the central nervous system. Am J Med 1984;76(1):101–8.

78. Sánchez-Portocarrero J, Pérez-Cecilia E, Corral O, et al. The central nervous system and infection by Candida species. Diagn Microbiol Infect Dis 2000;37(3):169–79.

79. Pendlebury WW, Perl DP, Munoz DG. Multiple microabscesses in the central nervous system: a clinicopathologic study. J Neuropathol Exp Neurol 1989 May;48(3):290–300.

80. Lai P, Lin S, Pan H, et al. Disseminated miliary cerebral candidiasis. AJNR Am J Neuroradiol 1997;18:1303–6.

81. Foreman NK, Mott MG, Parkyn TM, et al. Mycotic intracranial abscesses during induction treatment for acute lymphoblastic leukaemia. Arch Dis Child 1988;63:436–8.

82. Ilgren EB, Westmorland D, Adams CB, et al. Cerebellar mass caused by Candida species. J Neurosurg 1984;60:428–30.

83. Baker AS, Gang DL. Case records of the Massachusetts General Hospital, Case 45. N Engl J Med 1981;305:1135–46.

84. Fish DG, Ampel NM, Galgiani JN, et al. Coccidioidomycosis during human immunodeficiency virus infection. A review of 77 patients. Medicine (Baltimore) 1990;69(6):384–91.

85. Einstein HE. Coccidioidomycosis of the central nervous system. Adv Neurol 1974;6:101–5.

86. Erly WK, Bellon RJ, Seeger JF, et al. MR imaging of acute coccidioidal meningitis. AJNR Am J Neuroradiol 1999;20(3):509–14.

87. McGahan JP, Graves DS, Palmer PE, et al. Classic and contemporary Imaging of coccidioidomycosis. AJR Am J Roentgenol 1981;136:393–404.

88. Wrobel CJ, Meyer S, Johnson RH, et al. MR findings in acute and chronic coccidioidomycosis meningitis. AJNR Am J Neuroradiol 1992;13:1241–5.

89. Erly WK, Labadie E, Williams PL, et al. Disseminated coccidioidomycosis complicated by vasculitis: a cause of fatal subarachnoid hemorrhage in two cases. AJNR Am J Neuroradiol 1999;20:1605–8.

90. Bañuelos AF, Williams PL, Johnson RH, et al. Central nervous system abscesses due to Coccidioides species. Clin Infect Dis 1996;22(2):240–50.

91. Dismukes WE. Management of cryptococcosis. Clin Infect Dis 1993;17:S507–12.

92. Celso L, da Cruz H, Domingues RC. Intracranial infection. In: Atlas SW, editor. Magnetic resonance imaging of the brain and spine. 4th edition. Philadelphia: Locknut Williams & Wilkins; 2009. p. 989.

93. Mathews VP, Alo PL, Glass JD, et al. AIDS-related CNS cryptococcosis: radiologic-pathologic correlation. AJNR Am J Neuroradiol 1992;13(5):1477–86.

94. Kovoor JM, Mahadevan A, Narayan JP, et al. Cryptococcal choroid plexitis as a mass lesion: MR imaging and histopathologic correlation. AJNR Am J Neuroradiol 2002;23:273–6.

95. Eng RH, Bishburg E, Smith SM, et al. Cryptococcal infections in patients with acquired immunodeficiency syndrome. Am J Med 1986;81:19–23.

96. Kathuria MK, Gupta RK. Fungal infections. In: Gupta RK, Lufkin RB, editors. MR imaging and spectroscopy of central nervous system infections. New York: Kluwer Press; 2001. p. 177–203.

97. Miszkiel KA, Hall-Craggs MA, Miller RF. The spectrum of MRI findings in CNS cryptococcosis in AIDS. Clin Radiol 1996;51(12):842–50.

98. Andreula CF, Burdi N, Carella A. CNS cryptococcosis in AIDS: spectrum of MR findings. J Comput Assist Tomogr 1993;17(3):438–41.

99. Tien RD, Chu PK, Hesselink JR, et al. Intracranial cryptococcosis in immunocompromised patients: CT and MR findings in 29 cases. AJNR Am J Neuroradiol 1991;12:283–9.

100. Saigal G, Post MJ, Lolayekar S, et al. Unusual presentation of central nervous system Cryptococcal infection in an immunocompetent patient. AJNR Am J Neuroradiol 2005;26:2522–6.

Imaging of Rickettsial, Spirochetal, and Parasitic Infections

Ayca Akgoz, MD, Srini Mukundan, MD,
Thomas C. Lee, MD*

KEYWORDS

- Rickettsial Infections • Neurosyphilis • Lyme disease • CNS Toxoplasmosis

KEY POINTS

- Rickettsial, spirochetal and parasitic central nervous system (CNS) infections, although generally quite rare, are still being encountered in endemic regions around the world.
- Toxoplasmosis and neurosyphilis may manifest as opportunistic infections in immunocompromised patients, particularly in patients infected with human immunodeficiency virus.
- CNS involvement in spirochetal infections, particularly in neurosyphilis and Lyme disease, is quite varied in clinical presentation and imaging findings.
- A high index of suspicion and knowledge of the imaging features may lead to early diagnosis of the rickettsial, spirochetal, and parasitic CNS infections.

RICKETTSIAE

The Rickettsiae are small gram-negative bacteria, which are generally obligate intracellular parasites and transmitted to humans by arthropods.[1] The exception is Coxiella burnetii, which is transmitted by inhalation and has an endospore form that is capable of surviving in an extracellular environment.[2,3] The most common rickettsial infections are Rocky Mountain spotted fever, epidemic typhus, and Q fever. Rickettsial infections except for Q fever typically present with fever, rashes, and vasculitis. Imaging findings of central nervous system (CNS) involvement in Rocky Mountain spotted fever reported to date include diffuse cerebral edema, meningeal enhancement, arterial infarction, and signal abnormality within the distribution of perivascular spaces, which are dissimilar to the documented neuroimaging findings of Q fever consisting of (meningo) encephalitis, acute cerebellitis, and transverse myelitis.[4–9] To the authors' knowledge, there are no existing reports documenting neuroimaging findings of epidemic typhus or more commonly referred to as simply typhus. It should not be confused with typhoid fever, also known as typhoid, caused by the bacterium Salmonella typhi.

Owing to the small size of the bacteria, direct microscopic visualization of Rickettsiae is difficult and requires special stains such as Giemsa or Gimenez. Hence, serologic tests such as complement fixation test, indirect immunofluorescence, latex agglutination, and enzyme immunoassay tests, are commercially available and are used in the diagnosis of Rickettsial disease. Tetracyclines and chloramphenicol are effective in treatment, whereas sulfonamides enhance the disease and are contraindicated.

Department of Radiology, Brigham & Women's Hospital, Harvard Medical School, 75 Francis Street, Boston, MA 02115, USA
* Corresponding author. Dana-Farber Cancer Institute, Brigham & Women's Hospital, Harvard Medical School, 75 Francis Street, Boston, MA 02115.
E-mail address: tclee@post.harvard.edu

Neuroimag Clin N Am 22 (2012) 633–657
http://dx.doi.org/10.1016/j.nic.2012.05.015
1052-5149/12/$ – see front matter © 2012 Elsevier Inc. All rights reserved.

Rocky Mountain Spotted Fever

The causative agent in Rocky Mountain spotted fever is Rickettsia rickettsii, which is transferred to humans by the dog or wood tick bite. As opposed to the name that implies a mountainous predisposition, approximately 25% of the cases occur in North Carolina and more than 50% of the cases were reported in the South Atlantic region of the United States.[4,10] Rickettsia rickettsii spreads via the blood stream, proliferates, and injures endothelial and vascular smooth muscle cells, thereby causing damage to the microcirculation of virtually all organs.[5] Vascular lesions are prominent in the skin explaining the pathophysiologic basis for the rash found in Rocky Mountain spotted fever.[2,5] The skin rash initially appears on the wrists, ankles, soles, and palms and later spreads to the trunk.[3] The maculopapular skin lesions, later in the disease, may become petechial and eventually purpuric and ecchymotic and can rarely lead to skin necrosis or gangrene.[5] Other clinical manifestations include fever, headache, myalgias, confusion, meningismus, ataxia, aphasia, paralysis, seizures, and coma.[10] In the brain, vasculitis forms a characteristic pathologic appearance called typhus nodules, which are essentially perivascular infiltrates of lymphocytes, polymorphonuclear leukocytes, and macrophages.[2,5] Other pathologic lesions include white matter microinfarctions and a predominantly mononuclear cell leptomeningitis. Early recognition of the CNS involvement is critical, because such involvement often causes increased mortality.[5] Rocky Mountain spotted fever is still the most frequently reported life-threatening tick-borne infection, with mortality rates ranging from 2% to 10% even under adequate antibiotic therapy.[4,11] The largest case series reported in the literature was contributed by Bonawitz and colleagues[4] and reported the associated neuroimaging findings in patients with Rocky Mountain spotted fever. Of 34 patients, 28 had computed tomography (CT) of the brain (44 studies, 10 after contrast administration), 6 had contrast-enhanced brain magnetic resonance (MR) imaging, and 4 had both CT and MR studies of the brain. Four patients demonstrated abnormalities on CT imaging, including focal arterial basal ganglia infarction, diffuse cerebral edema, and diffuse meningeal enhancement (**Fig. 1**). MR imaging was abnormal in 4 patients with findings consisting of focal basal ganglia and frontal lobe arterial infarctions, diffuse edema, diffuse meningeal enhancement, and prominent perivascular spaces in the region of the basal ganglia. In addition, one patient had thoracolumbar contrast-enhanced spine MR imaging, which depicted abnormal enhancement along the surfaces

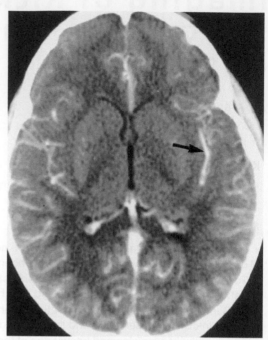

Fig. 1. Rocky Mountain spotted fever. Meningeal enhancement on CT. Axial post-contrast CT sections show enhancement of the subarachnoid space in both cerebral hemispheres, particularly at the level of the left Sylvian fissure (*arrow*). However, some of the enhancement may represent prominent vessels. At presentation, this patient was posturing and unresponsive and died during hospitalization. Autopsy showed meningitis with swollen and congested vessels in the leptomeninges and neuronal necrosis in the hippocampi. (*From* Bonawitz C, Castillo M, Mukherji SK. Comparison of CT and MR features with clinical outcome in patients with Rocky Mountain spotted fever. AJNR Am J Neuroradiol 1997;18(3):459–64; with permission.)

of the distal spinal cord as well as enhancement of the cauda equina (**Fig. 2**). Although the presence of abnormal neuroimaging is rare, its presence is associated with worse clinical prognosis. However, the neuroimaging findings are potentially reversible if appropriate treatment is initiated early in the course of the disease. Total resolution of MR imaging findings was also shown in a single case by Baganz and colleagues[5] in which there was reversal of extensive T2 signal abnormality in the distribution of the perivascular spaces without accompanying abnormal enhancement. Although nonspecific and also reported in diseases such as cryptococcosis and Lyme disease, the investigators postulated perivascular signal abnormality may reflect the underlying pathophysiology of Rocky Mountain spotted fever (**Fig. 3**).

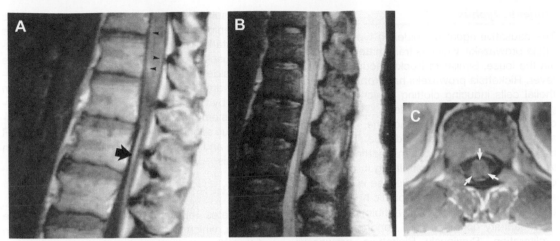

Fig. 2. Rocky Mountain spotted fever. Abnormal enhancement of the distal spinal cord, conus medullaris, and cauda equina. (A) Midsagittal T1-weighted MR image after contrast administration shows enhancement of the ventral and dorsal surface of the conus medullaris (arrowheads) and of the cauda equina (arrow). This patient presented with mental status changes, ataxia, aphasia, and bilateral lower extremity weakness. Residual paraparesis remained after treatment. (B) Corresponding T2-weighted MR image shows a questionable area of abnormally high signal intensity in the distal conus medullaris at the level of L-1. (C) Axial post-contrast T1-weighted MR image shows abnormal enhancement (arrows) on the surface of the distal thoracic spinal cord. Analysis of cerebrospinal fluid showed lymphocytosis and elevated proteins. Two years after presentation, the patient has mild residual bilateral lower extremity weakness. (From Bonawitz C, Castillo M, Mukherji SK. Comparison of CT and MR features with clinical outcome in patients with Rocky Mountain spotted fever. AJNR Am J Neuroradiol 1997;18(3):459–64; with permission.)

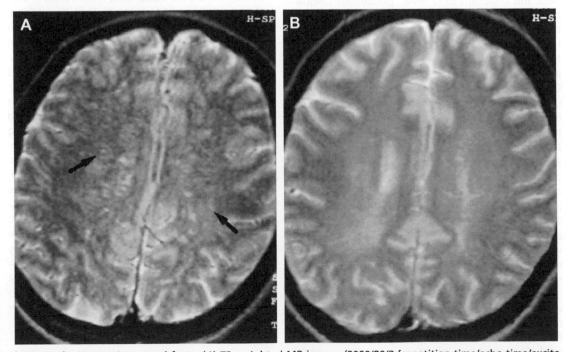

Fig. 3. Rocky Mountain spotted fever. (A) T2-weighted MR images (2000/80/2 [repetition time/echo time/excitations]) of the brain obtained at admission show numerous punctate regions of increased signal (arrows) in the distribution of perivascular (Virchow-Robin) spaces. (B) T2-weighted MR images (2000/80/2) of the brain obtained after clinical improvement show substantial resolution of the high signal, corresponding to resolution of the perivascular inflammation. (From Baganz MD, Dross PE, Reinhardt JA. Rocky Mountain spotted fever encephalitis: MR findings. AJNR Am J Neuroradiol 1995;16(Suppl 4):919–22; with permission.)

Epidemic Typhus

The causative agent of epidemic typhus is Rickettsia prowazekii, which is transmitted to humans via the louse. Similar to Rocky Mountain spotted fever, Rickettsia prowazekii has tropism to endothelial cells inducing clotting, which can lead to gangrene of the hands and feet.[3] The disease is characterized by fever, headache, and a rash sparing the palms, soles, and face. This disease is typically seen in an epidemic setting especially in overcrowded populations living in poverty and unsanitary conditions. The disease is still considered to be a major threat by public health authorities, despite the efficacy of antibiotics, because poor sanitary conditions are conducive to louse proliferation. Previously Rickettsia prowazekii, the causal agent, was thought to be confined to human beings and their body lice; however, in 1975, Rickettsia prowazekii infection in human beings was observed due to contact with the flying squirrel Glaucomys volans in the United States.[12]

Q Fever

This disease is recognized around the world and occurs mainly in people who come into contact with goats, sheep, and dairy cattle.[2] Coxiella burnetii, the organism of Q fever, possesses unique characteristics within the Rickettsiae family such as the ability to form an endospore that is resistant to heating and drying and does not need a vector to be transmitted to humans.[10] Transmission results from inhalation of dust contaminated with Coxiella burnetii from placenta, dried feces, urine, or milk or from aerosols in slaughterhouses.[2] This disease resembles influenza, nonbacterial pneumonia, endocarditis, hepatitis, and encephalopathy rather than typhus. CNS involvement is a rare manifestation documented in a few reports of (meningo) encephalitis that occurred in the late course of acute Q fever.[8] Sawaishi and colleagues[6] reported an 8-year-old child presenting with a 1-week history of moderate fever and headache and found to have acute cerebellitis on MR imaging with swelling and diffuse T2 signal abnormality of a cerebellar hemisphere. Serologic tests revealed positive titers for Q fever. The acute imaging findings resolved following treatment with only residual parenchymal volume loss of the affected cerebellar hemisphere. Sempere and colleagues[7] documented a case of Q fever encephalitis involving the temporal lobe, which created confusion at initial presentation with resemblance to herpes simplex encephalitis. In addition, there are a few reports in the literature concluding that infection with Coxiella burnetii can be associated with acute transverse myelitis as a result of direct infectious or parainfectious pathogenic mechanisms.[8,9] This central nervous manifestation of Coxiella burnetii adds to the treatable causes of acute myelitis and should therefore be considered as a differential diagnosis, especially in areas endemic for Q fever. Moreover, in a study by Garron and colleagues,[13] Coxiella burnetii was amongst the causative agents for nontuberculous spondylodiscitis in children in whom MR imaging and needle aspiration of the disc aided in diagnosis.

SPIROCHETES

Spirochetes are a phylum of gram-negative bacteria, which are distinguished by the location of their flagella that run lengthwise between the cell wall and outer membrane. These flagella cause a spiral motion that facilitates movement. Three genera whose members are human pathogens are Treponema, Borrelia, and Leptospira.[2] Syphilis and Lyme disease, which are caused by Treponema pallidum and Borrelia burgdorferi, respectively, are the most commonly encountered diseases in this pathogen group. Both diseases present in the form of well-recognizable clinical stages usually beginning with an initial skin lesion. However, CNS involvement in both diseases is quite varied in clinical presentation and imaging findings. In addition, imaging may be normal in both diseases even in the setting of known CNS involvement with evidence of positive cerebral spinal fluid (CSF) tests. Neurosyphilis may present with numerous findings including: meningeal and cranial nerve enhancement, arteritis and ischemia, mass lesions known as gummas, cortical atrophy, hydrocephalus, and mesial temporal signal abnormality mimicking herpes simplex encephalitis, mesial temporal sclerosis, and paraneoplastic limbic encephalitis. Hence, it is called "the great imitator".[14–26] Similarly, Lyme disease also acts as an imitator with various clinical and radiologic presentations. Imaging findings of CNS involvement of Lyme disease are also myriad including, meningeal and cranial nerve enhancement, white matter signal abnormality occasionally resembling multiple sclerosis, prominent Virchow-Robin spaces, enhancing masslike parenchymal lesions, arteritis, ischemia, hemorrhage, meningoradiculitis, acute transverse myelitis, and ocular myositis.[14,27–52]

Syphilis

Syphilis is a chronic venereal disease with multiple presentations. The causative spirochete, Treponema pallidum is a gram-negative corkscrew-shaped bacterium, which is too slender to be seen on Gram stain, but can be visualized by silver stains, dark-field examination, and immunofluorescence techniques.[53] Sexual contact is the usual mode of spread. However, there may be nonsexual transmission via skin contact with an infected skin ulcer. Transplacental transmission of Treponema pallidum occurs readily, and active disease during pregnancy results in congenital syphilis.

Syphilis is a chronic infection with 3 well-characterized stages. Cases of syphilis surged upward in the setting of AIDS.[14] Primary syphilis is characterized by a chancre (sore or ulcer) at the site of inoculation and painless regional lymphadenopathy. If left untreated, a secondary stage manifests during which a maculopapular rash is seen on the palms of the hand and soles of the feet with hematological dissemination of the bacteria. This rash is usually seen 2 to 8 weeks after the chancre appears, but in AIDS patients, there is much more rapid progression to secondary syphilis. About one-third of patients with secondary syphilis progress to tertiary syphilis and approximately one-third of those develop neurosyphilis. The tertiary stage usually occurs after a latent period of at least 5 years and has 3 main manifestations: cardiovascular syphilis, neurosyphilis, and syphilitic gummas. Cardiovascular disease is usually in the form of luetic aortitis which becomes apparent as aortic valve insufficiency and aneurysms of the proximal aorta. Gummas are nodular lesions likely related to the development of delayed hypersensitivity to the bacteria. These lesions may occur in various sites, most commonly in bone, skin, and the mucous membranes of the upper airway and mouth.[53]

Although neurosyphilis may appear at any stage of systemic infection, more commonly it occurs at late stages, primarily the tertiary stage.[14] CNS involvement can be asymptomatic, which accounts for about one-third of neurosyphilis cases and detected when CSF tests are abnormal with increased white cell counts, especially lymphocytes, increased protein, and decreased glucose.[53] Although symptomatic neurosyphilis may manifest in several ways, in general, 2 major clinical subtypes are recognized: (1) meningovascular disease and (2) parenchymal disease.[14]

Meningeal neurosyphilis usually appears within the first 2 years of infection and may result in headache, meningeal signs, and cranial nerve palsies, most frequently involving cranial nerves VII and VIII (**Fig. 4**). Pathologically, there is widespread thickening of the meninges, meningeal lymphocytic infiltrates, and perivascular lymphocytic infiltrates. Meningeal enhancement may be present and is usually better seen on MR imaging than CT.[14] Hydrocephalus may also occur. Involvement of cranial nerves VII and VIII in syphilitic basilar

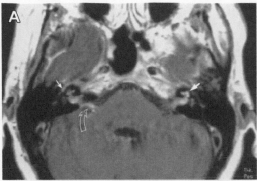

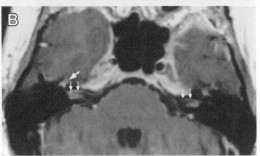

Fig. 4. Neurosyphilis. (*A*) Axial T1-weighted MR image (450/15/4), obtained after the administration of contrast medium, shows enhancement within the cisternal segment of the vestibulocochlear nerve complex on the right (*curved open arrow*), within both internal auditory canals, within the left cochlea (*curved solid arrow*), and within the tympanic portion of the right facial nerve (*small arrow*). The enhancement within the internal auditory canals involves both the nerves within the CSF and the meninges lining the canal. Enhancement is also seen within the middle turn of the right cochlea. (*B*) Axial T1-weighted MR image (450/15/4), obtained after the administration of contrast medium from a position that is slightly superior to that of **Fig. 4** (*A*), shows enhancement of the labyrinthine and geniculate portions of the right facial nerve (*large arrow*) and enhancement of the meninges lining both internal auditory canals (*small arrows*). Enhancement of the intracanalicular segments of the seventh and eighth cranial nerve complex is appreciated bilaterally. (*From* Smith MM, Anderson JC. Neurosyphilis as a cause of facial and vestibulocochlear nerve dysfunction: MR imaging features. AJNR Am J Neuroradiol 2000;21(9):1673–5; with permission.)

meningitis presents with facial paralysis, sensorineural hearing loss, and vertigo and radiologically, with enhancement of the seventh and eighth cranial nerves and cochlea as well as the meninges lining the internal auditory canals.[15] Involvement of the optic, oculomotor, and abducens nerves has also been reported (**Fig. 5**).[16,54]

Syphilitic gummas are another manifestation of meningovascular neurosyphilis and occur as the

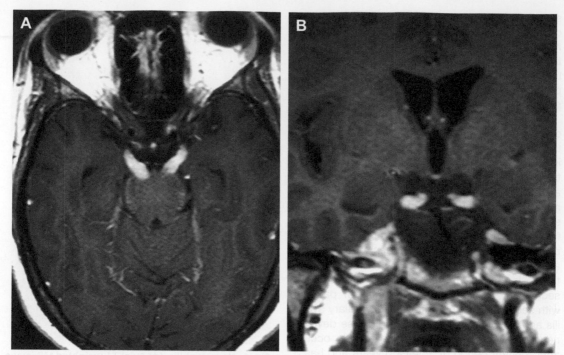

Fig. 5. Neurosyphilis. Contrast-enhanced T1-weighted (*A*) axial and coronal MR images (*B*) through the brainstem and proximal oculomotor nerves demonstrate bilateral thickening and contrast enhancement. (*From* Corr P, Bhigjee A, Lockhat F. Oculomotor nerve root enhancement in meningovascular syphilis. Clin Radiol 2004;59(3): 294–6; with permission.)

result of intense localized leptomeningeal inflammatory reaction early in the meningeal phase of neurosyphilis.[14] Pathologically, gummas appear as circumscribed masses of granulation tissue surrounded by mononuclear epithelial and fibroblastic cells with occasional giant cells and perivasculitis. They originate from the meningeal connective tissue and blood vessels extending to the adjacent parenchyma and leading to meningeal enhancement.[14] On imaging, gummas are seen as circumscribed solitary or multiple mass lesions with nodular or ring enhancement usually located overlying the cerebral convexities. However, they can be found anywhere in brain parenchyma that is adherent to dura. There may be an associated dural tail (**Fig. 6**).[55] Whereas cutaneous, mucosal, and skeletal gummatous lesions are not uncommon, neurosyphilitic gummas are rare.[56] The imaging findings of cerebral gumma may mimic those of other intracranial mass lesions, especially brain neoplasms, and definitive diagnosis has always been difficult (**Fig. 7**).[17–19] Moreover, gummas may demonstrate intense ^{18}F-2-fluoro-2-deoxy-D-glucose (FDG) avidity on positron emission tomography (PET)

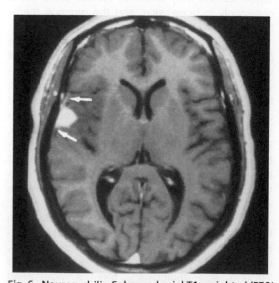

Fig. 6. Neurosyphilis. Enhanced axial T1-weighted (576/14/2) image shows intense enhancement of a 1.3-cm mass in the region of the right sylvian fissure, with enhancement of the adjacent dura (*arrows*). This is surgically proved syphilitic gumma. (*From* Bourekas EC, et al. The dural tail sign revisited. AJNR Am J Neuroradiol 1995;16(7):1514–6; with permission.)

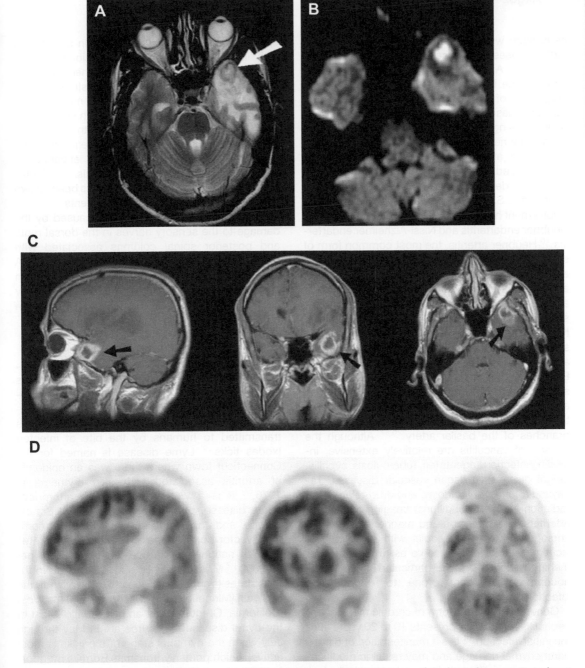

Fig. 7. Neurosyphilis. Neurosyphilitic gumma. (*A*) An axial T2-weighted MR image of the brain (Siemens Symphony 1.5T, Siemens Medical Systems, Erlangen, Germany) demonstrated edema in the left temporal lobe surrounding the lesion, which has a hypointense rim (*arrow*). (*B*) Diffusion-weighted axial MR image revealed restricted diffusion centrally within the lesion. The overall MR imaging appearances are suggestive of an abscess or a high-grade primary brain tumor such as glioblastoma multiforme with tumor necrosis. (*C*) The T1-weighted gadolinium-enhanced MR imaging in the sagittal (*left*), coronal (*middle*), and axial (*right*) planes showed an irregular ovoid lesion with a thick enhancing rim (*arrows*) and a hypointense center in the left temporal lobe associated with a significant midline shift and edema. There was also effacement of the left frontal horn of the lateral ventricle. (*D*) An ^{18}F-FDG PET of the brain using a Philips Allegro PET camera (Philips Medical systems, Milpitas, CA, USA) demonstrated an intensely FDG avid lesion at a metabolic activity similar to contralateral cortex, with a small central photon-deficient area, corresponding to the abnormality seen on MR imaging. There was also surrounding diffuse, mild-to-moderately reduced FDG uptake in the remainder of the left temporal lobe in keeping with associated edema. The overall appearances are suspicious for high-grade malignancy. ([D] *From* Lin M, Darwish BS, Chu J. Neurosyphilitic gumma on F18-2-fluoro-2-deoxy-D-glucose (FDG) positron emission tomography: an old disease investigated with a new technology. J Clin Neurosci 2009;16(3):410–2; with permission.)

as is seen with hypermetabolic tumors and this further poses challenges to diagnostic imaging (**Fig. 7**D).[56] A high index of suspicion and knowledge of the imaging features may lead to early diagnosis of this lesion, which is important because these lesions may regress or even disappear following penicillin treatment.[17]

Vascular neurosyphilis usually appears around 5 to 10 years after primary infection and is typically characterized by headache, vertigo, and focal neurologic deficit related to a vascular event, with abnormal CSF findings.[14] Two types of vascular involvement have been described in neurosyphilis: Heubner endarteritis and Nissl-Alzheimer endarteritis.[10] Heubner arteritis, the most common form of syphilitic arteritis, affects large- and medium-sized arteries and is characterized by fibroblastic proliferation of the intima, thinning of the media, and adventitial fibrous and inflammatory changes, resulting in an irregular luminal narrowing and ectasia. Nissl-Alzheimer type of arteritis typically affects small vessels and manifests as thickening of the adventitia to a greater degree than the endothelium. Both types of arteritis may lead to vascular occlusion.[14] The most common clinical presentation is an ischemic syndrome in a young adult, involving the middle cerebral artery or less commonly the branches of the basilar artery.[20,57] Although the causes of vasculitis are relatively extensive, including infectious agents (eg, tuberculosis, syphilis, fungal disease), collagen vascular diseases, Takayasu arteritis, sarcoidosis, and drug-related and radiation-induced conditions, imaging findings of arteritis on MR imaging and magnetic resonance angiography in young adults with symptoms of ischemic stroke should serve as an indicator for meningovascular syphilis, particularly in an immunocompromised host prone to opportunistic infection.[16,20]

General paresis is a form of chronic meningoencephalitis and usually presents 10 to 20 years after the initial infection.[14] It is a manifestation of diffuse parenchymal damage and may result in modifications of personality and affect, delusions, hallucinations, memory loss, loss of judgment and insight associated with speech disturbances, hyperactive reflexes, and the Argyll Robertson pupil. Argyll Robertson pupil, which is seen in both tabes dorsalis and general paresis, is a small irregular pupil that accommodates but does not react to light.[14] Neuropathologically, cortical atrophy and ependymitis are observed on gross examination associated with degenerative neuronal changes with gliosis and scattered microglia. Cortical atrophy is seen on MR imaging. There is often an associated hydrocephalus with damage to the ependymal lining and proliferation of subependymal glia called granular

ependymitis.[53] The hydrocephalus in association with impaired memory may occasionally mimic normal pressure hydrocephalus.[21] There are a few recent reports in the literature demonstrating unilateral or bilateral anterior temporal and mesiotemporal signal abnormality in patients with serologic or CSF evidence of neurosyphilis with or without accompanying abnormal enhancement mimicking mesial temporal sclerosis, herpes encephalitis, and paraneoplastic limbic encephalitis.[21–26] Partial clinical or radiologic improvement has been shown with penicillin treatment in some patients.

Tabes dorsalis is a myelopathy caused by the damage to the sensory nerves in the dorsal roots and posterior spinal columns associated with atrophy, degeneration, and demyelination.[14,53] A latent period of 15 to 20 years is usually seen with clinical tabes dorsalis, characterized classically by lightning pains, dysuria, ataxia, Argyll Robertson pupil, areflexia, and loss of proprioception.[16]

Lyme Disease

Lyme borreliosis is a multisystemic infectious disease caused by the spirochete Borrelia burgdorferi sensu stricto in the United States and Borrelia garinii and Borrelia afzelii in Europe, which is transmitted to humans by the bite of infected Ixodes ticks.[27] Lyme disease is named for the Connecticut town where there was an epidemic of arthritis associated with skin erythema in 1976.[53] It is a worldwide common arthropod-borne disease, particularly in the United States, Europe, and Japan and currently the most common vector-borne disease in the United States with a national incidence of 9.7 cases per 100,000.[27] Most cases occur in the coastal Northeast states (from Massachusetts to Maryland), the Midwest (Minnesota and Wisconsin), and the West (California, Oregon, Utah, and Nevada).[28] Most of the Lyme disease exposures are in May through July when the nymphal stage of the ticks is most active, which primarily transmits Borrelia burgdorferi to human beings.[2]

Similar to other spirochetal diseases such as syphilis, Lyme disease is clinically encountered in 3 main stages classified as early localized disease, early disseminated disease, and persisting late disease.[58] During the initial stage, spirochetes multiply in the dermis at the site of the tick bite and later spread centrifugally, which may result in an area of enlarging erythema, often associated with central clearing that resembles a bull's eye appearance.[53,58] This characteristic skin lesion is called erythema chronicum migrans and may be accompanied by flu-like symptoms and lymphadenopathy and usually disappears in 4 to

12 weeks. In the second stage, the early disseminated stage, spirochetes spread throughout the body via the blood stream, which may cause diverse clinical presentations, including arthralgia, arthritis, lymphocytic meningitis, cranial neuropathy most commonly Bell palsy, painful radiculopathy; and cardiac disease with conduction defects and myopericarditis.[2] If left untreated, a late disseminated stage may be seen generally 2 or 3 years after the initial bite, with a chronic arthritis sometimes with severe damage to large joints and a polyneuropathy and encephalitis that may vary from mild to debilitating.

The diagnosis of Lyme disease is essentially clinical based on a history of tick exposure, epidemiology, and clinical signs and symptoms at different stages of the disease, usually with use of serologic tests supporting the clinical diagnosis. Current standards for the serologic diagnosis of Lyme disease include a sensitive enzyme immunoassay (EIA), followed by confirmation of a positive or equivocal initial test by Western blot or immunoblot as Borrelia burgdorferi has extremely complex antigenic composition that may vary by host and stage of the infection.[27]

CNS symptoms are seen in about 15% to 20% of patients with the characteristic initial skin lesion.[14] However, CNS disease may occur without a preceding erythema chronicum migrans or may manifest as an isolated neurologic syndrome, which may pose a diagnostic challenge for practicing neurologists.[14] The genetic diversity and worldwide differential distribution of spirochete species affect the seasonal incidence and disease manifestations as well as the likelihood of a patient developing Lyme neuroborreliosis (LNB).[27,29] For instance, LNB is much more frequently seen in Europe in comparison to North America, which could be linked to probable greater neurotropism of Borrelia garinii, which has not been isolated in North America.[58] In addition, 86% of European LNB present as a painful radiculitis, which was first reported by Garin and Bujadoux in 1922 and is also known as Bannwarth syndrome.[30,59] The pain associated with Bannwarth syndrome is mostly described as a chronic pain lasting weeks or months, which can occasionally be severe and may increase in intensity at night. Moreover, lack of a recognizable erythema migrans is more frequently seen in Europe, which makes the diagnosis of LNB much more difficult.[27]

Despite increased knowledge and experience in diagnosis and treatment of LNB in common daily clinical neurologic practice, the underlying neuropathophysiology is still unclear. Several proposed mechanisms for CNS injury include direct cytotoxicity, neurotoxic mediators secreted by leukocytes and glial cells (indirect cytotoxicity), or triggered autoimmune reactions via molecular mimicry.[61] It is also a matter of debate how spirochetes reach the CNS and pass the blood-brain barrier. Given cultivation of Borrelia from plasma samples in approximately 35% to 45% of patients with early Lyme disease in the United States, hematogeneous dissemination of the spirochetes is considered frequent in patients with Lyme disease in the United States.[61] In contrast, it is hypothesized that migration of the spirochetes along the peripheral nerves is an alternative route to the CNS, particularly in European LNB. The initial and maximal radicular involvement in patients with meningoradiculitis (Bannwarth syndrome) is often linked to the location of the previous tick bite or the skin lesion.[61] Studies involving the nervous system in rhesus macaques localized LNB-associated inflammation within dorsal root ganglia, nerve roots, and leptomeninges with predominance of T-lymphocytes and plasma cells.[60] In addition, visualization of the spirochetes by immunohistochemistry in the leptomeninges, nerve roots, and dorsal root ganglia, but not in the CNS parenchyma, is consistent with the commonly encountered pattern of clinical involvement in infected human beings, with predominance of meningitis, radiculitis, and cranial nerve involvement, and, rarely, parenchymal brain and spinal cord involvement. On the other hand, there are a few case reports in the literature with presentation of findings from biopsy of tumefactive parenchymal lesions in patients with LNB with presence of a small number of spirochetes accompanied by microgliosis in 1 patient and presence of Borrelia burgdorferi DNA in tissue samples in 2 patients, which may indicate that direct invasion of Borrelia burgdorferi may be the pathogenetic mechanism for focal encephalitis in LNB.[31,62] Oksi and colleagues[31] detected perivascular or vasculitis lymphocytic inflammation in all 3 biopsy specimens suggestive of probable role of vasculitis in the pathogenesis of Lyme neuroborreliosis.

MR imaging findings of the brain in Lyme disease are often within normal limits, even in patients with known Lyme disease who have neurologic manifestations.[14,28] There are several studies in the literature that have evaluated MR neuroimaging findings in patients with Lyme disease and identified multiple bilateral periventricular and/or subcortical foci of T2 prolongation in patients with neurologic symptoms.[32,63–67] Some of the lesions are said to resemble multiple sclerosis plaques with involvement of the callososeptal interface (**Fig. 8**).[31,33] Although similar mechanisms of molecular mimicry and antigen-specific T-cell response have been identified in both multiple sclerosis and chronic LNB, T-cell

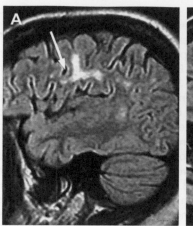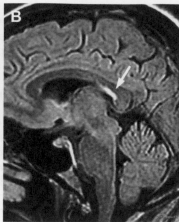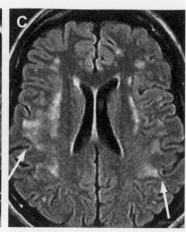

Fig. 8. Lyme disease. A 50-year-old woman with a history of tick bite and erythema migrans rash treated with doxycycline, who had recurrent erythema migrans rash with headache, fever, nausea, and nuchal rigidity. The patient had CSF pleocytosis with positive Lyme serum EIA and immunoglobulin M Western blot and negative Lyme antibodies in the CSF. Gradual symptomatic improvement occurred after intravenous ceftriaxone therapy. There has been stable MR imaging for 5 years. Sagittal (A and B) and axial (C) fluid-attenuated inversion recovery images show arcuate and confluent subcortical white-matter involvement and callososeptal interface involvement remarkably similar to that in multiple sclerosis, but without involvement of the periventricular white matter (arrows). (From Hildenbrand P, et al. Lyme neuroborreliosis: manifestations of a rapidly emerging zoonosis. AJNR Am J Neuroradiol 2009;30(6):1079–87; with permission.)

lines demonstrate only weak cross reactivity between myelin basic protein and Borrelia burgdorferi.[27] I addition, studies using diffusion tensor and magnetization transfer imaging demonstrated that contrary to what happens in multiple sclerosis, occult brain tissue damage and cervical cord pathology are not frequent findings in patients with neuroborreliosis.[67] Basal ganglia and the brainstem may also be involved.[14,32,34] Accompanying multifocal parenchymal enhancement has also been described.[35] Rare cases of parenchymal brain involvement have been reported, often either misdiagnosed initially as brain tumors or thought to represent encephalitis.[31,36,37] Recently, Agarwal and Sze[28] have retrospectively evaluated brain MR imaging findings of 66 patients who were proved to have LNB on the basis of clinical criteria, serologic results, and response to treatment. Of the 66 patients, 11 showed abnormal findings on MR imaging. Three patients showed nerve-root or meningeal enhancement, 7 patients demonstrated foci of T2-signal abnormality in the cerebral white matter without enhancement, and 1 patient had an enhancing lesion with edema. Of the 7 patients with white matter lesions, the blinded readings indicated that 3 of them had nonspecific lesions that, given the ages of the patients (ranging from 26 to 57 years), were probably small-vessel white matter disease. The remaining 4 patients had abnormalities that were considered unusual for their ages. The investigators concluded that

although Lyme disease has been generally reported to manifest as foci of T2 prolongation in the cerebral white matter, nerve root or meningeal enhancement is also frequently seen and may be equally common. In the literature, third, fifth, and seventh cranial nerve enhancements have all been documented as well as primary leptomeningeal enhancement (see Fig. 8).[27,38–42,68] Predominantly, seventh cranial nerve involvement is observed with a "tuft" of enhancement at the fundus of the internal auditory canal and enhancement of the labyrinthine and tympanic segments more than generalized fundal tuft-to-mastoid involvement (Fig. 9).[27] This enhancement correlates well with the fact that Lyme disease may be responsible for 25% of new-onset Bell palsy in endemic areas despite it being an infrequent cause of isolated facial palsy in patients without constitutional symptoms or additional neurologic findings.[27,69] Cranial neuropathies as well as motor or sensory radiculoneuritis have their highest incidence in children and adolescents with approximately 3% to 5% occurrence of facial nerve palsy during the course of pediatric Lyme neuroborreliosis.[27] Brain MR imaging findings in pediatric LNB include the presence of prominent Virchow-Robin spaces, T2 bright white matter lesions, pial and cranial nerve enhancement, and treatment-responsive lesion enhancement.

Another rare manifestation of LNB is vasculitis, which may be associated with ischemic stroke,

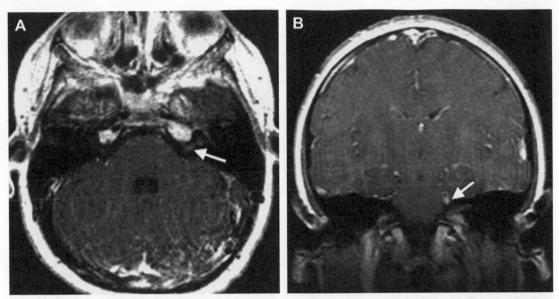

Fig. 9. Lyme disease. Manifestation of palsy of left seventh cranial nerve in a 10-year-old male patient with recent history of camping. (*A*) Transverse T1-weighted post-contrast MR image shows enhancement of left seventh cranial nerve (*arrow*). (*B*) Coronal T1-weighted post-contrast MR image demonstrates left trigeminal nerve enhancement (*arrow*). (*From* Agarwal R, Sze G. Neuro-lyme disease: MR imaging findings. Radiology 2009;253(1):167–73; with permission.)

subarachnoid hemorrhage, and intracerebral hemorrhage.[31,43–48,70]

Although most patients with LNB recover fully when treated with antibiotics, some patients who are treated months after the initial infection may still experience ongoing problems with fatigue, cognition, and pain despite receipt of a standard antibiotic treatment. These patients have been described as having chronic Lyme disease or post-treatment Lyme disease syndrome, which remains an ongoing focus of controversy.[27,71] Continuing symptoms have been attributed to persistent infection, pathogen-induced autoimmunity, or unrelated processes, such as depression, somatization, fibromyalgia, or chronic fatigue syndrome. Aalto and colleagues[72] conducted a study aiming to evaluate brain MR imaging findings of chronic neuroborreliosis with inclusion of age-matched healthy controls for comparison. White matter and basal ganglia lesions were observed in 12 of 16 patients; the findings, although, were nonspecific when compared with matched controls and did not correlate with disease duration. However, the investigators have also concluded that subependymal lesions may constitute a potential finding in chronic neuroborreliosis. Morgen and colleagues[73] analyzed the distribution of cerebral lesions in a cohort of 27 patients with post-treatment Lyme disease syndrome with further evaluation in a subgroup of 8 patients using whole-brain magnetization transfer imaging. They have found that in a portion of patients with post-treatment Lyme disease syndrome, white-matter lesions tend to occur in subcortical arteriolar watershed areas, although still nonspecific. Magnetization transfer ratio analysis did not provide evidence for structural abnormalities of the brain parenchyma in patients with nonfocal disease. Despite the lack of definitive imaging findings that may help identification of patients with chronic neuroborreliosis, a PET study conducted by Fallon and colleagues[71] has demonstrated objectively quantifiable topographic abnormalities in functional brain activity in patients with persistent Lyme encephalopathy with regional cerebral blood flow and regional cerebral metabolic rate reductions observed in all measurement conditions.

Rarely, ocular involvement is also seen during the course of Lyme disease at any clinical stage with conjunctivitis and episcleritis commonly seen during the early stage; optic neuritis and uveitis observed during the second stage; and keratitis, chronic intraocular inflammation, and orbital myositis seen in the third stage of Lyme disease (**Fig. 10**).[27] Although direct infection or a delayed immunologic response may be considered as the underlying mechanism, a hematogenous dissemination followed by an immunologically mediated reaction seems to be the most likely explanation for the muscle inflammation in orbital myositis.[74]

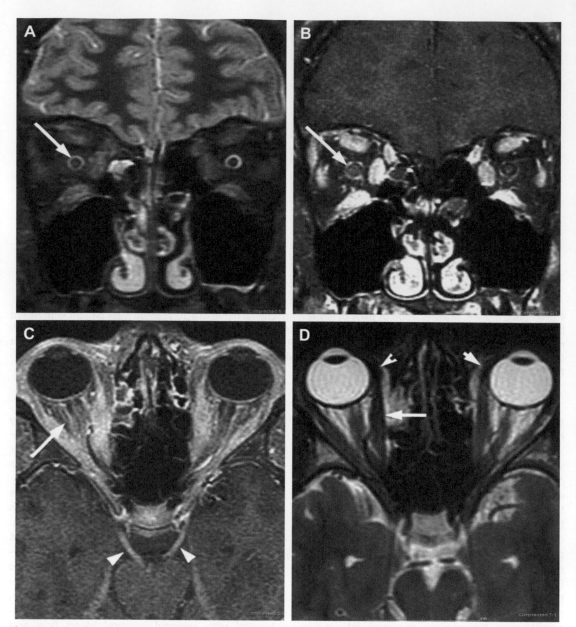

Fig. 10. Lyme disease. A 17-year-old boy with right papilledema and orbital pain and rule out pseudotumor. The patient had positive serum EIA and Western blot (IgM and IgG) and CSF Lyme IgM and IgG antibodies. Lyme PCR in the CSF was negative. Complete resolution of symptoms occurred after intravenous ceftriaxone therapy. Right optic nerve edema (*arrow*) on fat-saturated T2-weighted fast spin-echo images (*A*) and right-greater-than-left optic nerve enhancement (*arrow*) on coronal fat-saturated contrast-enhanced T1-weighted images (*B*). Bilateral third cranial nerve enhancement (*arrowheads*) and bilateral retrobulbar compartment congestion (*arrow*) (*C*). Note the generalized extraocular muscle enlargement and enhancement (*arrow*), including the insertions (*arrowheads*) (*D*). Additional imaging findings included enhancement of right fifth cranial nerve, optic chiasm, and intracanalicular right seventh nerve, all of which were occult to neurologic examination. (*From* Hildenbrand P, et al. Lyme neuroborreliosis: manifestations of a rapidly emerging zoonosis. AJNR Am J Neuroradiol 2009;30(6):1079–87; with permission.)

Lyme disease may closely mimic orbital pseudotumor. In the appropriate clinical presentation and lacking evidence of other disease conditions, Lyme disease should be considered in the differential diagnosis of ocular lesions, as initiation of antibiotic treatment is almost always followed by resolution of the clinical symptoms and radiologic findings.[74,75]

Although lymphocytic meningoradiculitis is the most common clinical manifestation of infection of the CNS in Europe, MR imaging findings of spinal cord involvement have only rarely been demonstrated. Demaerel and colleagues[30] has described diffuse intense enhancement along the thickened nerve roots of the cauda equina in a 10-year-old patient with lymphocytic meningoradiculitis (Bannwarth syndrome) (**Fig. 11**). Later, Pfefferkorn and colleagues[76] demonstrated similar findings in a 50-year-old patient with a post-treatment MR imaging study showing complete resolution of the findings. In addition, Hattingen and colleagues[77] reported cervical MR imaging findings of 2 children with bilateral intense enhancement along cervical nerve roots as a manifestation of Borrelia-associated radiculitis (**Fig. 12**). Mantienne and colleagues[49] described intense leptomeningeal enhancement along the surface of the distal thoracic spinal cord and conus medullaris without accompanying typical radiculitis in a patient with Lyme disease, with

improvement of these findings on follow-up study. Also, a few case reports of transverse myelitis associated with Lyme disease are present in the literature predominantly involving the cervical spinal cord with diffuse signal abnormality associated with enhancement.[50–52] Tullman and colleagues[78] described a case with cervical myelitis accompanied by bilateral cervical radiculitis. Hattingen and colleagues[77] noted lack of a close correlation between neurologic symptoms and imaging findings.[77]

Relapsing Fever

Relapsing fever in epidemic form is caused by Borrelia recurrentis, which is transmitted to humans by the human body louse and does not occur in the United States.[2] Endemic relapsing fever is caused by Borrelia transmitted by ticks of the genus Ornithodoros. After a short incubation period of 3 to 10 days, disease presents with sudden chills and an abrupt fever. The fever may persist for 3 to

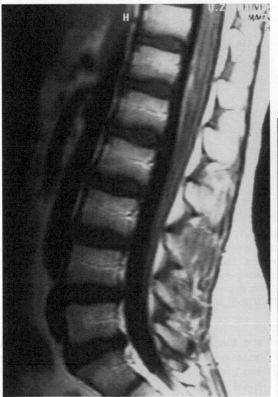
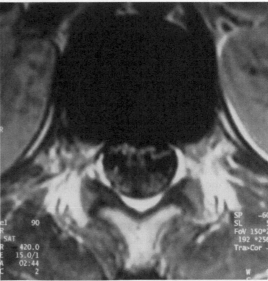

Fig. 11. Lyme disease. A 10-year-old boy presented with a 3-week history of right-sided low back pain radiating to the leg. There were no neurologic signs or fever at first presentation. There was progressive improvement of the symptoms. However, 2 months after his first presentation, the child was admitted with neurologic signs: weakness in the right leg with absent patellar and Achilles reflexes. Heel walking was limited whereas toe walking was normal. Lumbar spine MR imaging revealed enhancement of thickened nerve roots of the cauda equina on contrast-enhanced T1-weighted sagittal and axial images. (*From* Demaerel P, et al. Meningoradiculitis due to borreliosis presenting as low back pain only. Neuroradiology 1998;40(2):126–7; with permission.)

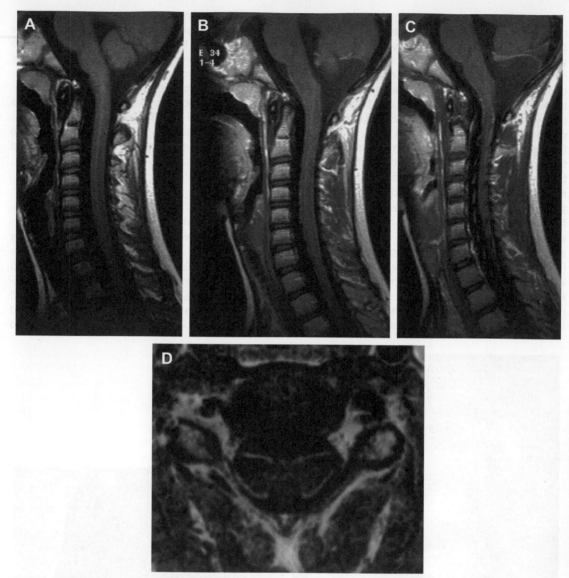

Fig. 12. Lyme disease. (*A–D*) Sagittal T1-weighted images (TR/TE = 870/18) before (*A*) and after (*B*) intravenous administration of 0.1 mmol/kg gadopentetate dimeglumine diethylene triamine pentaacetic acid in the midline of the cervical spinal cord revealing slight pial enhancement. Contrast-enhanced paramedian sagittal (*C*) and axial (*D*) T1-weighted images (TR/TE 513/12) demonstrate strong enhancement of the cervical and upper thoracic nerve roots. *Abbreviations:* TE, echo time; TR, repetition time. (*From* Hattingen E, et al. MR imaging in neuroborreliosis of the cervical spinal cord. Eur Radiol 2004;14(11):2072–5; with permission.)

5 days and then declines, followed by an afebrile period lasting approximately 4 to 10 days. Then, the cycle begins by a second attack of chills, fever, intense headache, and malaise repeating approximately 3 to ten times, generally of diminishing severity. During the febrile stages, organisms are present in the blood; however, while during the afebrile periods, they are absent. Fatal cases show spirochetes in great numbers in the spleen and liver, necrotic foci in other parenchymatous organs, and hemorrhagic lesions in the kidneys

and the gastrointestinal tract. Spirochetes have occasionally been demonstrated in the spinal fluid and brain of persons who have had meningitis.[2] There is no known corresponding neuroimaging finding documented in the literature.

Leptospirosis

The pathogenic species is Leptospira interrogans with a worldwide distribution. The leptospiroses are essentially animal infections; human infection is only accidental, following contact with water or other materials contaminated with the excreta of animal hosts, including rats, mice, wild rodents, dogs, swine, and cattle.[2] Leptospirae remain viable in stagnant water for several weeks; drinking, swimming, bathing, or food contamination may lead to human infection. Humans usually acquire infection from ingestion of water or food contaminated with leptospirae. More rarely, the organisms may enter through mucous membranes or breaks in the skin.[10] After an incubation period of 1 to 2 weeks, there is a variable febrile onset during which spirochetes are present in the bloodstream. Then, parenchymatous organs, particularly liver and kidneys, are involved with hemorrhage and tissue necrosis resulting in dysfunction of those organs (jaundice, hemorrhage, nitrogen retention). After initial improvement, the second phase develops when the immunoglobulin M (IgM) antibody titer rises. It manifests itself often as "aseptic meningitis" with intense headache, stiff neck, and pleocytosis of the cerebrospinal fluid. Nephritis and hepatitis may also recur, and there may be skin, muscle, and eye lesions. The degree and distribution of organ involvement vary in the different diseases produced by different leptospirae in various parts of the world. Many infections are mild or subclinical.

A few case reports are present in the literature describing rare occurrences of acute disseminated encephalomyelitis following leptospirosis.[79,80] Maldonado and colleagues[81] reported a patient who presented with bilateral Bell palsy on day 15 during the course of leptospirosis that he developed while returning from a 5-month trip to China. Given the delay of onset of facial palsy, investigators have suggested vasculitis rather than a direct neurotoxic effect as underlying mechanism. In addition, Habek and Brinar[82] documented an inhomogeneously enhancing pontomedullary brainstem lesion in a patient with central sleep apnea and ataxia who received diagnosis of neuroleptospirosis after 2 years from the initial disease presentation, and the brainstem lesion remained stable throughout those years under corticosteroid treatment.

EUKARYOTIC PARASITES
Amebiasis

Amoeba is a genus of protozoa (from the Greek words "proton" meaning first and "zoa" meaning animals). Protozoans are single-celled nonfungal eukaryotes, eukaryotes being distinguished from prokaryotes (Archaea and bacteria) by the presence of a nucleus.

CNS amebiasis is a rare condition that can be caused by several free living amoebic organisms including Naegleria fowleri and Acanthamoeba species.[14] Naegleria and Acanthamoeba organisms are responsible for causing primary amoebic meningoencephalitis and granulomatous amoebic meningoencephalitis (Fig. 13), respectively, with a distinctive epidemiology, pattern of presentation, clinical course, pathology, and imaging findings.[83] In contradistinction is Entamoeba histolytica, a relatively common intestinal parasite endemic to the Southern United States, South

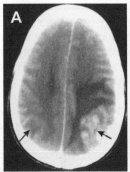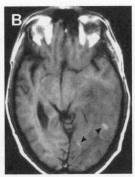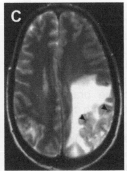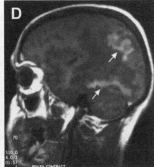

Fig. 13. Granulomatous amoebic meningoencephalitis. A 38-year-old man with deteriorating vision and persistent vomiting for a week (granulomatous amoebic encephalitis). (*A*) Contrast-enhanced CT scan of the brain shows an enhancing cortical-based lesion in the left parietal lobe with extensive perilesional edema. Another smaller hypoattenuated lesion is seen on the opposite side (*arrows*). (*B*) T1-weighted MR image shows hemorrhagic foci (*arrowheads*) in the left parietooccipital lesion with ill-defined gray-white matter distinction. (*C*) T2-weighted MR image shows heterogeneous signal intensity in the swollen cortex (*arrowheads*) with extensive white matter edema. The right-sided lesion also shows mild edema and cortical signal intensity changes. (*D*) Contrast-enhanced T1-weighted sagittal image shows gyriform enhancement of the affected cortex with nonenhancing edematous white matter. Similar enhancement is also seen in the undersurface of the occipital lobe (*arrows*). (*From* Singh P, et al. Amoebic meningoencephalitis: spectrum of imaging findings. AJNR Am J Neuroradiol 2006;27(6):1217–21; with permission.)

America, Latin America, Southeast Asia, and Africa, which is transmitted to humans via fecal-oral contamination and can rarely present with CNS involvement.[14,84] The organism is thought to reach the CNS via the blood stream through the hepatic, pulmonary, or vertebral veins.[10] Isolated CNS involvement is rare. Many patients with CNS disease may also have liver abscesses and/or concomitant gastrointestinal and pulmonary symptoms that may provide a clue for the diagnosis. Secondary cerebral amebiasis lesions could be single or multiple with central necrosis and often accompanied by hemorrhage.[14] Cortical and deep gray matter is frequently involved, particularly the frontal lobes and basal ganglia. Focal or generalized meningitis can also be observed.[14] Imaging findings described in a few case reports correlate well with pathologic findings with single or multiple ring-enhancing lesions demonstrated on CT and/or MR images. Although prognosis is poor, early treatment with metronidazole and if necessary prompt surgical intervention may improve the outcome.[14,84]

Naegleria fowleri is the causative agent for primary amoebic meningoencephalitis, which is a rapid onset fulminant infection of the brain, and meninges presenting with severe headache, fever, nausea, vomiting, ataxia, diplopia, photophobia, stiff neck with rapid progression to stupor and coma, and eventually death in several days in most cases.[83,85,86] Affected population is children and young adults without immunologic compromise.[83] The organism is found anywhere; however, the most frequent method of disease exposure for humans is by swimming in stagnant pools of warm freshwater, typically in summer months.[86] The organism gains access into the CNS via penetration of the olfactory neuroepithelium and then disseminates through the subarachnoid space and into the adjacent cerebral cortex at the base of the brain.[86] Corresponding pathologic changes include extensive damage to the brain parenchyma, ependyma, and meninges with congestion of the meningeal vessels, edematous cortex with herniation of uncus and cerebellum.[83] Microscopically, there is a purulent leptomeningeal exudate with hemorrhage and necrosis throughout the cerebral hemispheres, brain stem, cerebellum, and upper spinal cord. Imaging findings are rarely described and essentially nonspecific. CT and MR imaging findings may be normal during early disease with later development of brain edema (Fig. 14), hydrocephalus, and basilar meningeal enhancement.[83,86] Singh and colleagues[83] additionally documented basal ganglia infarction, which they linked to possible obliteration of the perforating vessels by the extensive exudates (Fig. 15).

The Acanthamoeba and Leptomyxa genera including Balamuthia mandrillaris can cause granulomatous amoebic encephalitis, which is a subacute to chronic infection and predominantly known to occur in patients who are debilitated or immunocompromised by AIDS, chemotherapy, or steroid therapy.[83,85] Unlike Naegleria fowleri, these amoebae secondarily infect the CNS, possibly from the lower respiratory tract, genitourinary tract, or skin.[86] Symptoms frequently resemble those of single or multiple space-occupying CNS lesions. Pathologically, infection is characterized by multifocal areas of hemorrhagic necrosis, edema, and abscess formation with predilection to the posterior fossa structures, the thalamus, and the brainstem with frequent involvement of the cerebral hemispheres. Microscopically, as the name implies, lesions demonstrate chronic granulomatous-type reaction with focal necrosis and hemorrhage. There may be severe necrotizing angiitis.[86] According to the published case reports to date, CT and MR imaging findings in granulomatous amoebic encephalomyelitis are either in the form of a multifocal pattern with discrete focal lesions in the corticomedullary junction, deep gray matter, or brainstem or as a larger solitary masslike lesion or a combination of the 2 findings.[83,85,87–91] Singh and colleagues[83] reported that a masslike lesion, which they called a pseudotumoral pattern, often demonstrates a linear and superficial gyriform pattern of enhancement, which could be a useful indicator of the diagnosis.

Schistosomiasis

Schistosomiasis, also known as bilharziasis, is a chronic human trematode infection affecting at least 200 million people worldwide. This infection is endemic to Africa, South America, Middle East, and most parts of Asia.[92] The disease typically involves urogenital, intestinal, and hepatolienal organs and may lead to severe liver disease with fibrosis and portal hypertension as well as bladder, liver, and rectal carcinoma.[93] Schistosoma haematobium, Schistosoma mansoni, and Schistosoma japonicum are the 3 main subspecies affecting humans. Schistosoma species have a complex life cycle beginning with the release of cercariae into streams or lakes by freshwater snails (the intermediate hosts), which then penetrate the human skin and migrate to the lungs and liver, where they mature to form mating pairs of male and female adult worms in the mesenteric veins.[94] Ectopic migration of the worms and oviposition can occur, resulting in a variety of lesions outside the gastrointestinal

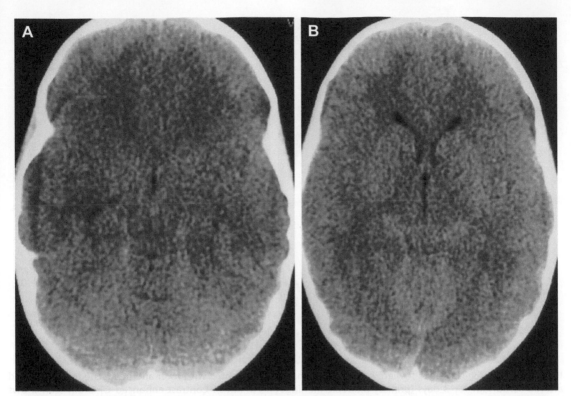

Fig. 14. Amebiasis_ Naegleria fowleri. (*A*) Noncontrast CT at the level of the temporal horns showing effacement of perimesencephalic cisterns. (*B*) Noncontrast CT at the level of the superior colliculus showing effacement of the quadrigeminal plate cistern. Sulci could not be identified anywhere in the cerebral cortex. At autopsy, Naegleria fowleri were identified in the subarachnoid space in this patient with panamebic meningoencephalitis. (*From* Schumacher DJ, Tien RD, Lane K. Neuroimaging findings in rare amoebic infections of the central nervous system. AJNR Am J Neuroradiol 1995;16(Suppl 4):930–5; with permission.)

system, including the lungs and CNS, with Schistosoma japonicum typically affecting the brain, whereas Schistosoma mansoni and Schistosoma hematobium infections characteristically result in spinal cord lesions.[93] The clinical manifestations of cerebral schistosomiasis are variable, including acute encephalopathy, seizures, paresis, headache, and visual disturbances.[10] Liu and colleagues[93] have investigated brain MR imaging findings in 33 patients with a presumptive diagnosis of cerebral schistosomiasis caused by Schistosoma japonicum, and discovered a common pattern of large discrete lesions with prominent perilesional edema with the lesions composed of multiple small enhancing nodules, sometimes with areas of linear enhancement (**Fig. 16**). Although not present in all cases, when this arborized pattern, which is also described by Wan and colleagues[94,95] as the Buddha's hand appearance, is observed, a diagnosis of cerebral schistosomiasis should be considered. This nodular pattern of contrast enhancement was also commonly documented in spinal schistosomiasis along with peripheral

enhancement and linear radicular enhancement in some patients and was correlated to multiple schistosomiasis microtubercles.[92] Saleem and colleagues[92] have concluded that schistosomiasis of the spinal cord should be considered in the differential diagnosis of lesions involving the lower thoracic cord, conus medullaris, and cauda equina in patients from endemic areas with history of exposure to schistosomal infestation particularly in the presence of intramedullary nodular enhancement described earlier (**Fig. 17**).

Toxoplasmosis

CNS toxoplasmosis is caused by Toxoplasma gondii, an intracellular protozoan that is found worldwide. It is transmitted to humans primarily by ingestion of cysts in undercooked pork or lamb or vegetables contaminated with cat feces or via transplacental infection.[14,96] Immunocompetent individuals with an acute infection are usually asymptomatic or may have a mononucleosis syndrome early in the disease. Following acute infection, a latent phase ensues that is

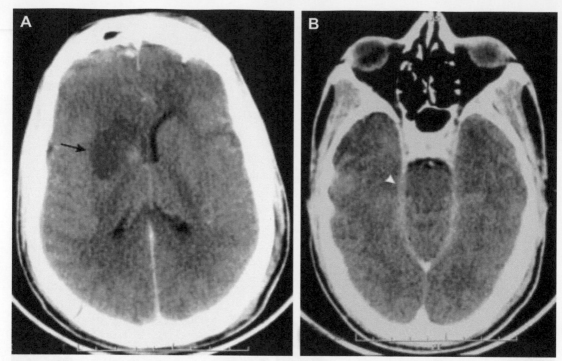

Fig. 15. Amebiasis_ Naegleria fowleri. A 40-year-old man who presented with fever and headache for a week and altered sensorium for 3 days (primary amoebic meningoencephalitis). Contrast-enhanced CT brain scan shows right basal ganglia infarction (*arrow, A*) and enhancing exudates in the perimesencephalic cistern (*arrowhead, B*). (*From* Singh P, et al. Amoebic meningoencephalitis: spectrum of imaging findings. AJNR Am J Neuroradiol 2006;27(6):1217–21; with permission.)

characterized by silent persistence of the organisms primarily in the brain, skeletal muscle, and heart.[96] Toxoplasma gondii seropositivity for adults in the United States varies between 20% and 70%.[14] These dormant organisms normally are not expected to reactivate unless these individuals develop defects in cell-mediated immunity such as in the presence of AIDS. Therefore, in clinical practice, toxoplasmic encephalitis cases are almost always secondary to reactivation of a latent

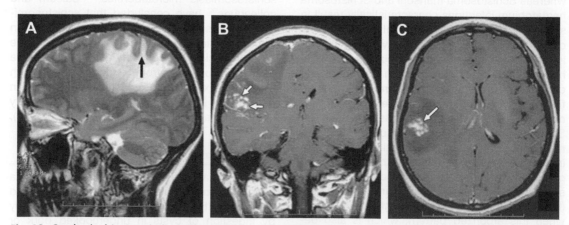

Fig. 16. Cerebral schistosomiasis. A 47-year-old woman with cerebral schistosomiasis and 2-week history of headache and seizures. Sagittal T2-weighted MR image shows prominent vasogenic edema in frontal and parietal lobes, with well-defined deep surface and fingerlike projections (*arrow, A*) into subcortical white matter. Axial and coronal T1-weighted images (*B, C*) after intravenous administration of contrast material show multiple intensely enhancing small nodules, 1 to 3 mm in diameter (*arrows*), clustered closely together. Second cluster in right frontal lobe superiorly is poorly seen because of partial volume effects. (*From* Liu H, et al. MRI in cerebral schistosomiasis: characteristic nodular enhancement in 33 patients. AJR Am J Roentgenol 2008;191(2):582–8; with permission.)

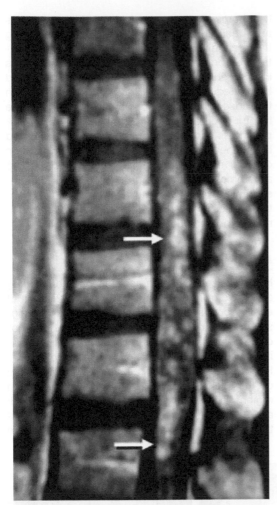

Fig. 17. Spinal schistosomiasis. Diffuse nodular enhancement form in spinal cord schistosomiasis. Post-contrast sagittal T1-weighted spin-echo MR image (TR/TE 520/20 ms) showing multiple small intramedullary enhancing nodules diffusely involving the distal thoracic cord and conus medullaris (*arrows*). (*From* Saleem S, Belal AI, el-Ghandour NM. Spinal cord schistosomiasis: MR imaging appearance with surgical and pathologic correlation. AJNR Am J Neuroradiol 2005;26(7):1646–54; with permission.)

disease. In fact, toxoplasmic encephalitis is the most common cause of brain space-occupying lesions in AIDS patients and may follow a progressive fatal course, if left untreated.[14] However, with the institution of prophylactic treatment against toxoplasmosis along with induction of highly active antiretroviral therapy, there has been decline in the occurrence of opportunistic infections.[97]

Pathologically, 3 types of focal lesions are described in toxoplasmic encephalitis including necrotizing abscesses, organizing abscesses, and chronic abscesses. In addition, 3 distinct

zones are recognized in parencyhmal toxoplasma lesions: (1) a central avascular zone reflecting coagulative necrosis; (2) an intermediate zone engorged with blood vessels and containing numerous tachyzoites, which corresponds to the enhancing ring seen on CT and/or MR images; (3) and a peripheral zone with few vascular changes and more encysted bradyzoites, which may appear as edema on neuroimaging studies.[14] Solitary lesions may occur in one-third of the cases; however, most commonly the lesions are multiple with predilection for the basal ganglia (in 75%–88% of cases), thalamus, and gray-white junction of cerebral hemispheres, particularly in the frontal and parietal lobes.[14] An "eccentric target sign" is described that is essentially a small eccentric nodule along the ring-shaped zone of peripheral enhancement and considered to be suggestive of cerebral toxoplasmosis, although not seen commonly in neuroimaging studies (**Fig. 18**). Ramsey and colleagues[98] suggested that it might be related to focal invagination or folding of the cyst wall on itself. According to them, toxoplasmosis lesions may lack obvious contrast enhancement in the brain of the

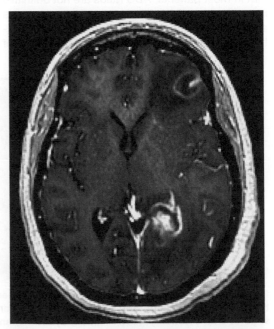

Fig. 18. Toxoplasmosis eccentric target sign. A 47-year-old woman presented with low grade fever and confusion. MR imaging demonstrated multiple rim enhancing lesions, which were found to be CNS toxoplasmosis in the setting of a newly diagnosed human immunodeficiency virus with a CD4 count of 14 and a viral load of 229,660. Contrast-enhanced T1-weighted 3D spoiled gradient recalled echo image shows left frontal and left medial occipital rim enhancing lesions with characteristic eccentric target signs.

immunocompromised patients, despite severe disease involvement (**Fig. 19**).[99,100]

Despite advances in imaging techniques, a correct diagnosis of mass lesion in an AIDS patient is still a dilemma, particularly with differentiation from primary brain lymphoma lesions.[14] Nuclear studies such as thallium-201 brain single-photon emission computed tomography and ^{18}F-FDG PET may aid in differentiation as toxoplasmosis lesions are not hypermetabolic.[101,102] Diffusion-weighted imaging may also be helpful in differentiating these 2 conditions, given the known hypercellular nature of lymphoma lesions that may result in reduction of apparent diffusion coefficient (ADC) values.[14,103] Furthermore, Chong-Han and colleagues[104] have evaluated ADC values in cerebral toxoplasmosis lesions and found that unlike pyogenic abscesses, the central core of rim-enhancing toxoplasma abscesses demonstrate facilitated water diffusion, which correlates well with the fact that the core of a toxoplasma abscess consists primarily of necrotic tissue and does not have the viscous, proteinaceous, and inflammatory debris of purulent fluid. However, in contrast, Schroeder and colleagues[105] have concluded that in most patients, ADC ratios are not definitive in making the distinction because toxoplasmosis exhibits a wide spectrum of diffusion characteristics that have significant overlap with those of

lymphoma. Dynamic perfusion MR imaging has also been proposed as a means of distinguishing these conditions with a relatively decreased relative cerebral blood volume in toxoplasma lesions in comparison to lymphoma lesions, which could be related to a relative lack of vasculature within the abscess.[106] MR spectroscopy may also be helpful in differentiation with the spectra in toxoplasmosis commonly revealing elevated lipid and lactate peaks in the absence or dramatic reduction of other normal brain metabolites, in contrast to a commonly seen spectra of lymphoma demonstrating mild-to-moderate increase in lipid and lactate peaks, a markedly elevated choline peak with relative preservation of the normal metabolites.[14]

Hydatid Disease

Hydatid disease is a parasitic infection caused by a tapeworm Echinococcus. There are 2 types of echinococcus infections: Echinococcus granulosus is the more common type, whereas Echinococcus multilocularis is less common but more invasive, usually mimicking a malignancy.[107] Hydatid disease remains endemic to some parts of the world, most notably the Mediterranean region, Middle East, South America, New Zealand, and Australia. Dogs or other carnivores are definitive hosts, whereas sheep or other ruminants are

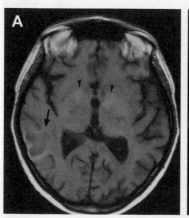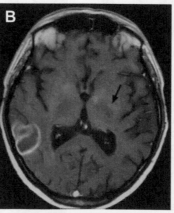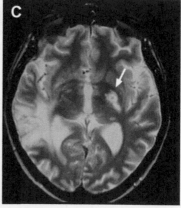

Fig. 19. Toxoplasmosis in immunosuppressed bone marrow transplant patient. A 31-year-old man had allogeneic bone marrow transplant (BMT) for treatment of chronic myeloid leukemia. On day 65, after BMT, he had focal seizures with secondary generalization, dysarthria, and mild cerebellar ataxia. MR imaging revealed: (*A*) Axial T1-weighted image reveals a low-signal temporal lesion with an incomplete high-signal ring suggesting a necrotic infectious lesion (*large arrow*). Bilateral foci of high signal in the basal ganglia (*arrowheads*) were thought to be due to calcium or manganese. (*B*) There is moderate ring enhancement of the right temporal lesion and only faint enhancement of a left basal ganglion lesion (*small arrow*). (*C*) Perifocal edema is better seen on T2 weighting (*white arrow*). This helped to distinguish between metabolic and infectious basal ganglion changes. Serologic tests were positive for IgG antibodies against Toxoplasma gondii but negative for IgM antibodies. Antitoxoplasmosis treatment was started with pyrimethamine and sulfadiazine. MR imaging 10 days later revealed only partial regression of the right temporal lesion, and stereotactic biopsy was performed to rule out other infectious agents. Histology confirmed necrotising encephalitis, suggestive of toxoplasmosis. (*From* Dietrich U, et al. MRI of intracranial toxoplasmosis after bone marrow transplantation. Neuroradiology 2000;42(1):14–8; with permission.)

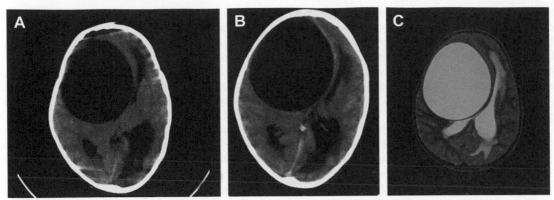

Fig. 20. Hydatid disease. (A) Plain CT, (B) contrast CT, and (C) T2-weighted MR image large cystic lesion with no evidence of enhancement or edema. The periventricular hyperintensity on the left is because of obstructive hydrocephalus. (From Kovoor JM, Thomas RD, Chandrashekhar HS, et al. Neurohydatidosis. Australas Radiol 2007;51(5):406–11. Copyright © 2007. This material is reproduced with permission of John Wiley & Sons, Inc.)

intermediate hosts. Humans are secondarily infected by the ingestion of food or water that has been contaminated by dog feces containing the eggs of the parasite.[107] The overall incidence of organ infestation is greatest in the liver (50%–77%) and lungs (8.5%–43%). Involvement of the CNS is rare and occurs in about 3% of all hydatid disease.[108] Cerebral hydatid disease is most commonly diagnosed in children (approximately 50%–70% of cases).[109] Histopathologically the wall of the Echinococcus granulosus cyst consists of an inner germinal layer (endocyst) and an outer laminated layer (ectocyst). The host reacts to the cyst by forming a fibrous capsule (pericyst), with vascularization thus providing nutrients for the parasite. In the brain, the pericyst is thin because of minimal host reaction.[110] Most Echinococcus granulosus cysts are usually solitary and most commonly supratentorial, within the middle cerebral artery territory.[14] Lesions usually appear as well-defined, smooth, thin-walled, spherical, homogeneous cystic lesions with the appearance of the cyst fluid similar to that of cerebrospinal fluid.[111] On unenhanced CT, the cyst wall is isodense or hyperdense to brain tissue. The cyst wall usually shows a rim of low signal intensity on both T1- and T2-weighted images; in particular, on T2-weighted MR imaging, the presence of a hypointense rim has been described as characteristic of cerebral hydatidosis.[14] Usually no enhancement or surrounding edema is evident unless the hydatid cyst is superinfected (Fig. 20). Calcification of the wall is rare, being less than 1%. The observation of daughter cysts is considered pathognomonic but has been very rarely reported.[111] Multiple cerebral hydatid cysts are relatively rare and result from spontaneous, traumatic, or iatrogenic rupture of a solitary cerebral cyst or as a consequence of a cyst rupture

elsewhere and hematogenous dissemination of organisms to the brain.[108,112] In contrast to Echinococcus granulosus cysts, the cyst of Echinococcus multilocularis grows by external budding of germinal membrane with progressive infiltration of the surrounding tissue. Furthermore, a multilocularis hydatid has little fluid with a semi-solid structure and many small vesicles are embedded in a dense connective tissue stroma.[110] Calcification and surrounding edema are common.[111]

Spinal hydatid disease is rarely seen and occurs in fewer than 1% of all cases of hydatid disease (Fig. 21). Thoracic disease is most commonly seen with mainly vertebral and paravertebral involvement as a result of portovertebral shunts.[108]

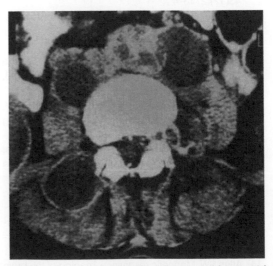

Fig. 21. Spinal hydatid disease. A 47-year-old man with left lower extremity pain attributed to lumbar hydatid disease. Enhanced CT scan shows multiple paravertebral hydatid cysts. (From Tuzun M, Hekimoglu B. Hydatid disease of the CNS: imaging features. AJR Am J Roentgenol 1998;171(6):1497–500; with permission.)

Usually, cysts are multiple with a cystic fluid resembling that of CSF without abnormal enhancement. Lack of lucency or sclerosis within the adjacent bone and absence of disc disease in vertebral hydatid disease may aid in differentiating from tuberculous spondylitis.[108]

REFERENCES

1. Smith AB, Smirniotopoulos JG, Rushing EJ. From the archives of the AFIP: central nervous system infections associated with human immunodeficiency virus infection: radiologic-pathologic correlation. Radiographics 2008;28(7):2033–58.

2. Brooks GF, Butel J, Morse S. Jawetz, Melnick, and Adelberg's medical microbiology. Lange Basic Science Series. 23rd edition. McGraw-Hill Companies; 2004. p. 704.

3. Gladwin M, Trattler B. Clinical microbiology made ridiculously simple. 3rd edition. Miami, Fl: Medmaster; 2004. p. 290.

4. Bonawitz C, Castillo M, Mukherji SK. Comparison of CT and MR features with clinical outcome in patients with Rocky Mountain spotted fever. AJNR Am J Neuroradiol 1997;18(3):459–64.

5. Baganz MD, Dross PE, Reinhardt JA. Rocky Mountain spotted fever encephalitis: MR findings. AJNR Am J Neuroradiol 1995;16(Suppl 4):919–22.

6. Sawaishi Y, Takahashi I, Hirayama Y, et al. Acute cerebellitis caused by Coxiella burnetii. Ann Neurol 1999;45(1):124–7.

7. Sempere AP, Elizaga J, Duarte J, et al. Q fever mimicking herpetic encephalitis. Neurology 1993; 43(12):2713–4.

8. Waltereit R, Kuker W, Jurgens S, et al. Acute transverse myelitis associated with coxiella burnetii infection. J Neurol 2002;249(10):1459–61.

9. Hwang YM, Lee MC, Suh DC, et al. Coxiella (Q fever)-associated myelopathy. Neurology 1993; 43(2):338–42.

10. Kornbluth CM, Destian S. Imaging of rickettsial, spirochetal, and parasitic infections. Neuroimaging Clin N Am 2000;10(2):375–90.

11. Walker DH. Rickettsiae and rickettsial infections: the current state of knowledge. Clin Infect Dis 2007;45(Suppl 1):S39–44.

12. Bechah Y, Capo C, Mege JL, et al. Epidemic typhus. Lancet Infect Dis 2008;8(7):417–26.

13. Garron E, Viehweger E, Launay F, et al. Nontuberculous spondylodiscitis in children. J Pediatr Orthop 2002;22(3):321–8.

14. Atlas SW. Magnetic resonance imaging of the brain and spine. In: Atlas SW, editor. 4th edition. Philadelphia: Lippincott Williams and Wilkins; 2009. p. 980–4, 998–1007, 1015–8.

15. Smith MM, Anderson JC. Neurosyphilis as a cause of facial and vestibulocochlear nerve dysfunction:

16. Brightbill TC, Ihmedian IH, Post MJ, et al. Neurosyphilis in HIV-positive and HIV-negative patients: neuroimaging findings. AJNR Am J Neuroradiol 1995;16(4):703–11.

17. Bandou N, Kamakura N, Yamanishi K, et al. Intracranial gumma mimicking a cerebral tumour. Aust N Z J Psychiatry 2008;42(9):838–9.

18. Darwish BS, Fowler A, Ong M, et al. Intracranial syphilitic gumma resembling malignant brain tumour. J Clin Neurosci 2008;15(3):308–10.

19. Lee CW, Lim MJ, Son D, et al. A case of cerebral gumma presenting as brain tumor in a human immunodeficiency virus (HIV)-negative patient. Yonsei Med J 2009;50(2):284–8.

20. Gaa J, Weidauer S, Sitzer M, et al. Cerebral vasculitis due to Treponema pallidum infection: MRI and MRA findings. Eur Radiol 2004;14(4):746–7.

21. Fadil H, Gonzales-Toledo E, Kelley BJ, et al. Neuroimaging findings in neurosyphilis. J Neuroimaging 2006;16(3):286–9.

22. Bash S, Hathout GM, Cohen S. Mesiotemporal T2-weighted hyperintensity: neurosyphilis mimicking herpes encephalitis. AJNR Am J Neuroradiol 2001;22(2):314–6.

23. Vieira Santos A, Matias S, Saraiva P, et al. Differential diagnosis of mesiotemporal lesions: case report of neurosyphilis. Neuroradiology 2005;47(9):664–7.

24. Hama K, Ishiguchi H, Tuji T, et al. Neurosyphilis with mesiotemporal magnetic resonance imaging abnormalities. Intern Med 2008;47(20):1813–7.

25. Jeong YM, Hwang HY, Kim HS. MRI of neurosyphilis presenting as mesiotemporal abnormalities: a case report. Korean J Radiol 2009;10(3):310–2.

26. Scheid R, Voltz R, Vetter T, et al. Neurosyphilis and paraneoplastic limbic encephalitis: important differential diagnoses. J Neurol 2005;252(9):1129–32.

27. Hildenbrand P, Craven DE, Jones R, et al. Lyme neuroborreliosis: manifestations of a rapidly emerging zoonosis. AJNR Am J Neuroradiol 2009;30(6): 1079–87.

28. Agarwal R, Sze G. Neuro-lyme disease: MR imaging findings. Radiology 2009;253(1):167–73.

29. Santino I, Comite P, Gandolfo GM. Borrelia burgdorferi, a great chameleon: know it to recognize it! Neurol Sci 2010;31(2):193–6.

30. Demaerel P, Crevits I, Casteels-Van Daele M, et al. Meningoradiculitis due to borreliosis presenting as low back pain only. Neuroradiology 1998;40(2):126–7.

31. Oksi J, Kalimo H, Marttila RJ, et al. Inflammatory brain changes in Lyme borreliosis. A report on three patients and review of literature. Brain 1996; 119(Pt 6):2143–54.

32. Fernandez RE, Rothberg M, Ferencz G, et al. Lyme disease of the CNS: MR imaging findings in 14 cases. AJNR Am J Neuroradiol 1990;11(3):479–81.

33. Curless RG, Schatz NJ, Bowen BC, et al. Lyme neuro-borreliosis masquerading as a brainstem tumor in a 15-year-old. Pediatr Neurol 1996;15(3):258–60.

34. Haene A, Troger M. Diffuse hyperintense brainstem lesions in neuroborreliosis. Neurology 2009;73(4):326.

35. Rafto SE, Milton WJ, Galetta SL, et al. Biopsy-confirmed CNS Lyme disease: MR appearance at 1.5 T. AJNR Am J Neuroradiol 1990;11(3):482–4.

36. Murray R, Morawetz R, Kepes J, et al. Lyme neuro-borreliosis manifesting as an intracranial mass lesion. Neurosurgery 1992;30(5):769–73.

37. Kalina P, Decker A, Kornel E, et al. Lyme disease of the brainstem. Neuroradiology 2005;47(12):903–7.

38. Savas R, Sommer A, Gueckel F, et al. Isolated oculomotor nerve paralysis in Lyme disease: MRI. Neuroradiology 1997;39(2):139–41.

39. Vanzieleghem B, Lemmerling M, Carton D, et al. Lyme disease in a child presenting with bilateral facial nerve palsy: MRI findings and review of the literature. Neuroradiology 1998;40(11):739–42.

40. Huisman TA, Wohlrab G, Nadal D, et al. Unusual presentations of neuroborreliosis (Lyme disease) in childhood. J Comput Assist Tomogr 1999;23(1):39–42.

41. Lell M, Schmid A, Stemper B, et al. Simultaneous involvement of third and sixth cranial nerve in a patient with Lyme disease. Neuroradiology 2003;45(2):85–7.

42. Kochling J, Freitag HJ, Bollinger T, et al. Lyme disease with lymphocytic meningitis, trigeminal palsy and silent thalamic lesion. Eur J Paediatr Neurol 2008;12(6):501–4.

43. Van Snick S, Duprez TP, Kabamba B, et al. Acute ischaemic pontine stroke revealing lyme neurobor-reliosis in a young adult. Acta Neurol Belg 2008;108(3):103–6.

44. Topakian R, Stieglbauer K, Nussbaumer K, et al. Cerebral vasculitis and stroke in Lyme neuroborre-liosis. Two case reports and review of current knowledge. Cerebrovasc Dis 2008;26(5):455–61.

45. Romi F, Krakenes J, Aarli JA, et al. Neuroborreliosis with vasculitis causing stroke-like manifestations. Eur Neurol 2004;51(1):49–50.

46. Heinrich A, Khaw AV, Ahrens N, et al. Cerebral vasculitis as the only manifestation of Borrelia burg-dorferi infection in a 17-year-old patient with basal ganglia infarction. Eur Neurol 2003;50(2):109–12.

47. Seijo Martinez M, Grandes Ibanez J, Sanchez Herrero J, et al. Spontaneous brain hemorrhage associated with Lyme neuroborreliosis. Neurologia 2001;16(1):43–5.

48. Defer G, Levy R, Brugieres P, et al. Lyme disease presenting as a stroke in the vertebrobasilar terri-tory: MRI. Neuroradiology 1993;35(7):529–31.

49. Mantienne C, Albucher JF, Catalaa I, et al. MRI in Lyme disease of the spinal cord. Neuroradiology 2001;43(6):485–8.

50. Bigi S, Aebi C, Nauer C, et al. Acute transverse myelitis in Lyme neuroborreliosis. Infection 2010;38(5):413–6.

51. Walid MS, Ajjan M, Ulm AJ. Subacute transverse myelitis with Lyme profile dissociation. Ger Med Sci 2008;6:Doc04.

52. Meurs L, Labeye D, Declercq I, et al. Acute trans-verse myelitis as a main manifestation of early stage II neuroborreliosis in two patients. Eur Neurol 2004;52(3):186–8.

53. Kumar V, et al. Robbins & cotran pathologic basis of disease. 8th edition. Saunders; 2010. p. 1464.

54. Corr P, Bhigjee A, Lockhat F. Oculomotor nerve root enhancement in meningovascular syphilis. Clin Ra-diol 2004;59(3):294–6.

55. Bourekas EC, Wildenhain P, Lewin JS, et al. The dural tail sign revisited. AJNR Am J Neuroradiol 1995;16(7):1514–6.

56. Lin M, Darwish BS, Chu J. Neurosyphilitic gumma on F18-2-fluoro-2-deoxy-D-glucose (FDG) positron emission tomography: an old disease investigated with a new technology. J Clin Neurosci 2009;16(3):410–2.

57. Flint AC, Liberato BB, Anziska Y, et al. Meningovas-cular syphilis as a cause of basilar artery stenosis. Neurology 2005;64(2):391–2.

58. Hengge UR, Tannapfel A, Tyring SK, et al. Lyme borreliosis. Lancet Infect Dis 2003;3(8):489–500.

59. Paralysie par les Tiques [Paralysis by Ticks]. J Med Lyon 1922;71:765–7 [in French].

60. Pachner AR, Steiner I. Lyme neuroborreliosis: infection, immunity, and inflammation. Lancet Neu-rol 2007;6(6):544–52.

61. Rupprecht TA, Koedel U, Fingerle V, et al. The pathogenesis of lyme neuroborreliosis: from in-fection to inflammation. Mol Med 2008;14(3–4):205–12.

62. Pachner AR, Duray P, Steere AC. Central nervous system manifestations of Lyme disease. Arch Neu-rol 1989;46(7):790–5.

63. Halperin JJ, Pass HL, Anand AK, et al. Nervous system abnormalities in Lyme disease. Ann N Y Acad Sci 1988;539:24–34.

64. Halperin JJ, Luft BJ, Anand AK, et al. Lyme neuro-borreliosis: central nervous system manifestations. Neurology 1989;39(6):753–9.

65. Kruger H, Heim E, Schuknecht B, et al. Acute and chronic neuroborreliosis with and without CNS involvement: a clinical, MRI, and HLA study of 27 cases. J Neurol 1991;238(5):271–80.

66. Belman AL, Coyle PK, Roque C, et al. MRI findings in children infected by Borrelia burgdorferi. Pediatr Neurol 1992;8(6):428–31.

67. Agosta F, Rocca MA, Benedetti B, et al. MR imaging assessment of brain and cervical cord damage in patients with neuroborreliosis. AJNR Am J Neurora-diol 2006;27(4):892–4.

68. Demaerel P, Wilms G, Van Lierde S, et al. Lyme disease in childhood presenting as primary leptomeningeal enhancement without parenchymal findings on MR. AJNR Am J Neuroradiol 1994;15(2): 302–4.

69. Halperin JJ. Nervous system Lyme disease. Infect Dis Clin North Am 2008;22(2):261–74.

70. Chehrenama M, Zagardo MT, Koski CL. Subarachnoid hemorrhage in a patient with Lyme disease. Neurology 1997;48(2):520–3.

71. Fallon BA, Lipkin RB, Corbera KM, et al. Regional cerebral blood flow and metabolic rate in persistent Lyme encephalopathy. Arch Gen Psychiatry 2009; 66(5):554–63.

72. Aalto A, Sjowall J, Davidsson L, et al. Brain magnetic resonance imaging does not contribute to the diagnosis of chronic neuroborreliosis. Acta Radiol 2007;48(7):755–62.

73. Morgen K, Martin R, Stone RD, et al. FLAIR and magnetization transfer imaging of patients with post-treatment Lyme disease syndrome. Neurology 2001;57(11):1980–5.

74. Fatterpekar GM, Gottesman RI, Sacher M, et al. Orbital Lyme disease: MR imaging before and after treatment: case report. AJNR Am J Neuroradiol 2002;23(4):657–9.

75. Nieto JC, Kim N, Lucarelli MJ. Dacryoadenitis and orbital myositis associated with lyme disease. Arch Ophthalmol 2008;126(8):1165–6.

76. Pfefferkorn T, Feddersen B, Schulte-Altedorneburg G, et al. Tick-borne encephalitis with polyradiculitis documented by MRI. Neurology 2007;68(15):1232–3.

77. Hattingen E, Weidauer S, Kieslich M, et al. MR imaging in neuroborreliosis of the cervical spinal cord. Eur Radiol 2004;14(11):2072–5.

78. Tullman MJ, Delman BN, Lublin FD, et al. Magnetic resonance imaging of meningoradiculomyelitis in early disseminated Lyme disease. J Neuroimaging 2003;13(3):264–8.

79. Chandra SR, Kalpana D, Anilkumar TV, et al. Acute disseminated encephalomyelitis following leptospirosis. J Assoc Physicians India 2004;52:327–9.

80. Lelis SS, Fonseca LF, Xavier CC, et al. Acute disseminated encephalomyelitis after leptospirosis. Pediatr Neurol 2009;40(6):471–3.

81. Maldonado F, Portier H, Kisterman JP. Bilateral facial palsy in a case of leptospirosis. Scand J Infect Dis 2004;36(5):386–8.

82. Habek M, Brinar VV. Central sleep apnea and ataxia caused by brainstem lesion due to chronic neuroleptospirosis. Neurology 2009;73(22):1923–4.

83. Singh P, Kochhar R, Vashishta RK, et al. Amebic meningoencephalitis: spectrum of imaging findings. AJNR Am J Neuroradiol 2006;27(6):1217–21.

84. Ohnishi K, Murata M, Kojima H, et al. Brain abscess due to infection with Entamoeba histolytica. Am J Trop Med Hyg 1994;51(2):180–2.

85. Kidney DD, Kim SH. CNS infections with free-living amebas: neuroimaging findings. AJR Am J Roentgenol 1998;171(3):809–12.

86. Schumacher DJ, Tien RD, Lane K. Neuroimaging findings in rare amebic infections of the central nervous system. AJNR Am J Neuroradiol 1995; 16(Suppl 4):930–5.

87. Zagardo MT, Castellani RJ, Zoarski GH, et al. Granulomatous amebic encephalitis caused by leptomyxid amebae in an HIV-infected patient. AJNR Am J Neuroradiol 1997;18(5):903–8.

88. Sell JJ, Rupp FW, Orrison WW Jr. Granulomatous amebic encephalitis caused by acanthamoeba. Neuroradiology 1997;39(6):434–6.

89. Mendez O, Kanal E, Abu-Elmagd KM, et al. Granulomatous amebic encephalitis in a multivisceral transplant recipient. Eur J Neurol 2006;13(3): 292–5.

90. Lowichik A, Rollins N, Delgado R, et al. Leptomyxid amebic meningoencephalitis mimicking brain stem glioma. AJNR Am J Neuroradiol 1995;16(Suppl 4): 926–9.

91. Cary LC, Maul E, Potter C, et al. Balamuthia mandrillaris meningoencephalitis: survival of a pediatric patient. Pediatrics 2010;125(3):e699–703.

92. Saleem S, Belal AI, el-Ghandour NM. Spinal cord schistosomiasis: MR imaging appearance with surgical and pathologic correlation. AJNR Am J Neuroradiol 2005;26(7):1646–54.

93. Liu HQ, Feng XY, Yao ZW, et al. Characteristic magnetic resonance enhancement pattern in cerebral schistosomiasis. Chin Med Sci J 2006;21(4): 223–7.

94. Liu H, Lim CC, Feng X, et al. MRI in cerebral schistosomiasis: characteristic nodular enhancement in 33 patients. AJR Am J Roentgenol 2008;191(2): 582–8.

95. Wan H, Masataka H, Lei T, et al. Magnetic resonance imaging and cerebrospinal fluid immunoassay in the diagnosis of cerebral schistosomiasis: experience in southwest China. Trans R Soc Trop Med Hyg 2009;103(10):1059–61.

96. Lee GT, Antelo F, Mlikotic AA. Best cases from the AFIP: cerebral toxoplasmosis. Radiographics 2009; 29(4):1200–5.

97. Berger JR. Mass lesions of the brain in AIDS: the dilemmas of distinguishing toxoplasmosis from primary CNS lymphoma. AJNR Am J Neuroradiol 2003;24(4):554–5.

98. Ramsey RG, Gean AD. Neuroimaging of AIDS. I. Central nervous system toxoplasmosis. Neuroimaging Clin N Am 1997;7(2):171–86.

99. Ionita C, Wasay M, Balos L, et al. MR imaging in toxoplasmosis encephalitis after bone marrow transplantation: paucity of enhancement despite fulminant disease. AJNR Am J Neuroradiol 2004; 25(2):270–3.

100. Dietrich U, Maschke M, Dorfler A, et al. MRI of intracranial toxoplasmosis after bone marrow transplantation. Neuroradiology 2000;42(1):14–8.

101. Ruiz A, Ganz WI, Post MJ, et al. Use of thallium-201 brain SPECT to differentiate cerebral lymphoma from toxoplasma encephalitis in AIDS patients. AJNR Am J Neuroradiol 1994;15(10):1885–94.

102. Love C, Tomas MB, Tronco GG, et al. FDG PET of infection and inflammation. Radiographics 2005; 25(5):1357–68.

103. Camacho DL, Smith JK, Castillo M. Differentiation of toxoplasmosis and lymphoma in AIDS patients by using apparent diffusion coefficients. AJNR Am J Neuroradiol 2003;24(4):633–7.

104. Chong-Han CH, Cortez SC, Tung GA. Diffusion-weighted MRI of cerebral toxoplasma abscess. AJR Am J Roentgenol 2003;181(6):1711–4.

105. Schroeder PC, Post MJ, Oschatz E, et al. Analysis of the utility of diffusion-weighted MRI and apparent diffusion coefficient values in distinguishing central nervous system toxoplasmosis from lymphoma. Neuroradiology 2006;48(10):715–20.

106. Ernst TM, Chang L, Witt MD, et al. Cerebral toxoplasmosis and lymphoma in AIDS: perfusion MR imaging experience in 13 patients. Radiology 1998;208(3):663–9.

107. Polat P, Kantarci M, Alper F, et al. Hydatid disease from head to toe. Radiographics 2003;23(2):475–94 [quiz: 536–7].

108. Tuzun M, Hekimoglu B. Hydatid disease of the CNS: imaging features. AJR Am J Roentgenol 1998;171(6):1497–500.

109. El-Shamam O, Amer T, El-Atta MA. Magnetic resonance imaging of simple and infected hydatid cysts of the brain. Magn Reson Imaging 2001;19(7):965–74.

110. Kovoor JM, Thomas RD, Chandrashektar HS, et al. Neurohydatidosis. Australas Radiol 2007;51(5): 406–11.

111. Tuzun M, Altinors N, Arda IS, et al. Cerebral hydatid disease CT and MR findings. Clin Imaging 2002; 26(5):353–7.

112. Turgut AT, Altin L, Topcu S, et al. Unusual imaging characteristics of complicated hydatid disease. Eur J Radiol 2007;63(1):84–93.

Imaging of Neurocysticercosis

Alexander Lerner, MD*, Mark S. Shiroishi, MD,
Chi-Shing Zee, MD, Meng Law, MD, MBBS, John L. Go, MD

KEYWORDS

- Computed tomography • Central nervous system • Neurocysticercosis
- Magnetic resonance imaging

KEY POINTS

- Neurocysticercosis (NCC) is the most common cause of acquired epilepsy in endemic regions.
- Parenchymal NCC lesions can be divided into 4 stages with unique imaging and clinical features.
- Intraventricular and subarachnoid NCC forms have a higher risk of complications.
- Evaluation of intraventricular and subarachnoid NCC is improved with magnetic resonance (MR) cysternography techniques.
- Advanced MR imaging can be helpful in differentiating of NCC lesions from metastatic disease and pyogenic abscesses.

INTRODUCTION

Neurocysticercosis is the result of the implantation of the cestode *Taenia solium* (pork tapeworm) in the human host. The larval stage of this organism may become disseminated throughout the central nervous system (CNS) of the affected individual. Neurocysticercosis is one of the most common causes of epilepsy in endemic regions throughout the world as well as in United States and European immigrant populations from these regions.[1] Endemic regions include Latin America, parts of Oceania, Asia, Eastern Europe, and Africa.[2,3] For a more thorough understanding of this disease, a full discussion of the complex life cycle of this parasite is necessary.

LIFE CYCLE AND PATHOGENESIS

The *T solium* life cycle includes humans as the definitive hosts and pigs as intermediate hosts. Sequential infection of both hosts is needed to complete the reproductive cycle of the tapeworm.

T solium is typically acquired by the human (definitive host) by ingestion of poorly cooked pork containing the larval form of the organism (cysticerci). The ingested larvae emerge in the gastrointestinal tract. The organism's head, known as the scolex, implants in the mucosa of the small intestine and the tapeworm grows by generating segments known as proglottids. The adult tapeworm may reach up to 4 m in length and has hundreds of proglottids. The oldest and most distal proglottids contain tens of thousands of mature eggs ready to infect a new host. These proglottids are shed and excreted in the human feces. The intestinal infection by this parasite is referred to as taeniasis, which in many cases is asymptomatic; however, it may occasionally cause mild diarrhea and abdominal pain. Consequently, many individuals with taeniasis are not aware of their disease.[2]

The pig (intermediate host) typically acquires the parasite by injection of feed contaminated with human fecal material containing *T solium* eggs (oncospheres). The larval forms of the parasite emerge from the eggs in the gastrointestinal tract,

Disclosures: None.
Department of Radiology, Keck school of Medicine, LAC+USC Medical Center, University of Southern California, 1200 North State Street, Los Angeles, CA 90033, USA
* Corresponding author. Division of Neuroradiology, LAC+USC Medical Center, 1200 North State Street, Room 3740A, Los Angeles, CA 90033.
E-mail address: alerner5@gmail.com

penetrate the wall of the bowel, and disseminate via the bloodstream throughout the muscle tissue of the pig, forming cysts in the surrounding tissue, known as cysticerci.

However, occasionally humans may become the intermediate hosts instead, which is manifested as cysticercosis. When humans ingest food contaminated with human feces containing *T solium* eggs, the larvae similarly invade the bloodstream of the humans and disseminate throughout the tissues of the body, forming cysticerci at terminal arterioles within the CNS, subcutaneous tissues, muscles, and so forth.[2,3]

Neurocysticercosis refers specifically to CNS involvement by cysticercosis. Although involvement of muscle and subcutaneous tissues by this disease is frequently asymptomatic, within the CNS cysticerci can produce a variety of clinical neurologic symptoms.

Initially, the tapeworm larvae invade the CNS and form viable cysticerci with minimal host-mediated inflammatory reaction in the surrounding brain parenchyma. Presumably, the blood-brain barrier and factors secreted by cysticerci inhibit a significant immune response to the lesion within the CNS.

Degeneration of the cyst may occur in several months to years with associated inflammatory response and edema, which can result in clinical symptoms. It is thought that degeneration of the cyst occurs when the larva fails to inhibit the immune response. The cyst may rupture, releasing antigens into surrounding tissue and resulting in more severe inflammation. The severity of associated inflammatory response and associated clinical manifestations vary extensively in each case.[2–4]

Cysticerci may also involve the subarachnoid space of the head and spine. Rarely, cysticerci may involve the spinal cord parenchyma.

The most common clinical manifestation of neurocysticercosis is seizure. In addition, cysticerci may cause obstructive hydrocephalus, intracranial hypertension, mass effect, and cerebral infarction. An acute encephalitis-like presentation has been described in the pediatric population, which is thought to represent a severe inflammatory response to cysticercal involvement of the CNS.[2,3,5]

DIAGNOSIS OF NEUROCYSTICERCOSIS

The clinical presentation of neurocysticercosis is often nonspecific and highly variable, depending on the number and location of the lesions. This variation may delay the correct diagnosis. Serologic tests are used to establish the diagnosis in suspected cases, including enzyme-linked immunoelectrodiffusion transfer blot (EITB). EITB has been used with different antigens and has demonstrated very high sensitivity and specificity for cysticercosis.[6,7] Imaging plays a critical role in confirming and fully characterizing CNS involvement by cysticercosis.

PARENCHYMAL NEUROCYSTICERCOSIS

Neurocysticercosis most commonly manifests in the parenchyma of the brain and typically involves the cerebral hemispheres, with lesions commonly found at the gray matter–white matter junction, presumably resulting from deposition of the larvae in terminal small vessels of this region. Multiple lesions are usually present, although the number is highly variable, with solitary lesions as well as innumerable lesions in a miliary pattern occasionally encountered.[8] Cerebellar, basal ganglia, or brainstem lesions may also be found in individuals with numerous lesions.

Computed tomography (CT) and magnetic resonance (MR) imaging excel at detecting acute and chronic forms of neurocysticercosis and its complications. Acute symptomatic lesions are best visualized on contrast-enhanced MR imaging. However, chronic lesions are best visualized on noncontrast CT as hyperdense calcifications, because MR imaging signal voids associated with chronic calcified lesions are difficult to identify on all sequences.[2]

The earliest form of larval invasion is noncystic and is usually not detectable on imaging, because of frequent lack of edema at that stage. However, occasionally lesions may develop associated edema and focal enhancement before cystic transformation.[9]

Four stages of neurocysticercosis lesions can be recognized on CT and MR imaging as they naturally evolve from the acute to the chronic form.

Vesicular Stage

Within a few weeks the larva transforms into a cysticercal cyst containing an invaginated scolex, representing a viable, active form of cysticercosis. The cyst matures over the course of several months and may subsequently enlarge to approximately 1 cm. Imaging hallmarks of this stage include visualization of the scolex within a cyst and absence of enhancement or thin linear enhancement of the cyst wall. The cyst fluid usually demonstrates the same signal intensity as cerebrospinal fluid (CSF) on all MR imaging sequences. On CT the cyst demonstrates attenuation, similar to the CSF (Fig. 1).

The scolex is identifiable in some lesions at this stage, as it has variable signal characteristics and may enhance (Fig. 2).[9–11] Fluid-attenuated

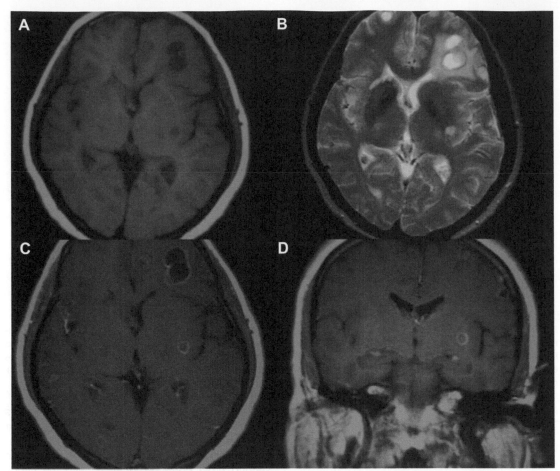

Fig. 1. Axial T1-weighted image (*A*), axial T2-weighted image (*B*), and axial and coronal T1-weighted images with contrast (*C, D*) of coexisting vesicular and colloidal vesicular stage neurocysticercosis. Two large left frontal lobe cysticerci lack identifiable scolices and demonstrate adjacent edema representing colloidal vesicular stage. Multiple smaller cysticerci with internal scolices and lack of associated edema are in the vesicular stage. Scolices can be best seen in these cysticerci on postcontrast images (*C* and *D*). Cyst contents demonstrate signal intensity similar to cerebrospinal fluid (CSF) on all sequences. Mild linear enhancement of cyst walls and punctate enhancement of the scolices is noted.

inversion recovery (FLAIR) imaging frequently improves the visualization of the T2-weighted hyperintense scolex immersed in CSF-like fluid of the cyst.[12]

Colloidal Vesicular Stage

As already described, the cyst usually begins to degenerate in several months. Early degeneration of the cysticercus results in destruction of the scolex, development of proteinaceous cyst contents, and associated inflammatory response in the surrounding brain parenchyma. This process represents a degenerating, active form of cysticercosis.

The process is manifest on CT, with hyperdense fluid within the cyst and ring enhancement of the lesion. MR imaging frequently reveals T1 hyperintensity of the cyst fluid and lack of a scolex. T1-weighted postcontrast images also reveal

a ring-enhancement pattern. T2-weighted images frequently demonstrate adjacent edema and may show a rim of the cyst of low signal intensity (**Fig. 3**).[5,9,10] However, absence of diffusion restriction is evident on diffusion-weighted (DW) imaging, helping to differentiate this lesion from an abscess (**Fig. 4**).[13] Occasionally a fluid-fluid level may be evident within, suggestive of internal debris.

Granular Nodular Stage

As degeneration of the cysticercus progresses, the cyst decreases in size and transforms into a smaller nodular lesion. This process represents a degenerating, active form of cysticercosis. CT and MR imaging demonstrate enhancement of the nodular lesion or a small ring-enhancing lesion at this stage. Mild associated edema may be identified in adjacent brain parenchyma (**Fig. 5**).[5,9]

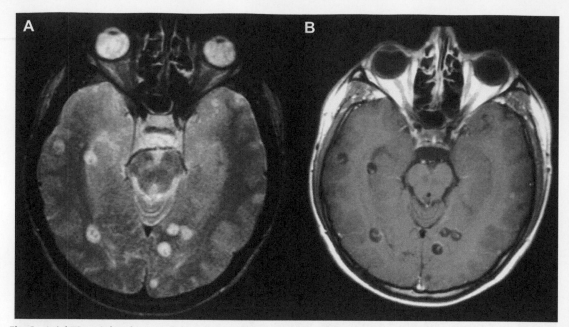

Fig. 2. Axial T2-weighted image (*A*) and axial T1-weighted image with contrast (*B*) of the vesicular stage of neurocysticercosis. There are multiple bilateral temporal and occipital lobe cysts, which are uniform in size and morphology. Scolices can be seen as hypointense foci within the cysticerci on T2-weighted imaging and as enhancing nodules on postcontrast T1-weighted imaging. Cyst contents reveal signal intensity similar to CSF on both sequences. No associated edema is seen. Minimal linear enhancement of cyst walls is present.

Nodular Calcified Stage

The nodular calcified stage is the end stage of cysticercal degeneration, with transformation into a small calcified granulomatous lesion. This process represents a degenerated, inactive form of cysticercosis. Usually no associated edema or enhancement is observed, representing a lack of immune response to this end-stage, nonviable lesion. CT is most sensitive for these lesions, revealing them as hyperdense parenchymal lesions (**Fig. 6**). The lesions are hypointense on T1- and T2-weighted imaging, and may be difficult to identify (**Fig. 7**).[5,9,10]

However, there have been recent reports of the reactivation of calcified neurocysticercosis manifesting as edema and enhancement associated with calcified lesions (see **Fig. 7**D). In addition, these patients may experience associated seizure activity. It is thought that residual antigens within calcified lesions may periodically induce an inflammatory response.[14–16]

INTRAVENTRICULAR NEUROCYSTICERCOSIS

The intraventricular form of neurocysticercosis may be seen in 10% to 21% of neurocysticercosis cases.[5,17,18] Although coexisting parenchymal lesions may be found, facilitating the radiologic diagnosis, up to 76% of patients may present with intraventricular lesion as the only detectable

disease.[19] This form of neurocysticercosis frequently manifests as a solitary intraventricular cyst. The fourth ventricle is the most common location for this cystic lesion. The third ventricle is the second most common location, with the lateral ventricle and cerebral aqueduct of Sylvius less frequently involved.[8,18] Migration of cystic lesions from one ventricle to another has been observed. Typically the cysts move from the lateral ventricle to the third ventricle, then to the aqueduct of Sylvius and the fourth ventricle. This form of neurocysticercosis may therefore result in obstructive hydrocephalus as the cyst blocks the flow of CSF through the ventricular system.[20] Follow-up imaging may be useful in following the movement of the cyst, especially if surgical intervention is planned. In addition, ependymal inflammation and subsequent adhesions may ensue, frequently in the cerebral aqueduct of Sylvius, resulting in CSF-flow obstruction and hydrocephalus.[8,19]

This form of neurocysticercosis may be challenging to identify on CT, especially if parenchymal calcified lesions are absent. The cysts are usually isointense to CSF on MR imaging with T2- and T1-weighted sequences (**Fig. 8**), and only infrequently demonstrate hyperintensity to CSF on T1-weighted imaging and FLAIR sequences (**Fig. 9**). The wall of the cyst may occasionally be seen as a thin linear structure on T2-weighted imaging, or demonstrate contrast enhancement. Because

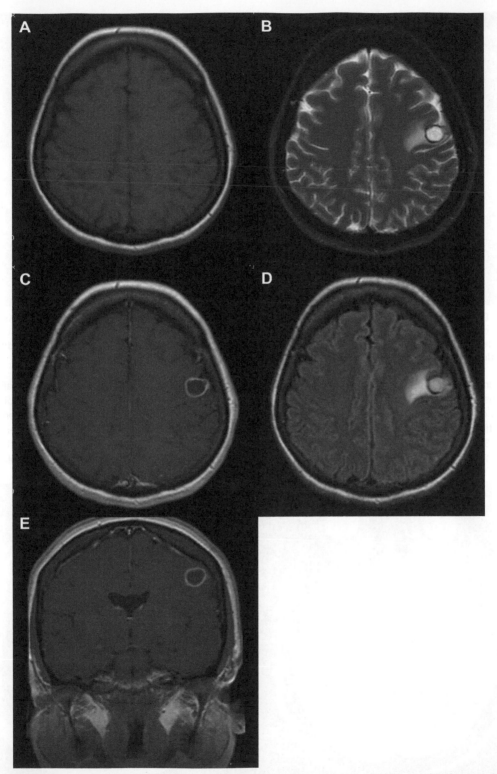

Fig. 3. MR imaging of left frontal lobe colloidal vesicular stage cysticercosis. (*A*) Axial T1-weighted image demonstrates cyst fluid as hyperintense relative to CSF. (*B*) Axial T2-weighted image reveals hypointense cyst wall and associated vasogenic edema. (*C, E*) Postcontrast T1-weighted image demonstrates ring enhancement of the cysticercus. (*D*) Axial fluid-attenuated inversion recovery (FLAIR) image demonstrates hyperintense cyst fluid and adjacent edema.

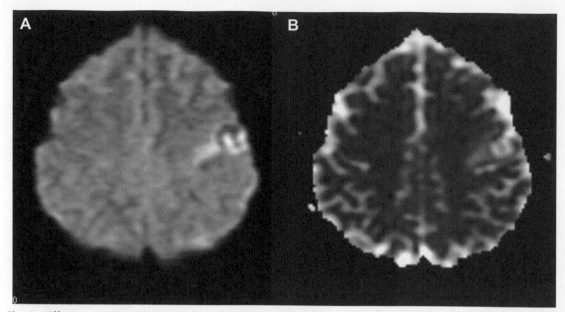

Fig. 4. Diffusion-weighted (DW) imaging of left frontal lobe colloidal vesicular stage cysticercosis. (*A*) Axial DW image demonstrates cyst as moderately hyperintense relative to CSF. (*B*) Axial apparent diffusion coefficient (ADC) map shows high ADC values in this region representing T2 shine-through effect and lack of diffusion restriction. This finding can be helpful in differentiation of cysticercus from pyogenic abscess.

many intraventricular neurocysticercosis cysts are isodense and isointense to CSF, they may be detected owing to presence of ventricular deformity, distention, and associated hydrocephalus (see **Fig. 8**). High-resolution MR cisternography sequences such as constructive interference in steady state (3D-CISS) may improve visualization of the intraventricular cyst and may resolve the internal scolex.[21] Ependymal enhancement may be seen in cases with inflammatory involvement of the adjacent ventricle. On rare occasions inflammatory changes may also involve the choroid plexus.[22]

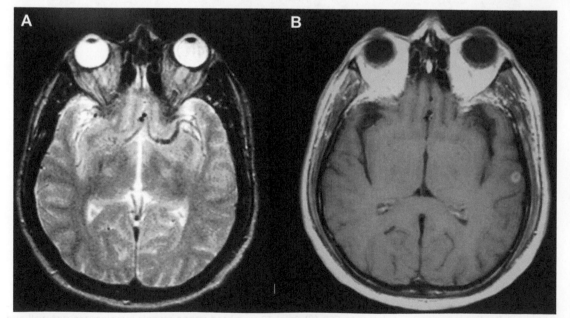

Fig. 5. Left temporal lobe granular nodular stage neurocysticercosis. (*A*) Axial T2-weighted image demonstrates a small nodular lesion with lack of significant associated edema. (*B*) Axial postcontrast T1-weighted image reveals corresponding small ring-enhancing lesion consistent with degenerating cysticercus in granular nodular stage. CT (not shown) demonstrated absence of calcification within the lesion.

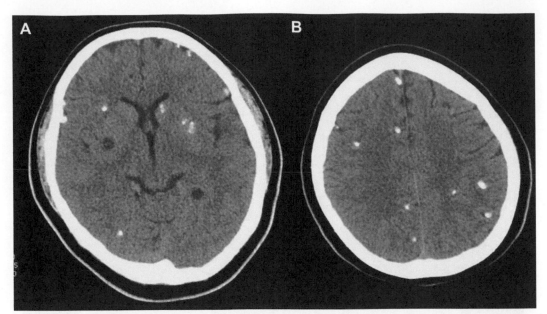

Fig. 6. (*A, B*) Noncontrast axial CT images of numerous nodular calcified stage cysticercosis lesions. Coexisting vesicular stage cysticerci can also be seen on image *A*, with hyperdense scolex demonstrated within the right basal ganglia cyst.

SUBARACHNOID AND MENINGEAL NEUROCYSTICERCOSIS

The subarachnoid form of neurocysticercosis is the third most common manifestation of this disease after parenchymal and intraventricular forms, and has been found in 3.6% of neurocysticercosis patients.[18] Neurocysticercosis of the subarachnoid spaces and the ventricular system is thought to result from hemotogenous dissemination of the larvae to these locations.[3] Involvement of the basal cisterns is frequently identified and has been referred to as the meningobasal form. The suprasellar cistern, prepontine cistern, and ambient cisterns are among the most commonly involved. In these regions the scolex is often absent or degenerated, and multiple complex cysts may form, filling the involved cisterns with associated mass effect and distortion of adjacent structures including brainstem and cranial nerves. The multiloculated appearance of these fluid-filled lesions lacking internal scolex has been likened to a cluster of grapes, and is termed the "racemose" cysticercosis. However, as it is now recognized that degenerated scolex can be found in these lesions, this designation has fallen out of favor.[5]

Cysticerci in this region are difficult to detect on CT. Even on MR imaging these lesions are often poorly visualized, owing to the isointensity of the lesions to CSF on all sequences similar to surrounding normal cisterns. Initially no enhancement may be detected within the basal cisterns, and the

cysts may be seen primarily as a result of distortion of the involved cisterns and adjacent structures (**Figs. 10** and **11**). The cyst walls may be identified as thin linear hypointensities on T2-weighted imaging (**Fig. 12**). Identification and characterization of these lesions is greatly improved with high-resolution MR cisternography sequences, such as 3D-CISS, through the basal cisterns. Cyst walls, degenerated scolex, and associated distortion of cranial nerves and vascular structures can be best visualized with this technique.[21]

This form of cysticercosis may elicit inflammation of the adjacent leptomeninges, with associated MR imaging findings of leptomeningeal enhancement and communicating hydrocephalus (**Fig. 13**). Over time leptomeningeal adhesions, thickening, and calcifications may be formed, increasing the conspicuity of subarachnoid disease on MR imaging and CT. Acute inflammation of the leptomeninges may also result in vasculitis involving the small perforating arterial branches in basal cisterns with secondary small focal infarctions. Occasionally arteritis of large vessels such as the middle cerebral artery may occur, with resulting large-territory cerebral infarction (**Fig. 14**).

Cysticerci in the basal cisterns and Sylvian fissures may become significantly larger than 1 cm in size (**Fig. 15**), with reported cases of lesions 10 cm and larger.[23] Subarachnoid cysts within the sulci of the cerebral convexities are more similar in size and appearance to parenchymal cysticerci, and may be difficult to distinguish from cortical lesions.[24]

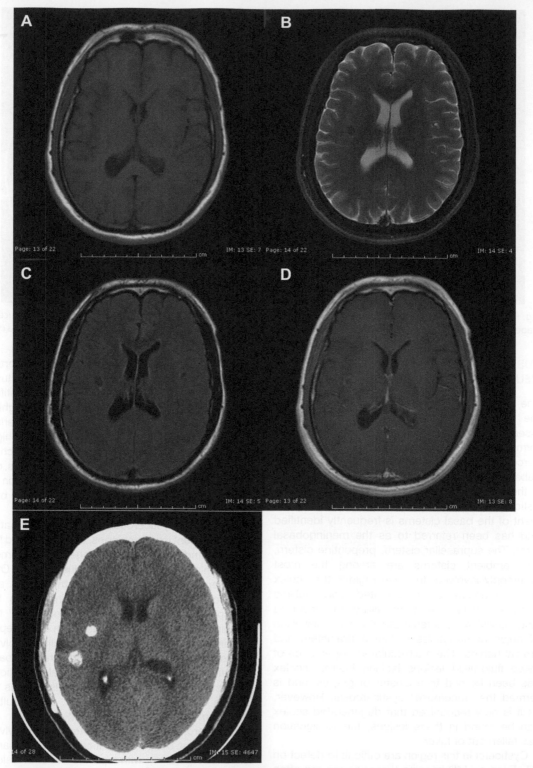

Fig. 7. Right insular nodular calcified stage cysticercosis. (*A*) Axial T1-weighted image demonstrates a hypointense nodular lesion. (*B, C*) Axial T2-weighted image and FLAIR image also demonstrate a hypointense lesion with lack of associated vasogenic edema. (*D*) Postcontrast T1-weighted image demonstrates thin, linear ring enhancement of the lesion. (*E*) Axial CT image shows dense calcification within the lesion.

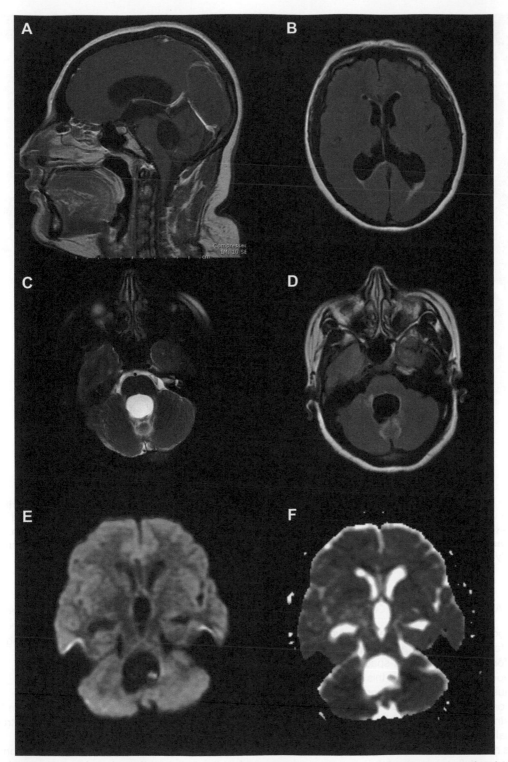

Fig. 8. Intraventricular neurocysticercosis of the fourth ventricle. (*A*) Sagittal postcontrast T1-weighted image shows a large nonenhancing cyst expanding the fourth ventricle, which is isointense relative to CSF. (*B*) Axial FLAIR image demonstrates associated enlargement of ventricular system representing associated hydrocephalus. (*C, D*) T2-weighted image and FLAIR image also reveal the fourth-ventricle cyst as isointense to CSF. FLAIR image shows a thin septation representing the cyst wall. (*E*) DW imaging also demonstrates fourth-ventricle fluid as iso-intense to CSF; however, hyperintense internal nodule is noted representing the scolex. (*F*) ADC map shows low values within the scolex consistent with diffusion restriction.

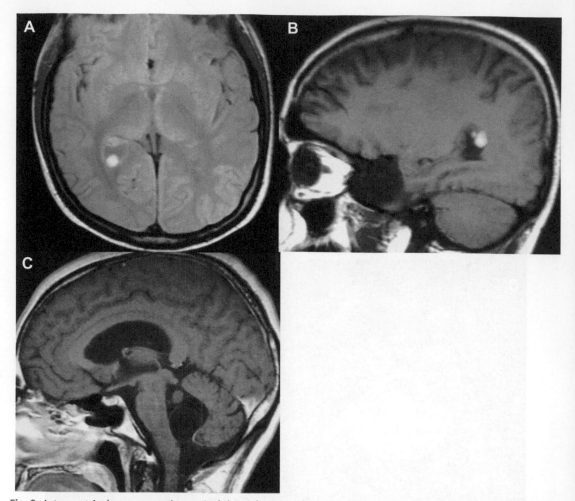

Fig. 9. Intraventricular neurocysticercosis. (*A*) Axial proton density–weighted image demonstrates a hyperintense lesion within the atrium of the right ventricle. (*B*) Sagittal T1-weighted image demonstrates high signal within this lesion. (*C*) Another patient's sagittal T1-weighted image demonstrates a large complex cystic lesion within the fourth ventricle with thin linear walls, small nodule isointense to gray matter, and internal cyst fluid predominantly isointense to CSF.

SPINAL NEUROCYSTICERCOSIS

Neurocysticercosis very rarely involves the spine, with fewer than 1% of all patients diagnosed with this form.[18] Subarachnoid-space neurocysticercosis represents most cases in this region, presumably because of migration of cysticerci from the intracranial compartment.[25] This form of spinal cysticercosis has similar imaging characteristics to those of intracranial subarachnoid neurocysticercosis, and the cysts may be mobile in this region (**Fig. 16**D).[5]

Intramedullary cysticerci are even more uncommon. These cysticerci arise from hemotogenous dissemination of the larva, in similar fashion to parenchymal cysticerci in the brain. The thoracic cord is more frequently involved because of the anatomy of its vascular supply. Similar to other forms of neurocysticercosis, intramedullary cysticercosis may cause direct mass effect and elicit inflammatory response, with resulting cord edema (**Fig. 16**A–C).[26,27]

ORBITAL CYSTICERCOSIS

This rare form of cysticercosis results from larval invasion of the orbit including the globe, extraocular muscles, and the optic nerve.[28,29]

The extraocular muscles are the most common location in the orbit involved by cysticercosis, and may result in myositis with secondary proptosis, diplopia, and pain.[30] Solitary or multiple lesions in this region have been described (**Fig. 17**). Multiple cysticerci in the extraocular muscle may have a "peas-in-the-pod" appearance.

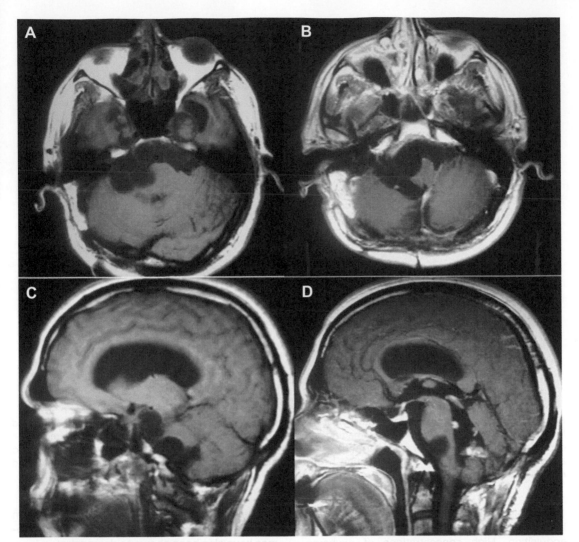

Fig. 10. Coexisting intraventricular and basal cistern neurocysticercosis with involvement of Meckel cave. (*A, B*) Axial T1-weighted images without and with contrast demonstrate numerous cysts distending and distorting the prepontine and perimedullary cisterns and bilateral Meckel caves without significant enhancement. (*C, D*) Sagittal T1-weighted images without and with contrast demonstrate coexisting fourth-ventricle lesions with enhancing components.

Intraocular cysticerci are typically found in the posterior wall of the globe, presumably because of dissemination of the larvae via the choroidal vasculature in this region. As the cyst matures retinal detachment and inflammation may occur, resulting in blindness. These lesions may be hyperintense on T1-weighted imaging and hypointense on T2-weighted imaging, with an MR imaging appearance similar to that of melanoma.

A cysticercus may also be found in the subconjunctival region and vitreous chamber.[29,30] Recently a case of anterior chamber cysticercus with secondary glaucoma has been described.[31]

ADVANCED IMAGING OF NEUROCYSTICERCOSIS
MR Cisternography

Detection of neurocysticercosis lesions can be challenging even on contrast-enhanced MR imaging of the brain, especially for the intraventricular and subarachnoid forms. As already mentioned, high-resolution MR cisternography sequences such as 3D-CISS can be instrumental in the identification and characterization of neurocysticercosis, and should be added to the MR imaging protocol for evaluation of neurocysticercosis.[21]

MR cisternography may also be performed using T2-FLAIR sequence with supplemental

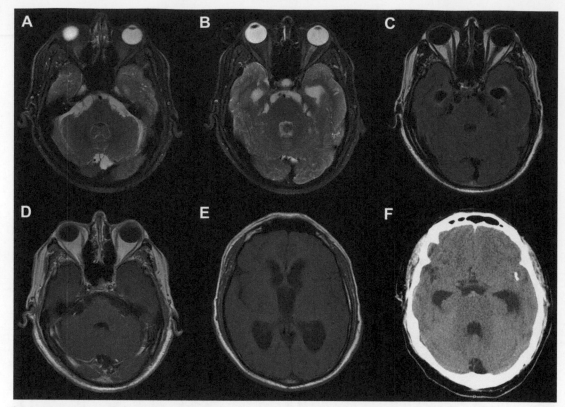

Fig. 11. Coexisting calcified nodular parenchymal and basal cistern "racemose" neurocysticercosis with associated hydrocephalus. (*A–C*) Axial T2-weighted imaging and FLAIR demonstrate distortion and expansion of prepontine cistern and cerebellopontine angle cisterns. (*D, E*) Axial T1-weighted images with and without contrast reveal no abnormal enhancement and communicating hydrocephalus. (*F*) Noncontrast CT reveals a coexisting calcified nodular parenchymal lesion.

100% O_2. Supplemental oxygen is administered to the patient for 5 minutes before FLAIR sequence acquisition. High concentrations of oxyhemoglobin within the CSF result in increased signal intensity of normal CSF on FLAIR images in basal cisterns and sulci of cerebral convexities.[32] This approach may allow visualization of subtle subarachnoid lesions in these locations.[33]

MR Spectroscopy

Neurocysticercosis may appear similar to metastatic disease on conventional MR imaging when multiple parenchymal lesions are identified in vesicular colloidal or granular nodular stages. [1]H nuclear MR spectroscopy of the cysticercal fluid has been shown to demonstrate elevated choline, lactate, succinate, alanine, lipid, and acetate, and decreased creatine and N-acetylaspartate.[34,35] However, similar MR spectroscopy findings may be seen in pyogenic abscesses and other infections.[34]

A large, sharp singlet resonance of pyruvate has been demonstrated in racemose neurocysticercosis.[36] Pyruvate may be further metabolized to acetate and lactate, producing the spectrum described in parenchymal cysticerci.[36] Tuberculomas have also been shown to demonstrate a large lipid resonance, as have some colloid cystic cysticerci.[37]

MR spectroscopy can be useful in differentiating neurocysticercosis from a necrotic neoplasm by sampling the nonenhancing portion of the lesion. In contrast to the cysticercal spectra already described, the necrotic regions in metastases and other neoplasms demonstrate only lactate and lipid peaks. However, when enhancing portions of the lesion are sampled, differentiation of cysticercus from neoplasm may be difficult because both lesions may demonstrate elevated choline and decreased N-acetylaspartate.[38,39] Differentiation of neurocysticercosis from other infections is difficult with MR spectroscopy; however, DW imaging can be used for this propose.

Diffusion-Weighted Imaging

A DW imaging sequence typically demonstrates marked hyperintensity within a pyogenic abscess.

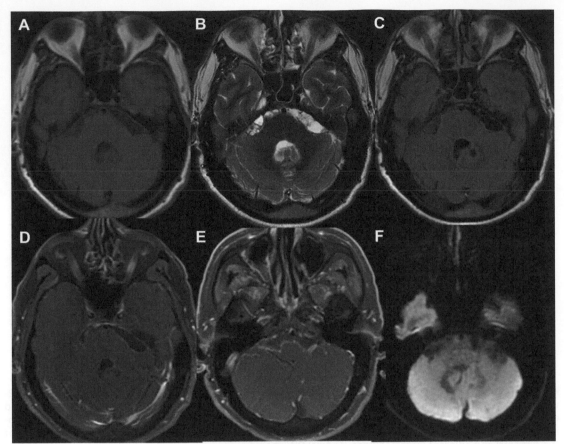

Fig. 12. MR imaging of basal cisterns racemose cysticercosis. (*A, C*) Axial T1-weighted image and FLAIR image reveal expansion and distortion of prepontine cistern. (*B*) Axial T2-weighted image reveals multiple septations within prepontine cisterns representing numerous subarachnoid cysts. (*D, E*) Postcontrast T1-weighted images demonstrate leptomeningeal enhancement of the pons and medulla representing meningeal inflammation. (*F*) Axial DW image shows no diffusion restriction.

Corresponding apparent diffusion coefficient (ADC) values are low, representing diffusion restriction within the abscess.[40]

Neurocysticercosis lesions on DW imaging sequence appear isointense to slightly hyperintense to CSF. ADC demonstrates high values, similar to CSF.[13,22] This finding represents absent diffusion restriction (see **Fig. 8**E, F), with occasional T2 shine-through effect (see **Fig. 4**).

Perfusion-Weighted Imaging

MR perfusion imaging using dynamic susceptibility contrast (DSC) techniques is a sensitive tool for analyzing microvascular pathology. Neoangiogenesis within the vascular network of a brain neoplasm can be detected as elevation of relative cerebral blood volume (rCBV) within the lesion.

By contrast, inflammatory lesions such as neurocysticercosis demonstrate no significant rCBV

elevation, reflecting absence of neoangiogenesis and hyperperfusion.[41,42]

When using this method, the enhancing portions of the lesion are sampled. This technique may help to differentiate a cysticercus from metastases or primary brain neoplasms.

Recently, the integration of multiple advanced imaging methods into a single imaging strategy was proposed.[43] This strategy may allow for differentiation of intracranial lesions by systematically applying advanced imaging techniques. Using a similar approach may allow neurocysticercosis to be differentiated from neoplasm and pyogenic abscess.

TREATMENT

Antiepileptic and anti-inflammatory medications are frequently used for symptomatic treatment.

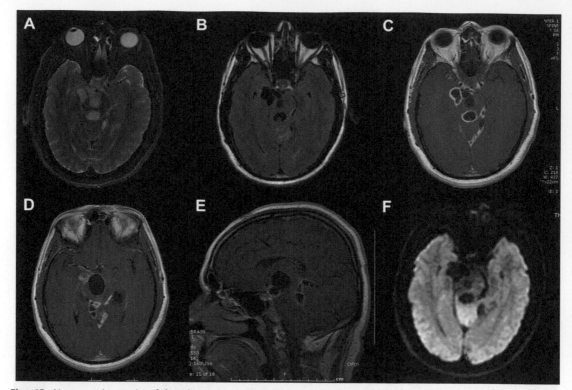

Fig. 13. Neurocysticercosis of basal cisterns with associated leptomeningeal inflammation. (*A, B*) Axial T2-weighted and FLAIR images demonstrate multiple cysts within interpeduncular, suprasellar, ambient, and quadrigeminal-plate cisterns with secondary displacement and distortion of adjacent structures. The cysts are iso-intense to CSF. (*C–E*) Axial and sagittal postcontrast T1-weighted imaging reveals ring enhancement of many of the cysticerci and adjacent leptomeninges. (*F*) Axial DW imaging sequence demonstrates lack of diffusion restriction within the cysts.

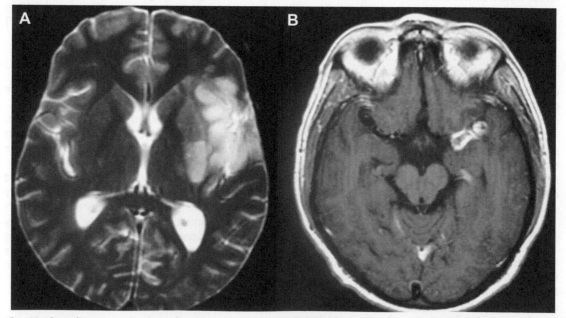

Fig. 14. Complications of subarachnoid cysticercosis. (*A*) Axial T2-weighted image demonstrates right middle cerebral artery (MCA)-territory acute infarct with associated T2 hyperintensity and sulcal effacement. (*B*) Postcontrast axial T1-weighted image demonstrates a region of enhancement of the left M1 segment of the MCA within the Sylvian fissure representing arteritis with secondary occlusion of the vessel.

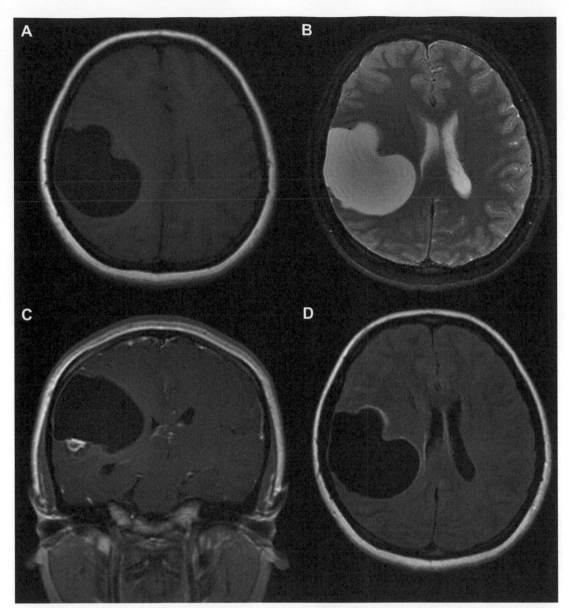

Fig. 15. Large right Sylvian fissure neurocysticercosis cyst. (*A, B, D*) Axial T1-weighted image, T2-weighted image, and FLAIR image demonstrate a very large cyst originating in the right Sylvian fissure with marked associated expansion of the fissure, mass effect, and midline shift. Cyst fluid is isointense relative to CSF. (*C*) Coronal post-contrast T1-weighted image demonstrates a small region of nodular enhancement at the inferior aspect of the cyst and lack of cyst wall enhancement.

Surgical intervention may be required in cases of hydrocephalus and intracranial hypertension.

The use of antiparasitic drugs in neurocysticercosis has been a subject of controversy. These agents are effective at destroying the parasites; however, dying larvae may induce an inflammatory response and result in complications.[6] For the parenchymal form with viable cysts (vesicular stage), albendazole or praziquantel are administered and may be combined with an anti-

inflammatory agent to reduce the edema generated by dying larvae. This therapy has been shown to reduce seizures.[4,44]

Degenerating cysticerci (colloid vesicular and granular nodular stages) may not need antiparasitic therapy and will improve with anti-inflammatory therapy alone. Calcified lesions usually require no treatment.

Subarachnoid cysticercosis may be treated with shunting, corticosteroids, and antiparasitic

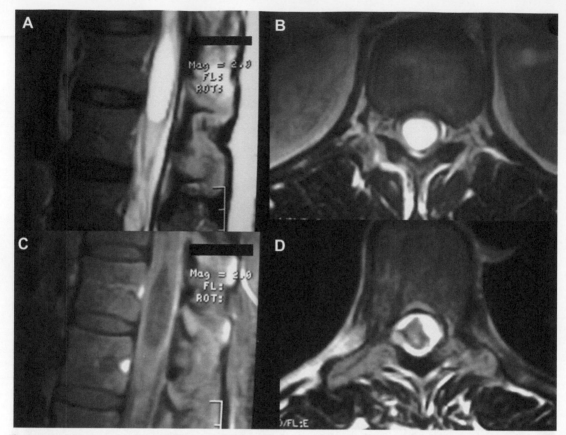

Fig. 16. MR imaging of intramedullary and subarachnoid spinal cysticercosis. (*A, B*) Sagittal and axial T2-weighted image demonstrates an intramedullary cyst in thoracic cord. (*C*) Postcontrast sagittal T1-weighted image demonstrates no enhancement of the cysticercus. (*D*) Axial T2-weighted image demonstrates multiple intradural extramedullary hyperintense cysticerci.

medication.[6,45] Intraventricular cysticercosis may be treated with shunting alone. However, surgical resection of intraventricular lesions may be necessary in selected cases.[20]

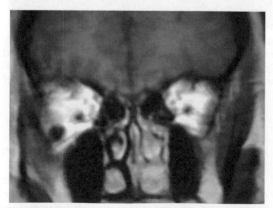

Fig. 17. MR imaging of orbital cysticercosis. Coronal T1-weighted postcontrast image demonstrates a nonenhancing hypointense lesion in the right orbit adjacent to the right lateral rectus muscle, which represents a calcified cysticercosis lesion.

REFERENCES

1. Wallin MT, Kurtzke JF. Neurocysticercosis in the United States: review of an important emerging infection. Neurology 2004;63:1559–64.
2. Garcia HH, Gonzalez AE, Evans CA, et al. *Taenia solium* cysticercosis. Lancet 2003;362:547–56.
3. White AC Jr. Neurocysticercosis: updates on epidemiology, pathogenesis, diagnosis, and management. Annu Rev Med 2000;51:187–206.
4. Garcia HH, Evans CA, Nash TE, et al. Current consensus guidelines for treatment of neurocysticercosis. 10.1128/CMR.15.4.747-756.2002. Clin Microbiol Rev 2002;15:747–56.
5. Castillo M. Imaging of neurocysticercosis. Semin Roentgenol 2004;39:465–73.
6. Garcia HH, Del Brutto OH, Nash TE, et al. New concepts in the diagnosis and management of neurocysticercosis (*Taenia solium*). Am J Trop Med Hyg 2005;72:3–9.
7. Garcia HH, Del Brutto OH. Neurocysticercosis: updated concepts about an old disease. Lancet Neurol 2005;4:653–61.

8. Amaral L, Maschietto M, Maschietto R, et al. Unusual manifestations of neurocysticercosis in MR imaging: analysis of 172 cases. Arq Neuropsiquiatr 2003;61:533–41.

9. Noujaim SE, Rossi MD, Rao SK, et al. CT and MR imaging of neurocysticercosis. AJR Am J Roentgenol 1999;173:1485–90.

10. Zee CS, Go JL, Kim PE, et al. Imaging of neurocysticercosis. Neuroimaging Clin N Am 2000;10:391–407.

11. Zoe CS, Segall HD, Boswell W, et al. MR imaging of neurocysticercosis. J Comput Assist Tomogr 1988; 12:927–34.

12. Tsuchiya K, Inaoka S, Mizutani Y, et al. Fast fluid-attenuated inversion-recovery MR of intracranial infections. AJNR Am J Neuroradiol 1997;18: 909–13.

13. Raffin LS, Bacheschi LA, Machado LR, et al. Diffusion-weighted MR imaging of cystic lesions of neurocysticercosis: a preliminary study. Arq Neuropsiquiatr 2001;59:839–42.

14. Sheth TN, Pillon L, Keystone J, et al. Persistent MR contrast enhancement of calcified neurocysticercosis lesions. AJNR Am J Neuroradiol 1998;19: 79–82.

15. Nash TE, Pretell EJ, Lescano AG, et al. Perilesional brain oedema and seizure activity in patients with calcified neurocysticercosis: a prospective cohort and nested case-control study. Lancet Neurol 2008;7:1099–105.

16. Nash TE, Pretell J, Garcia HH. Calcified cysticerci provoke perilesional edema and seizures. Clin Infect Dis 2001;33:1649–53.

17. Ginier BL, Poirier VC. MR imaging of intraventricular cysticercosis. AJNR Am J Neuroradiol 1992;13: 1247–8.

18. Shandera WX, White AC Jr, Chen JC, et al. Neurocysticercosis in Houston, Texas. A report of 112 cases. Medicine (Baltimore) 1994;73:37–52.

19. Zee CS, Segall HD, Destian S, et al. MRI of intraventricular cysticercosis: surgical implications. J Comput Assist Tomogr 1993;17:932–9.

20. Zee CS, Segall HD, Apuzzo ML, et al. Intraventricular cysticercal cysts: further neuroradiologic observations and neurosurgical implications. AJNR Am J Neuroradiol 1984;5:727–30.

21. Govindappa SS, Narayanan JP, Krishnamoorthy VM, et al. Improved detection of intraventricular cysticercal cysts with the use of three-dimensional constructive interference in steady state MR sequences. AJNR Am J Neuroradiol 2000;21:679–84.

22. do Amaral LL, Ferreira RM, da Rocha AJ, et al. Neurocysticercosis: evaluation with advanced magnetic resonance techniques and atypical forms. Top Magn Reson Imaging 2005;16:127–44.

23. Garcia HH, Del Brutto OH. Taenia solium cysticercosis. Infect Dis Clin North Am 2000;14:97–119, ix.

24. Creasy JL, Alarcon JJ. Magnetic resonance imaging of neurocysticercosis. Top Magn Reson Imaging 1994;6:59–68.

25. Torabi AM, Quiceno M, Mendelsohn DB, et al. Multilevel intramedullary spinal neurocysticercosis with eosinophilic meningitis. Arch Neurol 2004;61: 770–2.

26. Parmar H, Shah J, Patwardhan V, et al. MR imaging in intramedullary cysticercosis. Neuroradiology 2001;43:961–7.

27. Castillo M, Quoncer RM, Post MJ. MR of intramedullary spinal cysticercosis. AJNR Am J Neuroradiol 1988;9:393–5.

28. Kaufman LM, Villablanca JP, Mafee MF. Diagnostic imaging of cystic lesions in the child's orbit. Radiol Clin North Am 1998;36:1149–63, xi.

29. Chandra S, Vashisht S, Menon V, et al. Optic nerve cysticercosis: imaging findings. AJNR Am J Neuroradiol 2000;21:198–200.

30. Pushker N, Bajaj MS, Chandra M, et al. Ocular and orbital cysticercosis. Acta Ophthalmol Scand 2001; 79:408–13.

31. Chandra A, Singh MK, Singh VP, et al. A live cysticercosis in anterior chamber leading to glaucoma secondary to pupillary block. J Glaucoma 2007;16: 271–3.

32. Braga FT, da Rocha AJ, Hernandez Filho G, et al. Relationship between the concentration of supplemental oxygen and signal intensity of CSF depicted by fluid-attenuated inversion recovery imaging. AJNR Am J Neuroradiol 2003;24:1863–8.

33. Braga F, Rocha AJ, Gomes HR, et al. Noninvasive MR cisternography with fluid-attenuated inversion recovery and 100% supplemental O(2) in the evaluation of neurocysticercosis. AJNR Am J Neuroradiol 2004;25:295–7.

34. Chang KH, Song IC, Kim SH, et al. In vivo single-voxel proton MR spectroscopy in intracranial cystic masses. AJNR Am J Neuroradiol 1998;19: 401–5.

35. Pandit S, Lin A, Gahbauer H, et al. MR spectroscopy in neurocysticercosis. J Comput Assist Tomogr 2001;25:950–2.

36. Jayakumar PN, Chandrashekar HS, Srikanth SG, et al. MRI and in vivo proton MR spectroscopy in a racemose cysticercal cyst of the brain. Neuroradiology 2004;46:72–4.

37. Pretell EJ, Martinot C Jr, Garcia HH, et al. Differential diagnosis between cerebral tuberculosis and neurocysticercosis by magnetic resonance spectroscopy. J Comput Assist Tomogr 2005;29:112–4.

38. Law M. MR spectroscopy of brain tumors. Top Magn Reson Imaging 2004;15:291–313.

39. Lai PH, Ho JT, Chen WL, et al. Brain abscess and necrotic brain tumor: discrimination with proton MR spectroscopy and diffusion-weighted imaging. AJNR Am J Neuroradiol 2002;23:1369–77.

40. Ebisu T, Tanaka C, Umeda M, et al. Discrimination of brain abscess from necrotic or cystic tumors by diffusion-weighted echo planar imaging. Magn Reson Imaging 1996;14:1113–6.

41. Cha S, Knopp EA, Johnson G, et al. Intracranial mass lesions: dynamic contrast-enhanced susceptibility-weighted echo-planar perfusion MR imaging. Radiology 2002;223:11–29.

42. Lev MH, Rosen BR. Clinical applications of intracranial perfusion MR imaging. Neuroimaging Clin N Am 1999;9:309–31.

43. Al-Okaili RN, Krejza J, Woo JH, et al. Intraaxial brain masses: MR imaging-based diagnostic strategy—initial experience. Radiology 2007;243: 539–50.

44. Garcia HH, Gonzalez AE, Gilman RH. Diagnosis, treatment and control of *Taenia solium* cysticercosis. Curr Opin Infect Dis 2003;16:411–9.

45. Proano JV, Madrazo I, Avelar F, et al. Medical treatment for neurocysticercosis characterized by giant subarachnoid cysts. N Engl J Med 2001;345: 879–85.

Central Nervous System Tuberculosis
Pathophysiology and Imaging Findings

Deepak Patkar, MD[a,*], Jayant Narang, MD[a,b],
Rama Yanamandala, MD[a], Malini Lawande, MD[a],
Gaurang V. Shah, MD[c]

KEYWORDS

- CNS tuberculosis • Tuberculoma • Intracranial infection • Spinal tuberculosis

KEY POINTS

- Tuberculosis (TB) is a global clinical concern, particularly after the human immunodeficiency virus pandemic.
- Imaging, particularly magnetic resonance imaging, is a cornerstone in the diagnosis as well as follow-up of central nervous system (CNS) tuberculosis.
- Imaging appearance of CNS TB is becoming more and more complex and atypical with the onset of multidrug-resistant tuberculosis.
- Early, accurate diagnosis can help in preventing morbidity and mortality.
- Newer imaging techniques like magnetic resonance spectroscopy help to improve characterization and thus aid in diagnosis of atypical CNS TB.

INTRODUCTION

Tuberculosis (TB) remains a prominent global problem especially because of the increasing incidence of human immunodeficiency virus (HIV) and drug-resistant strains, although its incidence seems to have declined recently.[1] According to the World Health Organization report, 1.3 million deaths were caused by TB in 2008, which is equivalent to 20 deaths per 10,000 population.[2] Among all other forms of TB, central nervous system (CNS) TB accounts for approximately 1% and has the highest mortality.[3] Although diagnostic evaluation includes various microbiological, pathologic, molecular, and biochemical investigations,[4] imaging modalities have an important diagnostic role. Imaging helps in early diagnosis and helps in preventing morbidity and mortality. Imaging is essential in showing complications in addition to diagnosis of CNS TB.[5]

PATHOGENESIS

Mycobacterium TB is the most common organism causing tuberculous infection of CNS. Other species of mycobacteria may be involved in immunocompromised patients.[6] Based on the observations of Rich and McCordock,[6] a 2-step model has been proposed for the pathogenesis of CNS TB. During the initial pulmonary infection, tuberculous bacteria may enter the systemic circulation and subsequently reach the oxygen-rich CNS, establishing a focus called the Rich focus. This focus may be in the meninges, subpial or subependymal

[a] Department of MRI and CT scan, MRI Center, Dr Balabhai Nanavati Hospital, S.V. Road, Vile-Parle (West), Mumbai-400 056, India; [b] Department of Neuroradiology, Henry Ford Health System, 2799 West Grand Blvd, Detroit, MI 48202, USA; [c] Department of Radiology, University of Michigan Health System, 1500 E medical center Drive, Ann Arbor, MI 48109, USA
* Corresponding author.
E-mail address: drdppatkar@gmail.com

Neuroimag Clin N Am 22 (2012) 677–705
doi:10.1016/j.nic.2012.05.006

region of the brain, or the spinal cord. Later, this may rupture into the subarachnoid space or ventricular system leading to meningitis.[7] The probability of the organism reaching the brain depends on the extent of bacteremia and the immune response of the host.[8,9]

Meninges may be secondarily involved because of rupture of a tuberculoma into a vessel in the subarachnoid space, or rupture of miliary tubercles in miliary TB. There can be contiguous spread of infection from the adjacent bone. but this is uncommon. Cell-mediated immunity is responsible for the formation of dense, gelatinous, inflammatory exudate along the basal surface of the cerebrum. Severe cases may show leptomeningeal involvement over the cerebral convexities, and extension into the ventricular system can cause ependymitis and choroid plexitis. Parenchymal tuberculous focus can develop into tuberculoma or brain abscess in the absence of adequate immunity or in the presence of a sizable tuberculous focus.[10–15]

Imaging of CNS TB can be divided into types of involvement, as listed in **Box 1**.

TUBERCULOUS MENINGITIS
Tuberculous Leptomeningitis

After reaching the subarachnoid space, tuberculous focus leads to formation of thick, gelatinous, inflammatory exudate. It affects basal cisterns, sylvian fissures, and, rarely, leptomeninges over cerebral convexities. The exudate in the basal cisterns can cause obstruction to cerebrospinal fluid (CSF) flow, causing hydrocephalus, and can compress cranial nerves. Cerebral infarction can occur because of obliterative vasculitis, the vessels at the base of the brain being severely affected. Granulomas may coalesce to form tuberculomas or, rarely, an abscess.[1,14] Thus, common imaging triad includes abnormal meningeal enhancement predominantly in the basal regions of brain and its associated complications of hydrocephalus and infarcts. This triad is specific for the diagnosis of TBM.[16]

Kumar and colleagues[16] found that the presence of basal enhancement, hydrocephalus, tuberculoma, and infarction were more common in TBM than in children with pyogenic meningitis. They reported that basal enhancement, tuberculomas, or both were 100% specific and 89% sensitive for the diagnosis of TBM.[17] Andronikou and colleagues[17] suggested 9 criteria for the diagnosis of TBM on computed tomography (CT). Przybojewski and colleagues[18] evaluated these 9 criteria and showed high specificity for all the criteria, and 100% specificity for 4 individual

---

Box 1
Types of CNS TB involvement

Intracranial TB
- Meningeal TB
  - Tuberculous leptomeningitis
  - Pachymeningeal TB
- Complications of TB meningitis (TBM)
  - Hydrocephalus
  - Tuberculous vasculitis
  - Cranial nerve involvement
- Sequel of TBM
- Parenchymal TB
  - Tuberculomas
  - Tuberculous abscess
  - Tuberculous cerebritis
  - Tuberculous encephalopathy

Intraspinal TB
- Typical spinal TB
  - Spondylodiscitis
- Atypical spinal TB
  - Intramedullary TB
  - Solitary vertebral body involvement
  - Pure posterior-element TB
  - Tubercular arachnoiditis

---

criteria. It has been shown that sensitivity has been improved when more than 1 criterion was present.[19] Presence of hyperdensity on precontrast scans in the basal cisterns might be the specific sign of TBM in children.[18]

Magnetic resonance (MR) imaging has been shown to be superior to CT in evaluating patients with suspected meningitis and its associated complications.[20,21] In the early stages, noncontrast MR imaging shows little or no evidence of meningitis. Mild shortening of T1 and T2 relaxation times of CSF occurs as the disease progresses. Contrast-enhanced MR imaging has the added advantage of showing meningitis and its associated complications compared with contrast-enhanced CT and noncontrast MR imaging.[21–24] Abnormal meningeal enhancement is seen in the basal cisterns, and sylvian fissures, and severe and late-stage TBM can show enhancement over the convexities (**Fig. 1**). Tentorial and cerebellar meningeal involvement is less common.[22,25]

Minimal or absent meningeal enhancement has been reported in patients with acquired immune deficiency syndrome (AIDS) by some investigators, likely caused by the lack of immunologic response.[26] In contrast, others have reported no significant difference in the imaging appearances in these patients compared with immunocompetent patients.[27] Classic features of basal exudates, hydrocephalus, infarcts, and granulomas may not be seen in the elderly population, which has been attributed to age-related senescence of the immune system.[28]

Magnetic transfer (MT) MR imaging is an important technique and is considered superior to conventional MR imaging for showing abnormal meninges.[29] It also helps in differentiating tuberculous meningitis from other causes of meningitis.[29–31] On MT imaging, abnormal meninges appearing hyperintense on precontrast T1-weighted (T1W) MT images is considered to strongly suggest tuberculous meningitis. Also, the MT ratio (MTR) is significantly different from brain parenchyma and inflamed meninges, because the inflammatory exudate in TBM is composed of cellular infiltrate, degenerated and partially caseated fibrin, tubercles, and, less commonly, bacilli.[29]

Border Zone Encephalitis

The brain parenchyma immediately adjacent to the inflammatory exudate shows edema, perivascular infiltration, and a microglial reaction, known as border zone reaction (**Fig. 2**). Identification of border zone encephalitis is difficult because the hyperintense T2 signal in these regions merges with the bright signal of the leptomeningeal exudate.[11,13,32]

Complications of meningitis include hydrocephalus, vasculitis, cranial nerve involvement, and associated multiple tuberculomas.

HYDROCEPHALUS

Hydrocephalus can be communicating, noncommunicating, or complex in patients with TBM. Tubercular hydrocephalus is usually communicating, accounting for 80% of cases.[33] It occurs because of obstruction to CSF flow in the basal cisterns by inflammatory exudate (**Fig. 3**). Noncommunicating or obstructive hydrocephalus

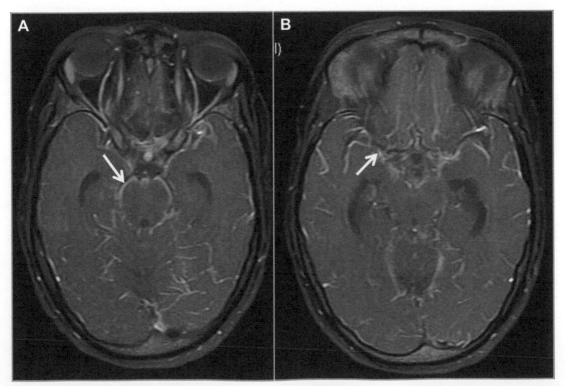

Fig. 1. Tuberculous meningitis. Fat-saturated postcontrast T1-weighted (T1W) images (*A* and *B*) show abnormal meningeal enhancement along the basal cisterns (*arrows*).

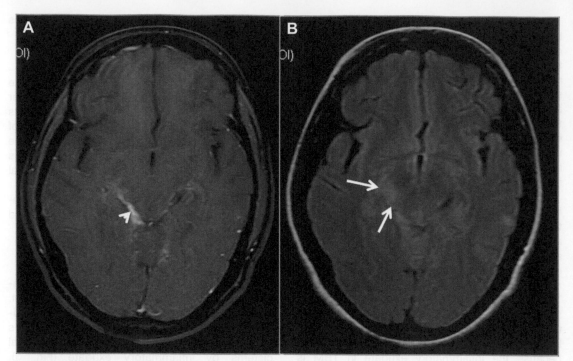

Fig. 2. Border zone encephalitis: postcontrast T1W image (*A*) shows abnormal enhancement along the right peri-mesencephalic cistern (*arrowhead*). Fluid-attenuated inversion recovery (FLAIR) image (*B*) shows the edema in the brain parenchyma immediately adjacent to the exudate (*arrows*), known as 'border zone reaction' or 'border zone encephalitis'.

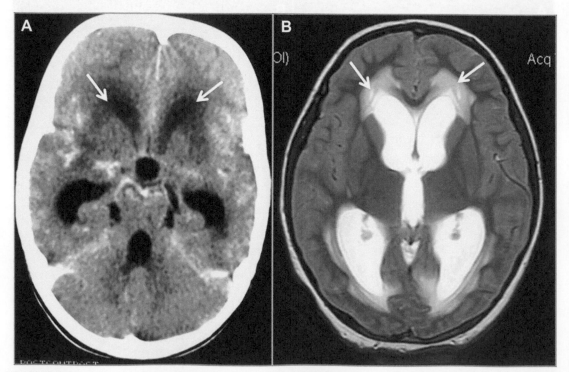

Fig. 3. Hydrocephalus. In a known case of TB meningitis, contrast-enhanced CT scan (*A*) and T2-weighted (T2W) MR imaging (*B*) show moderate communicating hydrocephalus with periventricular ooze (*arrows*).

can occur either because of obstruction of fourth ventricular outlet foramina by the basal exudates or mass effect by a focal parenchymal tuberculoma, because of brain abscess, or because of entrapment of part of a ventricle by ependymitis[14,34,35] (**Fig. 4**). Periventricular hypodensity on CT and periventricular hyperintense signal on proton density and T2-weighted (T2W) images on MR imaging indicate interstitial edema caused by periventricular ooze of CSF secondary to increase in intraventricular pressure.[13,36]

Complex hydrocephalus can be seen in TB with a combination of noncommunicating (obstructive) and communicating (defective absorption) hydrocephalus (**Fig. 5**). Yadav and colleagues[36] reported a high incidence of complex hydrocephalus in patients with TBM and found it to be a cause of failure of endoscopic third ventriculostomy.[37]

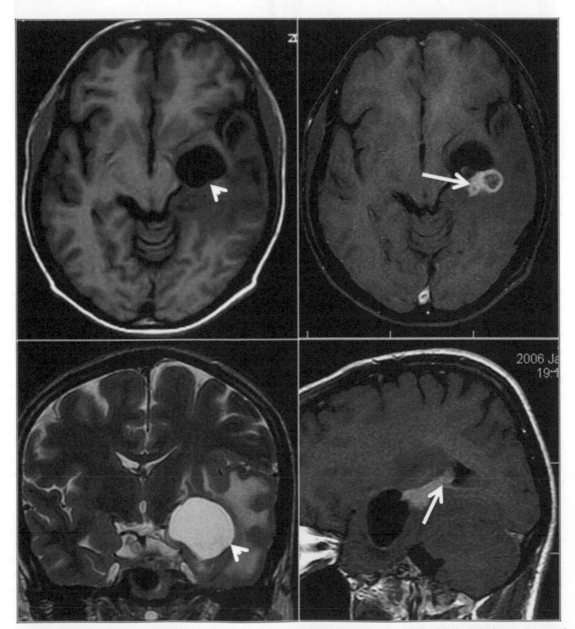

Fig. 4. Trapped ventricle: in a known case of TB meningitis with tuberculomas, MR scan reveals focal abnormal enhancement (*arrows*) representing a combination of conglomerate tuberculomas and ependymitis, leading to isolated dilatation of the temporal horn of the left lateral ventricle (*arrowheads*).

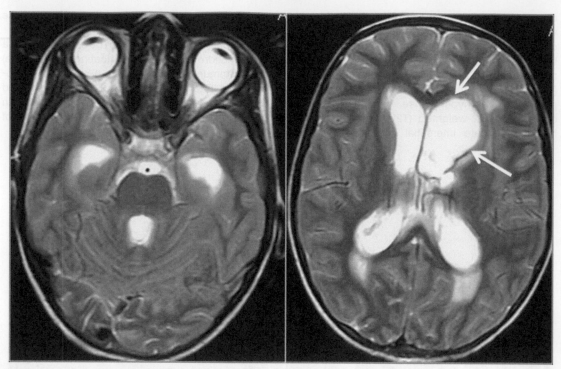

Fig. 5. Complex hydrocephalus. In a follow-up case of TB meningitis, T2W axial images show disproportionate enlargement of the left lateral ventricle (*arrows*) suggesting a complex hydrocephalus.

It is important to determine the type of hydrocephalus and the site of obstruction to define the optimal treatment option and also because of the possible complication of cerebral herniation in noncommunicating hydrocephalus. In addition, the type of hydrocephalus predicts the outcome of endoscopic third ventriculostomy.[38–41] CT cannot predict the level of CSF block in TBM because both types of hydrocephalus can present with panventricular dilatation.[42]

MR imaging, with its newer sequences, helps in differentiating the type of hydrocephalus and provides most details of brain and CSF pathways. Qualitative and quantitative information of CSF flow and dynamics can be obtained by MR imaging. The disadvantage of MR imaging is that the flow around the fourth ventricle may not easily be evaluated. In addition, MR imaging may not be readily available in resource-poor countries where TB is more common.[38,43] MR imaging also plays an important role in the postoperative evaluation of patients with endoscopic third ventriculostomy.[44]

Radiograph/CT pneumoencephalography or contrast-enhanced cisternography done via lumbar puncture may help in differentiating communicating and noncommunicating hydrocephalus. However, because these techniques are invasive and may be associated with complications, they should be used only if MR imaging is not available.[38] MR ventriculography has been used to evaluate CSF flow dynamics and in patients with hydrocephalus.[45,46]

VASCULITIS

The basal exudates cause inflammatory changes in the vessels predominantly involving the circle of Willis. At first, the vessel wall is involved, and later the lumen of the vessel, leading to complete occlusion by reactive subendothelial cellular proliferation and thrombus formation. Middle cerebral and lenticulostriate arteries are the most common vessels involved.[47,48] The conventional angiographic features of TBM include a triad of a hydrocephalic pattern, narrowing of arteries at the base of the brain, and narrowed or occluded small or medium-sized arteries with early draining veins.[49] CT or MR angiogram reveal small segmental narrowing, uniform narrowing of large segments, irregular beaded appearance of vessels, or complete occlusion (**Fig. 6**).[22,48] Gadolinium-enhanced MR angiogram is more sensitive to detect the involvement of smaller vessels.[50]

The reported incidence of infarcts on CT varies from 20.5% to 38%. MR imaging detects a greater

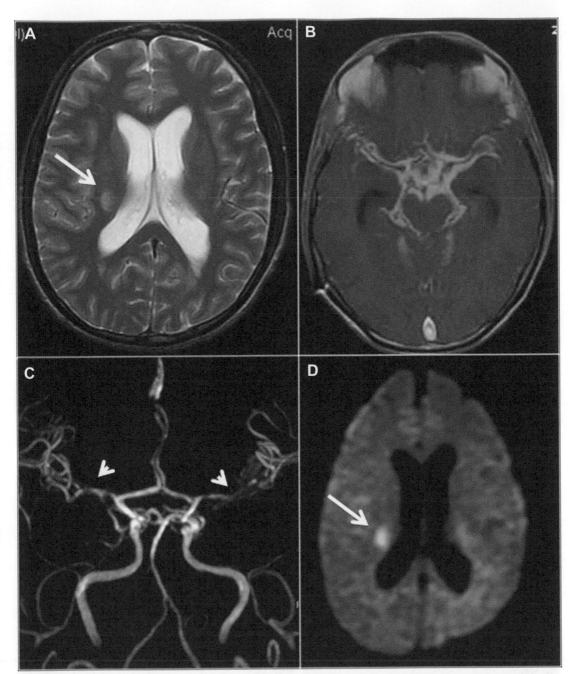

Fig. 6. TB vasculitis with acute infarct. A 32-year-old patient presented with severe headaches and left-sided hemiparesis. T2W images (*A*) show a small hyperintense area in the right corona radiata that shows restricted diffusion (*D*) suggesting an acute infarct (*arrows*). Postcontrast T1W axial image (*B*) shows extensive basal exudates encasing the circle of Willis. A maximum-intensity projection image of three-dimensional time-of-flight MR angiogram of circle of Willis (*C*) shows irregular narrowing of both middle cerebral arteries (*arrowheads*).

number of infarcts and hemorrhagic transformation of infarcts than CT.[50] Most infarcts involve thalamus, basal ganglia, and internal capsule regions.[48,51,52] Nair and colleagues[51] described the MR imaging pattern of infarcts in TB. Anterior

distribution, particularly in the caudate nucleus and in the presence of multiple infarcts, favored a tuberculous cause, and posterior distribution indicated the possibility of associated risk factors of stroke.[52] Diffusion-weighted MR imaging helps in early detection of infarction and in delineating the extent of infarction, which is of value in the management and prognostication of patients.[51]

CRANIAL NERVE INVOLVEMENT

Cranial nerve involvement in TBM is seen in 17% to 70% of patients. Nerve involvement occurs

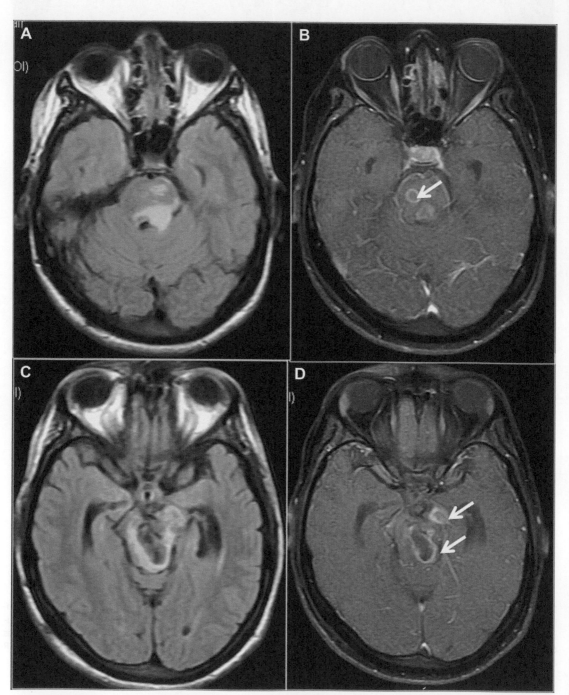

Fig. 7. TBM with cranial nerve involvement. A 43-year-old woman presenting with altered mental status and features of multiple cranial nerve involvement (in particular left fifth and seventh). Postcontrast T1W axial images (*B* and *D*) show multiple enhancing tuberculomas (*arrows*) in the brainstem as well in the adjoining cisterns. Corresponding FLAIR images (*A* and *C*) show extensive brainstem edema. Involvement of the cranial nerve nuclei or direct mass effect of a tuberculoma on the cisternal portion of the nerve may have been the mechanism of involvement.

because of ischemia of the nerve or entrapment of the nerve in basal exudates.[22,53] Direct mass effect of a tuberculoma on the nerve within the subarachnoid course or by direct involvement of the cranial nerve nuclei in the brain are the other mechanisms (**Fig. 7**).[22] Fibrotic changes in the late stage can cause permanent loss of function in these nerves.[13]

The affected nerve shows thickening and enhancement on postcontrast images. The

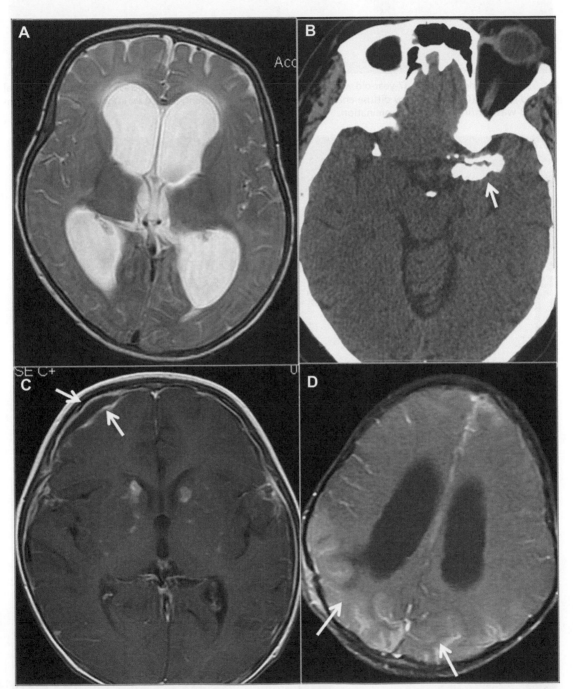

Fig. 8. Sequel of TB meningitis in 4 different patients. (*A*) T2W MR imaging showing moderate communicating hydrocephalus. (*B*) Nonenhanced CT scan showing calcifications in the suprasellar cistern regions (*arrow*). (*C*) Postcontrast T1W MR imaging reveals subdural empyema (*arrows*) separate from evidence of TB meningitis and bilateral basal ganglia tuberculomas. (*D*) Postcontrast T1W MR imaging reveals gyral enhancement caused by subacute infarcts in bilateral parieto-occipital region (*arrows*).

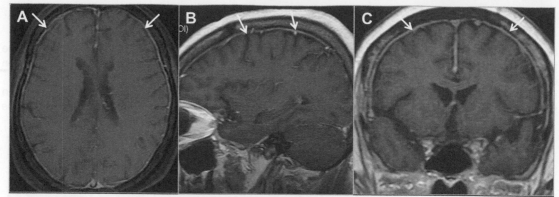

Fig. 9. TB pachymeningitis. A 37-year-old woman presented with headaches. Postcontrast T1W axial (*A*), sagittal (*B*), and coronal (*C*) images show diffuse enhancement of the pachymeninges (*arrows*) suggesting pachymeningitis. TB was confirmed on CSF examination.

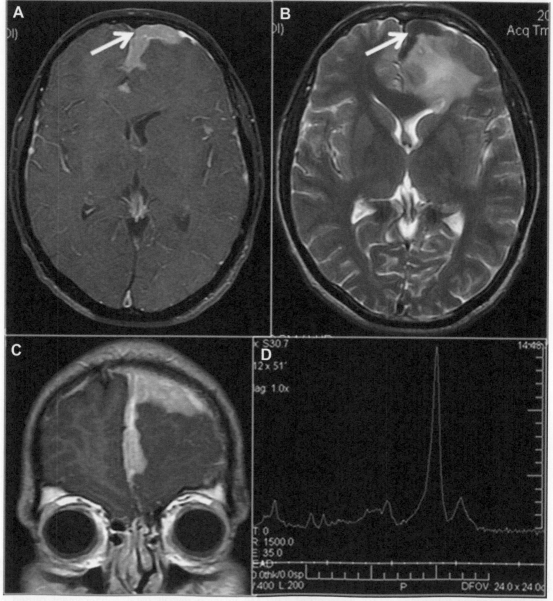

Fig. 10. Epidural en plaque tuberculoma. Axial (*A*) and coronal (*C*) postcontrast T1W images show focal pachymeningeal thickening along the left frontal convexity and interhemispheric fissure (*arrow*). It appears hypointense on T2W images (*B*, *arrow*) and single-voxel MR spectroscopy (*D*) shows a predominant lipid peak.

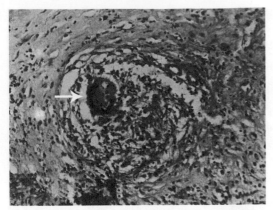

Fig. 11. Photomicrograph of tuberculous granuloma. Multiple large, pale histiocytes with plump cytoplasm are seen in the center. A large central Langhans giant cell (*arrow*) reveals multiple nuclei arranged peripherally in a horseshoe pattern. Areas of caseating necrosis are seen as empty spaces together with mononuclear inflammatory cells. A peripheral collar of fibrocytes and collagen fibers is seen.

proximal portion of the nerve near its root entry is most commonly affected.[22,54] Localization of the cause of cranial nerve involvement, whether confined to the nerve or its brain stem nucleus, may help in prognostication of patients. Brain stem infarcts are less likely to show significant improvement, whereas the disorder confined to the nerve (neuritis/perineuritis) may improve with treatment.[48]

SEQUELAE OF TBM

Focal or diffuse cerebral atrophy and areas of encephalomalacia secondary to infarcts and hydrocephalus (Fig. 8), meningeal or ependymal calcifications, and occasionally syringomyelia or syringobulbia, are the sequelae of TBM.[11,22]

Tuberculous Pachymeningitis

Tuberculous pachymeningitis can be localized or diffuse. Pachymeningeal TB can occur as either isolated dural involvement (Fig. 9) or with associated pial or parenchymal lesions. The term en plaque tuberculoma has been used to describe the focal pachymeningeal lesion (Fig. 10). However, this terminology is used to describe all types of tuberculomas with en plaque morphology, including primary intraparenchymal lesions. The lesions are hyperdense on noncontrast CT scans, isointense to brain on T1W MR imaging, and isointense to hypointense on T2W images with homogeneous postcontrast enhancement. However, similar imaging findings can be seen in various causes of inflammatory and noninflammatory conditions, especially meningioma.[55,56] It is important to diagnose pachymeningeal TB because it responds well to antitubercular treatment and thus should be considered in the differential diagnosis of pachymeningeal abnormalities. If there is evidence of TB elsewhere in the body, it may further suggest the diagnosis.[55,57]

Parenchymal TB

Parenchymal TB can occur in the form of tuberculoma, brain abscess, tuberculous encephalopathy, and tuberculous cerebritis.

Tuberculoma

Tuberculomas are among the most common intracranial mass lesions and the most common

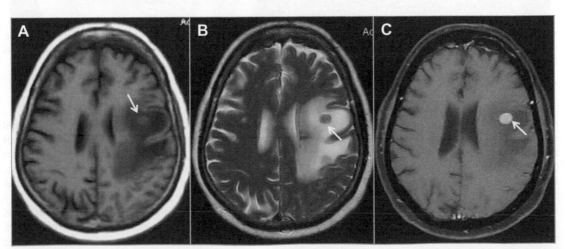

Fig. 12. Noncaseating disc-enhancing tuberculoma. Axial T1W (*A*) and T2W (*B*) images show an oval isointense lesion in the left frontal lobe that shows solid disc enhancement on postcontrast axial T1W image (*C*) (*arrows*).

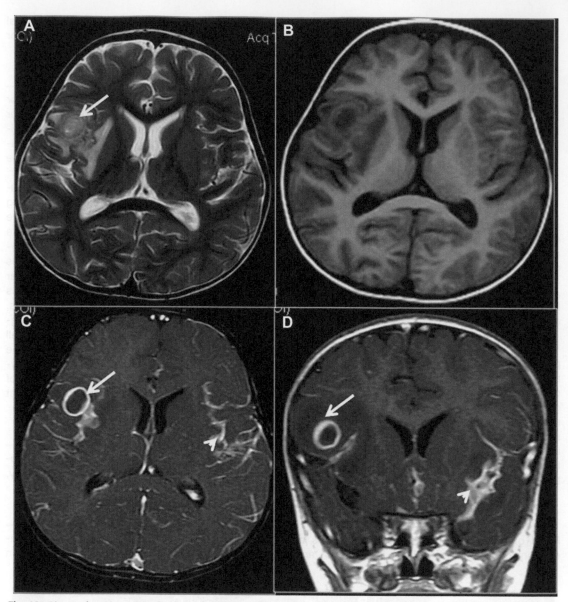

Fig. 13. Ring-enhancing typical tuberculoma. Axial T2W (*A*) and T1W (*B*) images show an oval hypointense lesion in the right perisylvian region. It shows ring enhancement on postcontrast axial (*C*) and coronal (*D*) T1W images (*arrows*).

manifestation of parenchymal TB. Tuberculomas can occur at any age. They can be solitary or multiple and can occur anywhere in the brain parenchyma. In children, they predominate in the infratentorial compartment, whereas, in adults, the supratentorial compartment is more commonly affected.[11,58] Tuberculomas arise when tubercles in the parenchyma of brain enlarge without rupturing into the subarachnoid space. They usually occur in the absence of TBM, but may occur with meningitis because of the extension of CSF

infection into the adjacent parenchyma via cortical veins or Virchow-Robin spaces.[13,34] Presence of tuberculomas at the corticomedullary junction suggests the hematogenous spread of infection, because there is narrowing of the arterioles at the gray/white matter junction.[13,24]

Tuberculomas show typical granulomatous reaction consisting of epithelioid cells, giant cells mixed with mononuclear inflammatory cells (predominantly lymphocytes) forming a noncaseating granuloma. It subsequently develops a central area of caseating necrosis. The central area of necrosis is initially solid and later may liquefy (**Fig. 11**).[11,22,59]

Patients usually present with headache, seizures, focal neurologic deficit, and features of raised intracranial tension. Infratentorial tuberculomas may present with brainstem syndromes, cerebellar symptoms, and multiple cranial nerve palsies.[12,13,60,61]

Imaging findings depend on the stage of tuberculoma, whether it is noncaseating or caseating with solid or liquid center.

On CT, solid noncaseating granuloma is isodense or slightly hypodense to the surrounding brain parenchyma. On MR imaging, it is hypointense on both T1W and T2W images. They show homogeneous enhancement on post contrast scans (**Fig. 12**). A caseating granuloma is isointense to

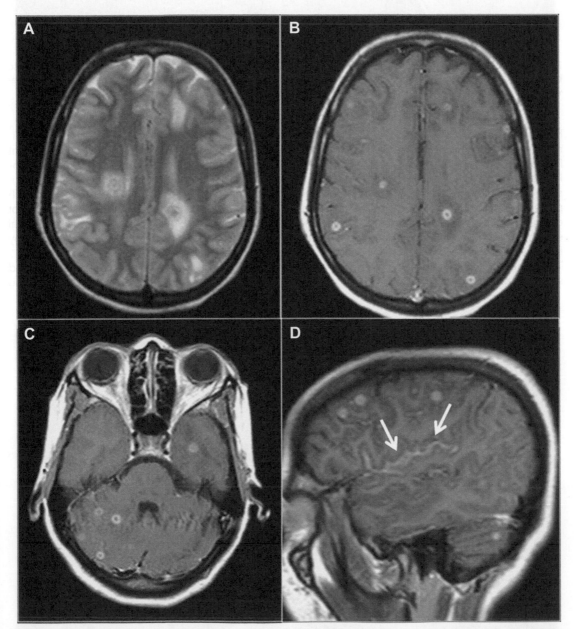

Fig. 14. Miliary TB of the brain: Postcontrast axial T1W images (*B*) and (*C*) show multiple small discs of 2 to 3 mm and ring-enhancing lesions in both cerebral and cerebellar hemispheres. On axial T2W imaging (*A*), these appear isointense to hypointense and show variable mild to no associated vasogenic edema. Postcontrast sagittal T1W image (*D*) shows associated meningeal enhancement as well (*arrows*).

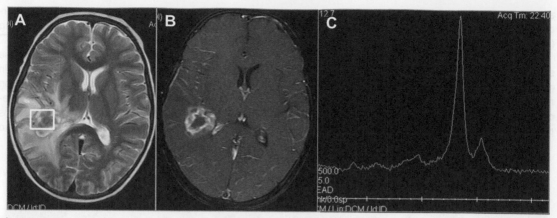

Fig. 15. Spectroscopy signature of tuberculoma. Axial T2W image (*A*) shows a predominantly T2 hypointense lesion (box) with vasogenic edema showing rim enhancement on postcontrast axial T1W image (*B*). Single-voxel MR spectroscopy (*C*) from the center of the lesion shows predominant lipid peak at 1.3 ppm.

hypointense on both T1W and T2W images and shows isointense to hyperintense rim on T2W images. It shows rim enhancement on postcontrast images (**Fig. 13**). The complex relationship between solid caseation, fibrosis/gliosis, macrophages, and perilesional cellular infiltrate dictates the degree of central hypointensity on T2W images. When the solid center liquefies, the center of the granuloma becomes hypodense on CT and hyperintense on T2W images with a peripheral hypointense rim and shows peripheral enhancement.[1,13,22,62]

On CT, presence of target sign, a central calcification or nidus surrounded by ring enhancement on postcontrast images, was considered pathognomonic of tuberculoma.[63] However, recently it has been shown that only the target sign with central calcifications is pathognomonic of tuberculoma, whereas the sign with a central enhancing dot is not necessarily be caused by tuberculoma.[64]

Miliary tuberculomas are usually associated with meningitis and most of these patients have

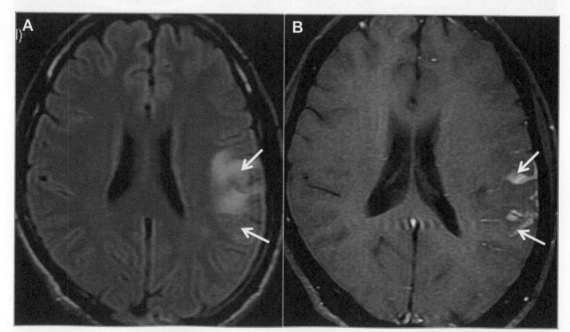

Fig. 16. Tuberculous cerebritis. A 48-year-old man presented with a history of recent-onset generalized convulsions. Axial FLAIR image (*A*) shows an area of vasogenic edema in the left parietal lobe. Postcontrast axial T1W image (*B*) shows patchy gyral enhancement (*arrows*).

a primary pulmonary focus of infection.[1,13,22] They are usually less than 2 to 5 mm in size (**Fig. 14**) and are usually seen as tiny hyperintense foci on T2W images or may not be seen on conventional spin echo images. They show homogeneous enhancement on administration of gadolinium. The lesions may be invisible on spin echo images and may or may not enhance on contrast administration but are usually clearly seen on MT-SE T1W images. Thus, the true disease load can be defined on MT-SE imaging.[31]

Numerous conditions can mimic tuberculomas on conventional imaging, including neurocysticercosis, fungal granulomas, and tumors like lymphomas, glioma, and metastases. Newer imaging techniques, like diffusion imaging, MR spectroscopy and MT imaging may help in differentiating these conditions.[65–72]

The cellular components of the noncaseating tuberculomas appear brighter on MT T1W imaging. This feature is specific for the disease and thus helps in differentiating these lesions from metastases, lymphomas, and other infective granulomas.[65] Solid caseating granulomas with T2 hypointense center can be confused with lymphoma and fungal and cysticercus granulomas. These lesions appear hypointense on T1W MT images surrounded with a hyperintense rim. MTRs of 23.8 ± 1.76 and 24.2 ± 3.1 are reported from the rim and the core of the lesions, respectively.[30,31] The high lipid content of the tuberculomas contributes to the lower MTR of these lesions. Fluid-attenuated inversion recovery (FLAIR) and MT imaging has been used to evaluate

the patients with tuberculomas by Saxena and colleagues.[72] They found that FLAIR is not as useful as MT imaging either in the characterization of the lesions or in assessing the true disease load.[67]

Liquid caseating lesions show restricted diffusion, whereas solid caseating lesions do not reveal restriction of diffusion. Thus T2 hypointense solid caseating lesions can be differentiated from lymphoma and medulloblastoma, which show restricted diffusion.[71]

MR spectroscopy is specific for the diagnosis of tuberculoma. Fingerprinting of the metabolites of *Mycobacterium tuberculosis* was performed by Gupta and colleagues[73] using in vivo, ex vivo, and in vitro MR spectroscopy. In vivo MR spectroscopy with stimulated echo acquisition mode (STEAM) sequence reveals lipid resonances at 0.9, 1.3, 2.0, 2.8, and 3.7 ppm, corresponding with various components of the lipid molecule. Ex vivo spectroscopy reveals many other peaks in addition to those seen on in vivo spectroscopy. In vivo spectroscopy shows only a lipid peak in lesions with a T2 hypointense center (**Fig. 15**), whereas those with heterogeneous appearance reveal a choline peak at 3.22 ppm in addition to lipid. These lesions have a large cellular component appearing bright on MT imaging and with a choline peak on spectroscopy.[73]

Dynamic contrast enhancement (DCE) MR imaging has been used by Gupta and colleagues[73] to correlate the relative cerebral blood volume values with the cellular and necrotic components of tuberculomas and also with the expression of various immunohistochemical markers.[74] In

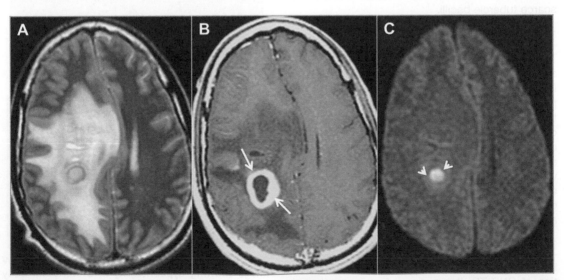

Fig. 17. Tuberculous abscess. Axial T2W image (*A*) shows a hyperintense lesion with hypointense rim and marked vasogenic edema in the right parietal lobe. It shows thick rim enhancement (*arrows*) on postcontrast axial T1W image (*B*) and restricted diffusion (*arrow heads*) on diffusion-weighted image (*C*).

a different study, tuberculomas showed varying degrees of vascularity on perfusion MR imaging and the investigators concluded that it may be difficult to differentiate tuberculomas and tumors on perfusion MR imaging alone.[75] Haris and colleagues[75] assessed the role of the DCE MR imaging index to evaluate the therapeutic response in brain tuberculomas. They found that changes in volume transfer coefficient (K^{trans}) and edema volume are associated with a therapeutic response even when there is a paradoxic increase in the lesion volume.[76]

Serial diffusion tensor imaging (DTI) has been used to evaluate brain tuberculomas by Gupta and colleagues,[76] who correlated the indices of DTI with matrix metalloproteinase-9 (MMP-9) expression. There was strong correlation of DTI indices with MMP-9 and they concluded that it may be of value in assessing the therapeutic response of tuberculomas that are treated only with specific antituberculous drugs.[77]

Fluorodeoxyglucose positron emission tomography can be helpful in differentiating an atypical tuberculoma from other neoplastic and nonneoplastic CNS lesions.[78] It can also be used in the follow-up of tuberculomas.[79]

Tuberculous Cerebritis

Tuberculous cerebritis is a less common clinicoradiological pattern reported in patients who do not have AIDS. It is seen as intense focal gyral enhancement[80] with associated edema (**Fig. 16**). Microscopically, it is characterized by microgranulomata, lymphocytic infiltrate, Langerhans giant cells, epithelioid cells, and variable evidence of scarce tubercle bacilli.[11]

Tuberculous Encephalopathy

Tuberculous encephalopathy occurs because of an immunologic mechanism with a delayed type IV hypersensitivity reaction caused by tuberculous protein. This condition leads to extensive damage to the white matter along with the infrequent onset of perivascular demyelination. Infants and young children with pulmonary TB are commonly affected. Imaging shows extensive brain edema, which sometimes severely affects 1 cerebral hemisphere. Death usually occurs within 1 to 2 months of onset of illness despite antituberculous medication.[5,14]

Tubercular Abscess

Intracranial abscess formation is a rare complication of CNS TB. It can occur from parenchymal tuberculous granulomas or via the spread of tuberculous foci in the meninges to the brain

parenchyma in patients with TBM. It is an encapsulated collection of pus with abundant viable tubercle bacilli without classic tubercular granuloma formation. Tuberculous brain abscess has a thicker wall than pyogenic abscess.[81] Brain abscesses can be solitary or multiple. According

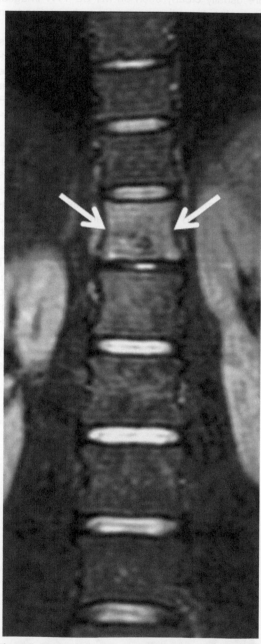

Fig. 18. Early TB spine. Coronal fat-saturated T2W image showing hyperintensity in L1 vertebral body (*arrows*) representing marrow edema, the earliest sign of infection. There is no associated soft tissue or disc involvement at this stage.

to the Whitener[81] criteria for tuberculous abscess, it should reveal macroscopic evidence of abscess formation within the brain parenchyma, and, on histologic confirmation, the abscess wall should be composed of vascular granulation tissue containing acute and chronic inflammatory cells and tubercle bacilli.[82]

TB abscesses clinically present acutely and with a more rapidly deteriorating course than tuberculomas, with symptoms of fever, headache, and focal neurologic signs.[12]

Imaging findings are usually nonspecific. They present as large, frequently multiloculated, ring-enhancing lesions with perilesional edema and mass effect.[83] Tuberculous abscess may mimic granuloma with central liquid caseation. On imaging, abscesses are generally larger in size (usually >3 cm

in diameter), with thin walls, are multiloculated, and are usually solitary.[34,84,85]

Diffusion-weighted imaging shows restricted diffusion (Fig. 17) with low apparent diffusion coefficient (ADC) values because of the presence of inflammatory cells in the pus.[72] MR spectroscopy helps in differentiating tuberculous abscess from those of pyogenic and fungal causes. MR spectroscopy shows lipid, lactate, and phosphoserine without evidence of cytosolic amino acids, in contrast with pyogenic abscess. MT imaging can differentiate tuberculous from pyogenic abscesses. The rim of tuberculous abscesses (19.89 ± 1.55) show lower MTR (MTR) values compared with pyogenic abscesses (24.81 ± 0.03). The high lipid content of tuberculous bacilli is responsible for this low MTR.[86–88]

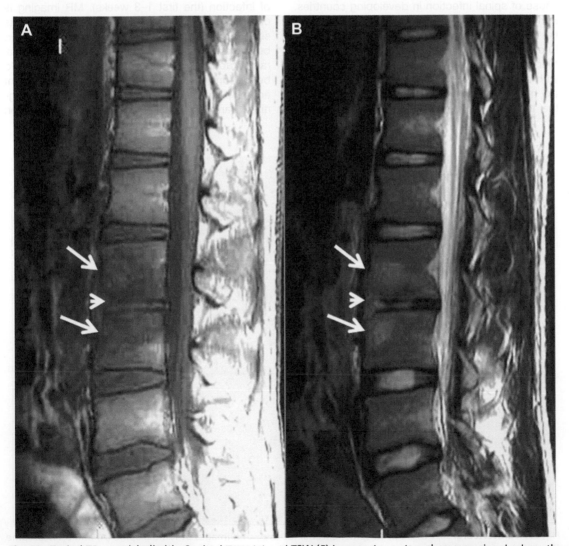

Fig. 19. Typical TB spondylodiscitis. Sagittal T1W (A) and T2W (B) images show altered marrow signals along the adjoining portions of L2 and L3 vertebral bodies (arrows) and the intervening L2 to L3 disc (arrowheads).

Intraspinal TB

TB involves the spine in multiple ways with varied imaging appearances. Although the imaging features of typical spondylodiscitis are well known, other presentations may be misleading. This article reviews the typical imaging features of spondylodiscitis as well as some more atypical and unusual imaging features including intramedullary TB, myelitis, spinal meningitis, and arachnoiditis. TB spondylitis, also called as Pott disease, was first described by Percival Pott in 1779. However, TB spondylitis has been detected in ancient mummies in Egypt and Peru, and is hence one of the oldest diseases known.

Tuberculous spondylodiscitis

Tuberculous spondylodiscitis is an important cause of spinal infection in developing countries. Early diagnosis and prompt treatment are essential to avoid morbidity. Infective spondylitis constitutes 2% to 4% of all cases of osteomyelitis.[89] Men are more frequently affected than women, with a ratio of 2:1 to 3:1.[90] The lumbar spine is the most commonly affected region, followed by the thoracic and cervical spine and, rarely, the sacrum.[89] The thoracolumbar junction is a common site involved in tuberculous spondylitis.[90] Potential routes of infection include hematogenous spread, both arterial and venous; direct contamination; and direct spread from adjoining abscess.[91] The arteries at the anterior aspect of the vertebra possess the richest supply, accounting for the initial infective focus in the anterior subchondral bone.[92] The Batson paravertebral venous plexus of valveless veins provides a potential route of retrograde spread from abdominal veins.[89–91] Direct contamination of the spine may occur after surgery or after spinal canal puncture, although the incidence is low. Mycobacterium TB is the most common cause of a spondylodiscitis in developing countries, and shows an increasing incidence worldwide, followed by brucella.

Radiographs are often normal in the early stage of infection (the first 1–3 weeks). MR imaging is currently the imaging modality of choice, given its superior ability in the detection of soft tissue and bone marrow changes even in patients with normal radiographs. MR imaging of the entire spine should be performed to exclude multilevel involvement and skip lesions. Bone marrow edema is a recognized early sign of infection (**Fig. 18**) that is seen

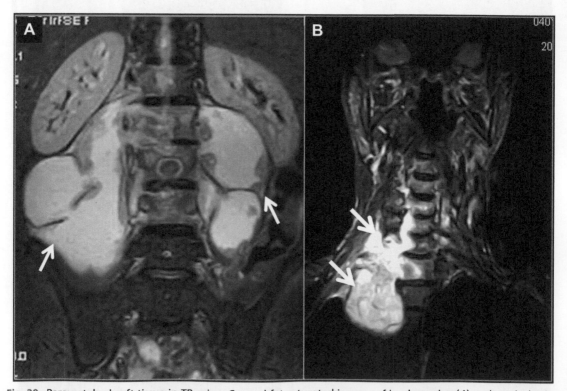

Fig. 20. Paravertebral soft tissue in TB spine. Coronal fat-saturated images of lumbar spine (A) and cervical spine (B) showing paravertebral soft tissue abscesses (*arrows*) in 2 different cases of TB spine. MR imaging is the imaging modality of choice to accurately delineate the extent of these soft tissue masses.

as areas of hypointensity on T1W images, and hyperintense areas on T2W, short tau inversion recovery (STIR), and proton density fat-suppressed sequences.[89–91] T1W images are the most sensitive in detecting marrow edema. Performing contrast-enhanced T1W sequences with fat suppression provides valuable additional information and is highly recommended.

Other MR imaging changes evident in the acute phase include T1 hypointensity with loss of definition of the end plates and adjacent vertebral bodies, and T2-hyperintense intervertebral discs and adjacent vertebral bodies (Fig. 19). Vertebral end plate erosion is seen as loss of the normal T1-hypointense line on sagittal MR images.[89] Increased conspicuity of the end plates from pseudosparing has been described, caused by marrow fat replacement and loss of the chemical

shift artifact.[92] The intervertebral disc space may show homogeneous T2 hyperintensity with loss of the normal intranuclear cleft, although this sign may be inconsistent.[5] Discal enhancement patterns include homogeneous disc enhancement, patchy nonconfluent areas of disc enhancement, and varying areas of peripheral disc enhancement.[92] Reduced disc height and finding of T1 hypointensity, rather than the usual isointensity, are additional findings.[89] MR imaging is also superior in the demonstration of paravertebral soft tissue masses (Fig. 20), most often being T1 hypointense, T2-heterogeneously hyperintense, and epidural masses, which are slightly T1 hypointense and T2 hyperintense. Compression or displacement of the spinal cord should be looked for in the presence of epidural masses, which may show craniocaudal migration (Fig. 21). MR imaging findings with good

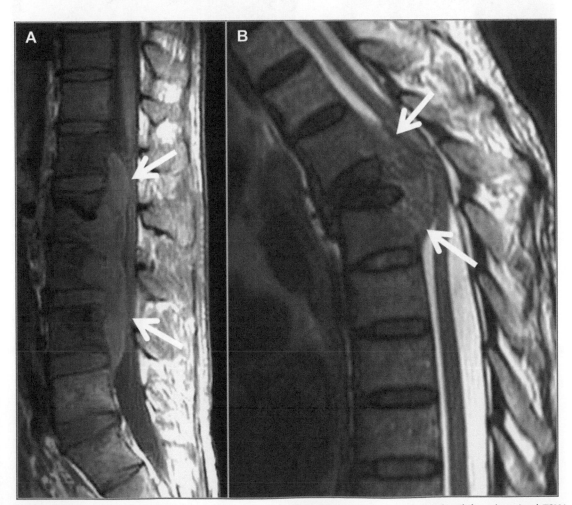

Fig. 21. Epidural soft tissue in TB spine. Postcontrast sagittal T1W image of lumbar spine (A) and sagittal T2W image of thoracic spine (B) in 2 different cases of TB spine showing the extent of epidural soft tissue component (arrows). Cord compression with cord edema is also visualized in (B).

to excellent sensitivity for infective spondylitis include the presence of paravertebral or epidural inflammatory tissue, intradiscal contrast enhancement, T2 signal hyperintensity or fluid-equivalent intensity, and erosion or destruction of the vertebral end plates on T1W images (**Fig. 22**). MR findings with low sensitivity include finding of a T1-hypointense disc, decrease in intervertebral disc height, and effacement of the intranuclear cleft.[93]

Differential Diagnosis

TB of the spine should be considered in the differential diagnosis of any patient presenting with back pain. It is important to be able to diagnose TB because it can be successfully treated, especially if detected early. The radiological differential diagnosis includes pyogenic and fungal infections. Although differentiation between pyogenic and TB infection is often difficult in individual cases, some general guidelines may be helpful. Patients with pyogenic spondylitis may be more toxic compared with TB. TB of the spine is usually more chronic and is slower in progression compared with pyogenic spondylitis. This difference is reflected radiographically as increased areas of sclerosis.[94] The soft tissue abscesses and paravertebral extension in TB are usually larger compared with

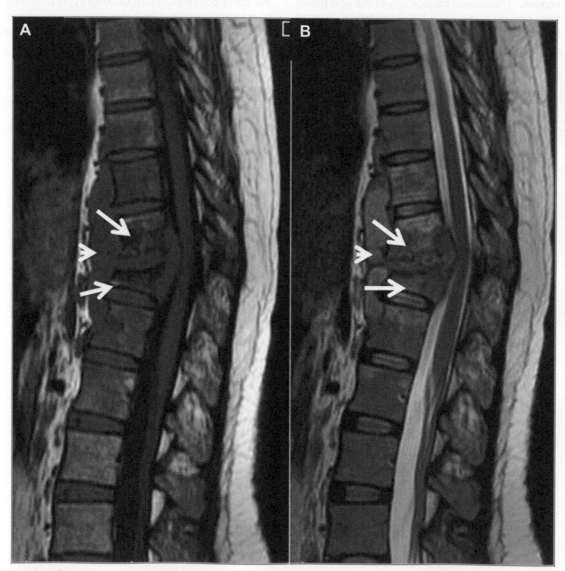

Fig. 22. Advanced TB spine. Sagittal T1W (*A*) and T2W (*B*) images show advanced spinal TB with destruction of end plates (*arrows*), reduced intervertebral disc height, and curvature deformity. Prevertebral (*arrowheads*) and epidural soft tissue with mild cord indentation are also noted.

pyogenic spondylitis. Soft tissue calcifications are more characteristic of TB than of pyogenic spondylitis.[95] TB more commonly involves more than one vertebral level. Subligamentous spread is a particular feature of TB and is frequent, occurring in a craniocaudal manner, and leads to skip vertebral involvement (4%) or noncontiguous multilevel involvement. Anterior vertebral scalloping with relative disc space preservation is a sign of subligamentous spread on lateral radiographs and CT.[90,96] The 2 most reliable MR imaging findings that suggest tuberculous spondylitis are thin and smooth abscess wall enhancement and well-defined paravertebral abnormal signal intensity.[97] Because of its slower disease progression, sclerosis and bony destruction are more common, with gibbus deformity (marked forward kyphosis of the spine), secondary to infective compression fracture, being frequently seen.[96]

In metastatic disease, lymphoma and multiple myeloma, subligamentous spread, and disc involvement are not typically seen. The disc height is usually preserved in such cases but may rarely be involved in lymphoma and multiple myeloma. The vertebral end plates are also distinct and usually regular.[98] Adjacent surrounding inflammatory collections are usually not present in tumor infiltration. Other differentials include degenerative disc disease, pseudoarthrosis in ankylosing spondylitis, hemodialysis amyloid spondyloarthropathy, and neuropathic spondyloarthropathy. Imaging, particularly MR imaging, remains essential for an accurate diagnosis, and is useful in follow-up for monitoring disease progression. In all cases, obtaining tissue for culture and sensitivity may be essential in arriving at a definitive diagnosis, and spinal biopsy may be best done under CT guidance.

Atypical presentations of spine involvement by TB include solitary vertebral body involvement (**Fig. 23**), multifocal skip lesions (**Fig. 24**), pure posterior-element involvement (**Fig. 25**),

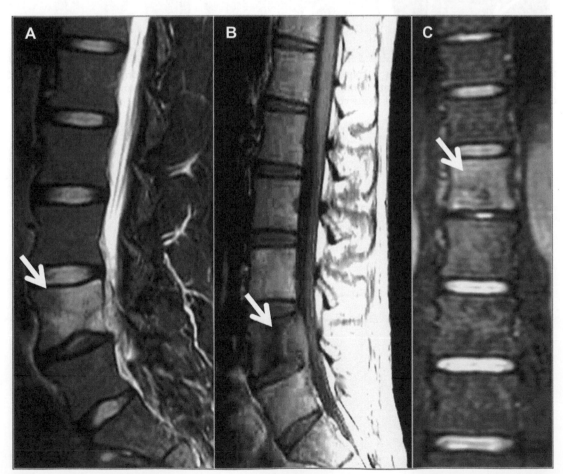

Fig. 23. Solitary vertebral body involvement. Sagittal T2W (*A*), T1W (*B*), and coronal fat-saturated T2W (*C*) images show solitary vertebral body involvement (*arrows*) of L4 vertebral body without disc involvement or significant soft tissue component.

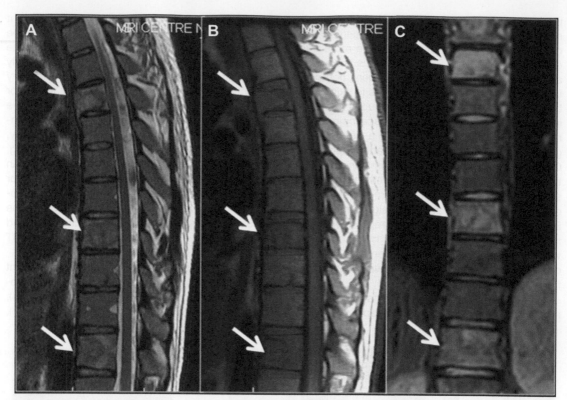

Fig. 24. Multiple-level skip lesions in spine TB. Sagittal T2W (*A*), T1W (*B*), and coronal fat-saturated T2W (*C*) images show altered signal intensity in multiple noncontiguous vertebral bodies (*arrows*). There is no obvious disc involvement or associated soft tissue component.

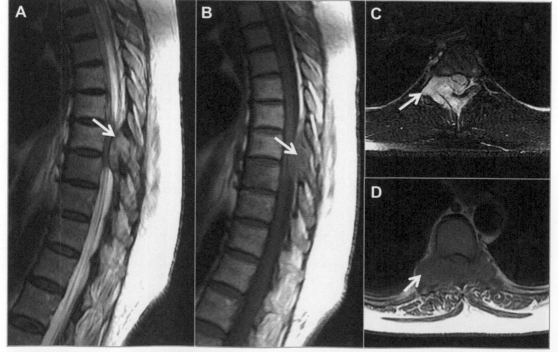

Fig. 25. Posterior-element TB. In a 55-year-old man presenting with back pain and paraparesis, sagittal T2W (*A*), T1W (*B*), axial fat-saturated T2W (*C*), and T1W (*D*) images show pure posterior-element involvement (*arrows*) with associated epidural soft tissue component causing cord compression.

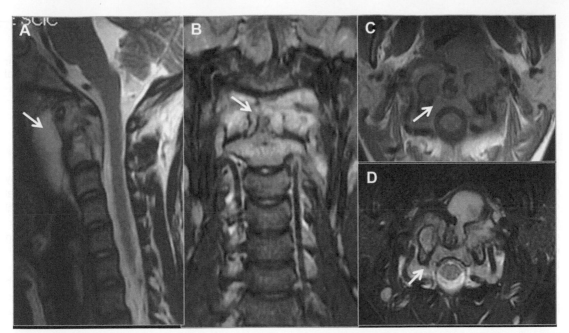

Fig. 26. In a 37-year-old man with history of neck pain, sagittal T2W (*A*), coronal fat-saturated T2 (*B*), axial T1W (*C*), and fat-saturated T2W (*D*) images show erosion of C2 vertebral body and anterior arch of atlas with associated preparavertebral and epidural soft tissue components (*arrows*). Histopathology confirmed atlantoaxial TB.

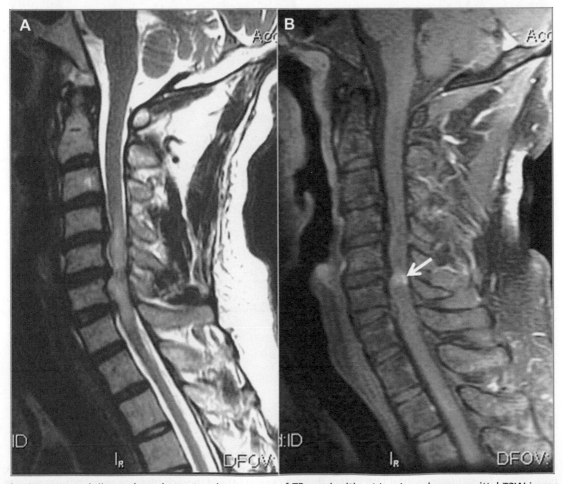

Fig. 27. Intramedullary tuberculoma. In a known case of TB meningitis with tuberculomas, sagittal T2W image (*A*) shows cord edema in the mid and lower cervical spinal cord. Fat-saturated postcontrast sagittal T1W image (*B*) shows a disc-enhancing intramedullary tuberculoma at C5 to C6 level (*arrow*).

craniovertebral involvement (**Fig. 26**), and tubercular myelitis, arachnoiditis, and intramedullary tuberculomas.

TB Myelitis and Intramedullary Tuberculomas

The MR imaging features of TB myelitis are similar to those of cerebritis. One week after initiation of treatment, the region of myelitis becomes less diffusely hyperintense on T2W images, with more clearly defined marginal enhancement on postcontrast T1W images.[99,100] The surrounding edema continues to be more extensive than the margins of enhancement. These findings suggest the beginning of intramedullary tuberculoma formation (**Fig. 27**). The central cavitary portions of the intra-axial necrotic areas are seen as hypointense and hyperintense foci on T1W and T2W

images, respectively.[100] Although the abnormalities visible on T2W images subside after several weeks, foci of contrast enhancement on postcontrast images may persist for several months.[100]

SPINAL MENINGITIS AND SPINAL ARACHNOIDITIS

These are inflammatory spinal diseases caused by *M tuberculosis*.[101] The pathophysiology of spinal meningitis is similar to that of TBM: a submeningeal tubercle forms during primary infection and ruptures into the subarachnoid space, eliciting mediators of delayed hypersensitivity.[55] As with intracranial lesions, there is granulomatous inflammation with areas of caseation and tubercles with eventual development of fibrous tissue in chronic or treated cases. MR imaging features include

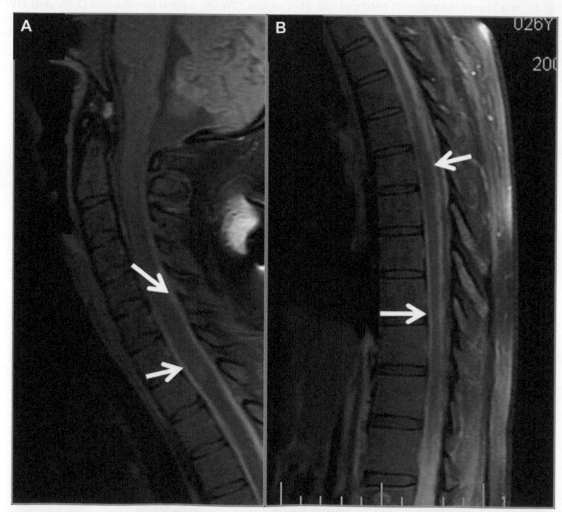

Fig. 28. Tuberculous spinal meningitis. In a 27-year-old man with history of progressive weakness of all 4 limbs, postcontrast fat-saturated sagittal T1W images through cervical (*A*) and thoracic (*B*) spine reveal diffuse, nodular, thick, linear, intradural enhancement filling the subarachnoid space (*arrows*), consistent with spinal meningitis.

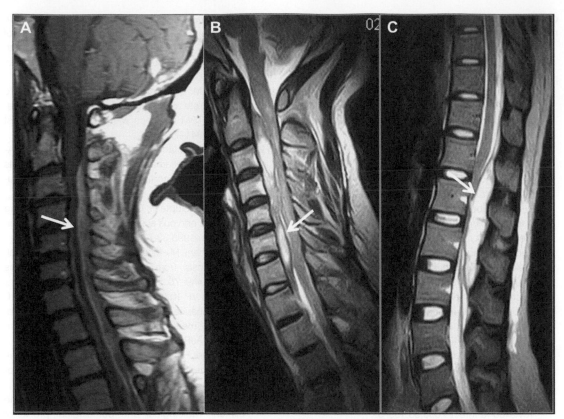

Fig. 29. Epidural spinal TB. Three different cases of epidural spinal TB. Postcontrast sagittal T1W image through cervical spine (A), sagittal T2W image through cervical spine (B), and sagittal T2W image through thoracolumbar spine (C) reveal large epidural soft tissue components/abscesses causing cord compression (*arrows*). There is no other associated involvement in (A) and (C), whereas multiple vertebral bodies are involved in (B).

CSF loculation and obliteration of the spinal subarachnoid space with a loss of outline of the spinal cord in the cervicothoracic spine and matting of the nerve roots in the lumbar region. Patients who appear normal on unenhanced MR imaging images may show nodular, thick, linear, intradural enhancement (Fig. 28), often completely filling the subarachnoid space on postcontrast images.[100] In chronic stages of the disease, the postcontrast images may not show any enhancement even when unenhanced images show signs of arachnoiditis.[100,101] Spinal cord involvement in the form of infarction and syringomyelia may occur as a complication of arachnoiditis.

Tuberculous pus formation may occur between the dura and the leptomeninges and may appear loculated. It appears hyperintense on T2W and isointense to hypointense on T1W images. The dural granulomas appear hypointense to isointense on T2W and isointense on T1W images. Rim enhancement can be seen on postcontrast images.[100] Epidural TB lesions generally appear to be isointense to the spinal cord on T1W images and have mixed intensity on T2W images (Fig. 29). In postcontrast images, uniform enhancement can be seen if the TB inflammatory process is phlegmonous, whereas peripheral enhancement is seen if true epidural abscess formation or caseation has developed.[57,58] Epidural tuberculous abscess may occur as primary lesions or may be seen in association with arachnoiditis, myelitis, spondylitis, and intramedullary and dural tuberculomas.[100,101]

SUMMARY

CNS TB is a common clinical concern in developing countries, with increasing incidence in developed countries because of the HIV pandemic. Imaging, particularly MR imaging, is a cornerstone in the diagnosis of CNS TB and its associated complications as well as in monitoring response to treatment. A thorough knowledge of typical and atypical imaging characteristics help in accurate diagnosis as well as in the differential diagnosis. The newer imaging modalities help in improved characterization and thus aid in better diagnosis and management.

REFERENCES

1. Shah GV. Central nervous system tuberculosis: imaging manifestations. Neuroimaging Clin North Am 2000;10(2):355–74.
2. Iseman MD. A clinician's guide to tuberculosis. Philadelphia: Lippincott Williams & Wilkins; 2000. p. 173–81.
3. Rock RB, Olin M, Baker CA, et al. Central nervous system tuberculosis: pathogenesis and clinical aspects. Clin Microbiol Rev 2008;21(2):243–61.
4. Bernaerts A, Vanhoenacker FM, Parizel PM, et al. Tuberculosis of the central nervous system: overview of neuroradiological findings. Eur Radiol 2003;13:1876–90.
5. Jacob CN, Henein SS, Heurich AE, et al. Nontuberculous mycobacterial infection of the central nervous system in patients with AIDS. South Med J 1993;86:638–40.
6. Rich AR, McCordock HA. Pathogenesis of tubercular meningitis. Bull John Hopkins Hosp 1933;52:5–13.
7. Donald PR, Schaaf HS, Schoeman JF. Tuberculous meningitis and miliary tuberculosis: the rich focus revisited. J Infect 2005;50:193–5.
8. Rajajee S, Narayanan PR. Immunological spectrum of childhood tuberculosis. J Trop Pediatr 1992;21:490–6.
9. Engin G, Acuna B, Acuna G, et al. Imaging of extrapulmonary tuberculosis. Radiographics 2000; 20:471–88.
10. de Castro CC, de Barros NG, Campos ZM, et al. CT scans of cranial tuberculosis. Radiol Clin North Am 1999;33:753–69.
11. Garcia-Monco JC. Central nervous system tuberculosis. Neurol Clin 1999;17:737–59.
12. McGuinness FE. Intracranial tuberculosis. In: Clinical imaging in non-pulmonary tuberculosis. Berlin, Heidelberg, New York: Springer; 2000. p. 5–25.
13. Dastur DK, Manghani DK, Udani PM. Pathology and pathogenetic mechanisms in neurotuberculosis. Radiol Clin North Am 1995;33:733–52.
14. Sheller JR, Des Prez RM. CNS tuberculosis. Neurol Clin 1986;4:143–58.
15. Bullock MR, Welchman JM. Diagnostic and prognostic features of tuberculous meningitis on CT scanning. J Neurol Neurosurg Psychiatry 1982; 45:1098–101.
16. Kumar R, Kohli N, Thavnani H, et al. Value of CT scan in the diagnosis of meningitis. Indian Pediatr 1996;33:465–8.
17. Andronikou S, Smith B, Hatherhill M, et al. Definitive neuroradiological diagnostic features of tuberculous meningitis in children. Pediatr Radiol 2004; 34:876–85.
18. Przybojewski S, Andronikou S, Wilmshurst J. Objective CT criteria to determine the presence of abnormal basal enhancement in children with suspicious tuberculous meningitis. Pediatr Radiol 2006;36:687–96.
19. Pienaar M, Andronikou S, van Toorn R. MRI to demonstrate diagnostic features and complications of TBM not seen with CT. Childs Nerv Syst 2009;25:941–7.
20. Chang KH, Han MH, Roh JK, et al. Gd-DTPA-enhanced MR imaging of the brain in patients with meningitis: comparison with CT. Am J Neuroradiol 1990;11:69–76.
21. Jinkins JR, Gupta R, Chang KH, et al. MR imaging of central nervous system tuberculosis. Radiol Clin North Am 1995;33:771–86.
22. Harisinghani M, McLoud TC, Shepard JA, et al. Tuberculosis from head to toe. Radiographics 2000;20:449–70.
23. Mathews VP, Kuharik MA, Edwards MK, et al. Gd-DTPA-enhanced MR imaging of experimental bacterial meningitis: evaluation and comparison with CT. AJR Am J Roentgenol 1989;152:131–6.
24. Kioumeher F, Dadsetan MR, Rooholamini SA, et al. Central nervous system tuberculosis: MRI. Neuroradiology 1994;36:93–6.
25. Katrak SM, Shembalkar PK, Bijwe SR, et al. The clinical, radiological and pathological profile of tuberculous meningitis in patients with and without human immunodeficiency virus infection. J Neurol Sci 2000;181:118–26.
26. Villoria MF, de la Torre J, Fortea F, et al. Intracranial tuberculosis in AIDS: CT and MRI findings. Neuroradiology 1991;34:11–4.
27. Srikanth SG, Taly AB, Nagarajan K, et al. Clinicoradiological features of tuberculous meningitis in patients over 50 years of age. J Neurol Neurosurg Psychiatry 2007;78:536–8.
28. Kamra P, Azad R, Prasad KN, et al. Infectious meningitis: prospective evaluation with magnetization transfer MRI. Br J Radiol 2004;77:387–94.
29. Gupta R. Magnetization transfer MR imaging in central nervous system infections. Indian J Radiol Imaging 2002;12:51–8.
30. Gupta RK, Kathuria MK, Pradhan S. Magnetization transfer MR imaging in CNS tuberculosis. AJNR Am J Neuroradiol 1999;20:867–75.
31. Nogami K, Nomura S, Kashiwagi S, et al. Fluid-attenuated inversion-recovery imaging of cerebral infarction associated with tuberculous meningitis. Comput Med Imaging Graph 2000;24:333–7.
32. Lamprecht D, Schoeman JF, Donald P, et al. Ventriculo peritoneal shunting in childhood tuberculous meningitis. Br J Neurosurg 2001;15:119–25.
33. Atlas SW. Intracranial infections. In: Magnetic resonance imaging of the brain and spine. Philadelphia: Lippincott-Raven; 1996. p. 738–42.

34. van Well GT, Paes BF, Terwee CB, et al. Twenty years of pediatric tuberculous meningitis: a retrospective cohort study in the Western Cape of South Africa. Pediatrics 2009;123(1):e1–8.

35. Schroth G, Kretzschmar K, Gawehn J, et al. Advantage of magnetic resonance imaging in the diagnosis of cerebral infections. Neuroradiology 1987; 29:120–6.

36. Yadav YR, Mukerji G, Parihar V, et al. Complex hydrocephalus (combination of communicating and obstructive type): an important cause of failed endoscopic third ventriculostomy. BMC Res Notes 2009;2:137. DOI:1186/1756-0500/2/137.

37. van Lindert EJ, Beems T, Grotenhuis JA. The role of different imaging modalities: is MRI a conditio sine qua non for ETV? Childs Nerv Syst 2006;22: 1529–36.

38. Bharucha PE, Iyer CG, Bharucha EP, et al. Tuberculous meningitis in children: a clinicopathological evaluation of 24 cases. Indian Pediatr 1969;6(5):282–90.

39. Visudhiphan P, Chiemchanya S. Hydrocephalus in tuberculous meningitis in children: treatment with acetazolamide and repeated lumbar puncture. J Pediatr 1979;95(4):657–60.

40. Thwaites GE, Schoeman JF. Update on tuberculosis of the central nervous system: pathogenesis, diagnosis, and treatment. Clin Chest Med 2009; 30(4):745–54.

41. Bruwer GE, Van der Westhuizen S, Lombard CJ, et al. Can CT predict the level of CSF block in tuberculous hydrocephalus? Childs Nerv Syst 2004;20(3):183–7.

42. Karachi C, Le Guerinel C, Brugieres P, et al. Hydrocephalus due to idiopathic stenosis of the foramina of Magendie and Luschka. Report of three cases. J Neurosurg 2003;98:897–902.

43. Lev S, Bhadelia RA, Estin D, et al. Functional analysis of third ventriculostomy patency with phase-contrast MRI velocity measurements. Neuroradiology 1997;39:175–9.

44. Joseph VB, Raghuram L, Korah IP, et al. MR ventriculography for the study of CSF flow. AJNR Am J Neuroradiol 2003;24:373–81.

45. Singh I, Haris M, Husain M, et al. Role of endoscopic third ventriculostomy in patients with communicating hydrocephalus: an evaluation by MR ventriculography. Neurosurg Rev 2008;31: 319–25.

46. Dastur DK, Lalitha VS, Udani PM, et al. The brain and meninges in TBM. Gross pathology and pathogenesis in 100 cases. Neurol India 1970;20: 1015–23.

47. Gupta RK, Gupta S, Singh D, et al. MR imaging and angiography in tuberculous meningitis. Neuroradiology 1994;36(2):87–92.

48. Lehrer H. The angiographic triad in tuberculous meningitis. A radiographic and clinicopathologic correlation. Radiology 1966;87:829–35.

49. Chang KH, Han MH, Roh JK, et al. Gd-DTPA enhanced MR imaging in intracranial tuberculosis. Neuroradiology 1990;32:19–25.

50. Shukla R, Abbas A, Kumar P, et al. Evaluation of cerebral infarction in tuberculous meningitis by diffusion weighted imaging. J Infect 2008;57:298–306.

51. Nair PP, Kalita J, Kumar S, et al. MRI pattern of infarcts in basal ganglia region in patients with tuberculous meningitis. Neuroradiology 2009;51:221–5.

52. Uysal G, Kose G, Guven A, et al. Magnetic resonance imaging in diagnosis of childhood central nervous system tuberculosis. Infection 2001;29:148–53.

53. Saremi F, Helmy M, Farzin S, et al. MRI of cranial nerve enhancement. AJR Am J Roentgenol 2005; 185:1487–97.

54. Goyal M, Sharma A, Mishra NK, et al. Imaging appearance of pachymeningeal tuberculosis. Am J Roentgenol 1997;169:1421–4.

55. Brismar T, Hugosson C, Larsson SG, et al. Tuberculosis as a mimicker of brain tumour. Acta Radiol 1996;37:496–505.

56. Callebout J, Dormont D, Dubois B, et al. Contrast enhanced MR imaging of tuberculous pachymeningitis cranialis hypertrophica: case report. AJNR Am J Neuroradiol 1990;11:821–2.

57. Villoria MF, Fortea F, Moreno S, et al. MR imaging and CT of central nervous system tuberculosis in the patient with AIDS. Radiol Clin North Am 1995; 4:805–20.

58. Gupta RK, Kohli A, Gaur V, et al. MRI of the brain in patients with miliary pulmonary tuberculosis without symptoms or signs of central nervous system involvement. Neuroradiology 1997;39:699–704.

59. Talamas O, Del Brutto OH, Garcia-Ramos G. Brainstem tuberculoma. Arch Neurol 1989;46:529–35.

60. Rajshekhar V, Chandy MJ. Tuberculomas presenting as isolated intrinsic brain stem masses. Br J Neurosurg 1997;11:127–33.

61. Gupta RK, Lufkin RB. MR imaging and spectroscopy of central nervous system infection. In: tuberculosis and other nontuberculous bacterial granulomatous infection. New York: Kluwer Academic/Plenum Publishers; 2001. p. 95–145.

62. Van Dyk A. CT of intracranial tuberculomas with special reference to the "target sign". Neuroradiology 1988;30:329.

63. Bargalló J, Berenguer J, García-Barrionuevo J, et al. The "target sign": is it a specific sign of CNS tuberculoma? Neuroradiology 1996;38:547–50.

64. Gupta RK, Husain N, Kathuria MK, et al. Magnetization transfer MR imaging correlation with histopathology in intracranial tuberculomas. Clin Radiol 2001;56:656–63.

65. Poptani H, Gupta RK, Roy R, et al. Characterization of intracranial mass lesions with in vivo proton MR spectroscopy. AJNR Am J Neuroradiol 1995;16: 1593–603.

66. Gupta RK, Poptani H, Kohli A, et al. In vivo localized proton magnetic resonance spectroscopy of intracranial tuberculomas. Indian J Med Res 1995;101:19–24.

67. Gupta RK, Roy R, Dev R, et al. Finger printing of *Mycobacterium tuberculosis* in patients with intracranial tuberculomas by using in vivo, ex vivo, and in vitro magnetic resonance spectroscopy. Magn Reson Med 1996;36:829–33.

68. Gupta RK, Roy R. MR imaging and spectroscopy of intracranial tuberculoma. Curr Sci 1999;76: 783–8.

69. Poptani H, Kaartinen J, Gupta RK, et al. Diagnostic assessment of brain tumours and non-neoplastic brain disorders in vivo using proton magnetic resonance spectroscopy and artificial neural networks. J Cancer Res Clin Oncol 1999;125:343–9.

70. Schaefer PW, Grant PE, Gonzalez RG. Diffusion-weighted MR imaging of the brain. Radiology 2000;217:331–45.

71. Gupta RK, Prakash M, Mishra AM, et al. Role of diffusion weighted imaging in differentiation of intracranial tuberculoma and tuberculous abscess from *Cysticercus* granulomas – a report of more than 100 lesions. Eur J Radiol 2005;55:384–92.

72. Saxena S, Prakash M, Kumar S, et al. Comparative evaluation of magnetization transfer contrast and fluid attenuated inversion recovery sequences in brain tuberculoma. Clin Radiol 2005;60:787–93.

73. Gupta RK, Haris M, Husain N, et al. Relative cerebral blood volume is a measure of angiogenesis in brain tuberculoma. J Comput Assist Tomogr 2007; 31:335–41.

74. Batra A, Tripathi RP. Perfusion magnetic resonance imaging in intracerebral parenchymal tuberculosis. J Comput Assist Tomogr 2003;27:882–8.

75. Haris M, Gupta RK, Husain M, et al. Assessment of therapeutic response on serial dynamic contrast enhanced MR imaging in brain tuberculomas. Clin Radiol 2008;63:562–74.

76. Gupta RK, Haris M, Husain N, et al. DTI derived indices correlate with immunohistochemistry obtained matrix metalloproteinase (MMP-9) expression in cellular fraction of brain tuberculoma. J Neurol Sci 2008;275:78–85.

77. Villringer K, Jäger H, Dichgans M, et al. Differential diagnosis of CNS lesions in AIDS patients by FDG-PET. J Comput Assist Tomogr 1995;19(4): 532–6.

78. Park IN, Ryu JS, Shim TS. Evaluation of therapeutic response of tuberculoma using F-18 FDG positron emission tomography. Clin Nucl Med 2008;33(1):1–3.

79. Jinkins JR. Focal tuberculous cerebritis. Am J Neuroradiol 1988;9:121–4.

80. Kumar R, Pandey CK, Bose N, et al. Tuberculous brain abscess: clinical presentation, pathophysiology and treatment (in children). Childs Nerv Syst 2002;18:118–23.

81. Whitener DR. Tuberculous brain abscess. Report of a case and review of the literature. Arch Neurol 1978;35:148–55.

82. Farrar DJ, Flanigan TP, Gordon NM, et al. Tuberculous brain abscess in a patient with HIV infection: case report and review. Am J Med 1997;102:297–301.

83. Palmer PE. Tuberculosis of the central nervous system. In: The imaging of tuberculosis. Berlin Heidelberg, New York: Springer; 2002. p. 125–33.

84. Provenzale JM, Jinkins JR. Brain and spine imaging findings in AIDS patients. Radiol Clin North Am 1997;35:1127–66.

85. Luthra G, Parihar A, Nath K, et al. Comparative evaluation of fungal, tubercular, and pyogenic brain abscesses with conventional and diffusion MR imaging and proton MR spectroscopy. AJNR Am J Neuroradiol 2007;28:1332–8.

86. Kapsalaki EZ, Gotsis ED, Fountas KN. The role of proton magnetic resonance spectroscopy in the diagnosis and categorization of cerebral abscesses. Neurosurg Focus 2008;24(6):E7.

87. Gupta RK, Vatsal DK, Husain N, et al. Differentiation of tuberculous from pyogenic brain abscesses with in vivo proton MR spectroscopy and magnetization transfer MR imaging. AJNR Am J Neuroradiol 2001;22:1503–9.

88. James SLJ, Davies AM. Imaging of infectious spinal disorders in children and adults. Eur J Radiol 2006;58:27–40.

89. Jetvic V. Vertebral infection. Eur Radiol 2004;14: E43–52.

90. Howard SA, Seldomridge JA. Spinal infections. Diagnostic tests and imaging studies. Clin Orthop 2006;444:27–33.

91. Varma R, Lander P, Assaf A. Imaging of pyogenic infectious spondylodiskitis. Radiol Clin North Am 2001;39:203–13.

92. Ledermann HP, Schweitzer ME, Morrison WB, et al. MR imaging findings in spinal infections: rules or myths? Radiology 2003;228:506–14.

93. Buchelt M, Lack W, Kutschera HP, et al. Comparison of tuberculous and pyogenic spondylitis. An analysis of 122 cases. Clin Orthop 1993;296: 192–9.

94. Magnus KG, Hoffman EB. Pyogenic spondylitis and early tuberculous spondylitis in children: differential diagnosis with standard radiographs and computed tomography. J Pediatr Orthop 2000;20:39–43.

95. Gouliamos AD, Kehagias DT, Lahanis S, et al. MR imaging of tuberculous vertebral osteomyelitis: pictorial review. Eur Radiol 2001;11:575–9.

96. Jung NY, Jee WH, Ha KY, et al. Discrimination of tuberculous spondylitis from pyogenic spondylitis on MRI. Am J Roentgenol 2004;182: 1405–10.

97. Moore SL, Rafii M. Imaging of musculoskeletal and spinal tuberculosis. Radiol Clin North Am 2001;39: 329–42.

98. Gupta RK, Gupta S, Kumar S, et al. MRI in intraspinal tuberculosis. Neuroradiology 1994;36:39–43.

99. Murphy KJ, Brunberg JA, Quint DJ, et al. Spinal cord infection: myelitis and abscess formation. AJNR Am J Neuroradiol 1998;19:341–8.

100. Brooks WD, Fletcher AP, Wilson RR. Spinal cord complications of tuberculous meningitis; a clinical and pathological study. Q J Med 1954;23:275–90.

101. Kumar A, Montanera W, Willinsky R, et al. MR features of tuberculous arachnoiditis. J Comput Assist Tomogr 1993;17:127–30.

Pediatric Intracranial Infections

Hemant Parmar, MD*, Mohannad Ibrahim, MD

KEYWORDS

• Pediatric • Intracranial • Infection • Congenital • Complications

KEY POINTS

- As in adults, imaging is crucial to look for complications of intracranial infection.
- In very young children, the clinical features of intracranial infection are nonspecific and imaging may help in suggesting a diagnosis.
- Cytomegalovirus is the commonest type of congenital infection.
- Infectious bacterial meningitis is the commonest type of intracranial infection in children.
- In patients with recurrent episodes of meningitis, it is important to look for a possible osteodural break, like spinal dermal sinus or nasal dermal sinus.

INTRODUCTION

Infection of the central nervous system (CNS) in children is an important entity and early recognition is paramount to avoid long-term brain injury, especially in very young patients. The causal factors are different in children compared with adults and so are the clinical presentations. However, imaging features of CNS infection show similar features to those of adults. This article reviews some of the common types of pediatric infections, starting with the congenital (or in utero) infections followed by bacterial infections of the meninges and brain parenchyma. The viral infections are also reviewed. CNS tuberculosis and fungal and parasitic infections are discussed separately in this issue and are not discussed in this article.

CONGENITAL INFECTIONS

Congenital infections are transmitted to the fetus from the mother through the transplacental route or during birth. The mnemonic TORCH is often used to describe these entities, which stands for toxoplasmosis, others (syphilis, human immunodeficiency

virus [HIV]), rubella, cytomegalovirus (CMV), and herpes simplex virus (HSV) type 2. All these are transmitted to the fetus from primary maternal infections, except for herpes, which is acquired during parturition. It is important to realize that infections of the fetus have long-term effects and sequelae on the developing brain. These sequelae depend on the fetal age at the time of infections, the cellular susceptibility to the infecting agent and host immune responses. Insults in the first or second trimesters typically result in CNS malformations (like microcephaly, lissencephaly, or polymicrogyria), whereas infections in the third trimester result in destructive lesions like aqueductal stenosis and hydrocephalus, porencephaly, multicystic encephalomalacia, calcifications, demyelination, and atrophy.[1-3]

Toxoplasmosis

Toxoplasmosis is caused by *Toxoplasma gondii*, an intracellular parasite that infects birds and mammals. Cats usually serve as primary hosts for the parasites. Domestic animals like pigs and cattle serve as intermediate hosts. Human infection occurs through consumption of undercooked,

Disclosure: The authors report no conflicts of interest.
Division of Neuroradiology, Department of Radiology, University of Michigan Health System, 1500 East Medical Center Drive, Ann Arbor, MI 48109-0302, USA
* Corresponding author.
E-mail address: hparmar@umich.edu

Neuroimag Clin N Am 22 (2012) 707–725
http://dx.doi.org/10.1016/j.nic.2012.05.016
1052-5149/12/$ – see front matter © 2012 Elsevier Inc. All rights reserved.

infected meat or by ingestion of infectious oocysts. When primary infection happens during pregnancy, the parasites are disseminated hematogenously to the placenta and the fetus. Although the transmission rate from the mother to the fetus increases with each trimester, the severity of infection decreases with each trimester.[2] It has been estimated that the rate of transmission of *Toxoplasma* in first trimester is 17%, in the second trimester it is 25%, and 65% in the third trimester.[4] Early first-trimester infection by *Toxoplasma* causes spontaneous abortions, infections in the second trimester lead to fetal death or severe disease, whereas infection in the last trimester are often mild and subclinical. Approximately 10% of infected patients presents with clinical symptoms.[1] Symptoms are either present at the time of birth or present several days afterward. Patients exhibit hepatosplenomegaly, jaundice, and rash. They have chorioretinitis (bilateral in 85%), hydrocephalus, microcephaly, and intracranial calcifications. In children affected with CNS toxoplasmosis, the prognosis is poor with overall mortality ranging from 11% to 14%.[1] Those who survive have long-term sequelae like seizures, spasticity, and developmental delay.[5] Within the cranium there is diffuse inflammation of the meninges, with varying sized granulomatous lesions. Inflammation of the ependyma (ependymitis) causes obstruction of the cerebral aqueduct leading to hydrocephalus. Unlike CMV infection, there is no malformation of cortical development seen with toxoplasmosis. On imaging, calcifications are common. These calcifications are seen in the basal nuclei, periventricular regions, or cerebral parenchyma (**Fig. 1**). If hydrocephalus is present, it is characterized by marked dilatation of the lateral and third ventricles. In infants with severe infection, there is marked destruction with hydrocephalus, porencephaly, and extensive basal ganglia calcifications.[1,4] In cases with mild infection (typically after the 30th week of gestation) there is mild ventricular enlargement and few intracranial calcifications.

HIV

Since the first description of neonatal acquired immunodeficiency syndrome (AIDS) in 1982, HIV infection and AIDS has become a significant public health problem because of the large number of HIV-positive women of childbearing age. Approximately 78% of childhood HIV infection is maternally transmitted and about 40% of HIV-positive mothers pass on their infection to the fetus.[6] This has been shown to reduce dramatically with antiretroviral treatment of mothers and delivery by cesarean section.[7] Mother-to-child transmission can occur in utero,

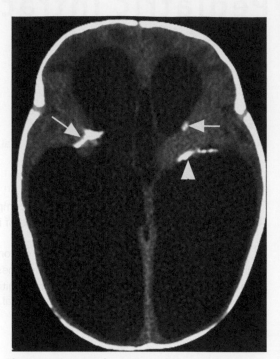

Fig. 1. Brain toxoplasmosis. Axial computed tomography (CT) head in a 11-week-old patient with congenital toxoplasmosis show massive hydrocephalus caused by aqueductal stenosis. There are calcifications in bilateral basal nuclei (*arrows*) and calcification of the ependyma (*arrowhead*). (*Courtesy of* Dr Charles Raybaud, Toronto, Canada.)

intrapartum during birth, or postpartum during breast-feeding. Children with congenital HIV infection are often asymptomatic at birth and manifest neurologic signs or symptoms between 2 months and 5 years of age. They usually show progressive developmental delay, microcephaly, generalized lymphadenopathy, hepatosplenomegaly, recurrent diarrhea, or oral candidiasis.[8] Two major neurological syndromes have been described. In progressive encephalopathy, patients become demented, spastic, and show decreased rates of head growth. In static encephalopathy, there is a delay in cognitive and motor development.[1,8] In contrast with adults, children rarely develop opportunistic CNS complications like lymphoma or toxoplasmosis. On pathology, HIV encephalitis is associated with glial and microglial nodules in the basal ganglia, brain stem, and white matter with multinuclear giant cells. Perivascular calcifications are seen most prominently in the basal ganglia. Perivascular inflammation with demyelination is also seen.[9] On imaging, there is cerebral atrophy with ventricular and sulcal prominence. Intracranial calcifications are seen caused by vasculitis in which calcium is deposited around small affected blood vessels. Children with higher viral loads show more calcifications.[10] White matter abnormality is seen as decrease in attenuation of computed tomography (CT) and increased T2 signal on magnetic resonance (MR) imaging (**Fig. 2**A, B). Corticospinal tract degeneration and demyelination is sometimes seen.[9] Parenchymal hemorrhage and infarction are rare complications of congenital HIV infection.[1]

Syphilis

Congenital syphilis is caused by a spirochete, *Treponema pallidum*. Humans are the only natural host of the spirochete and transmit the organism with intimate contact or contact with bodily fluids. The fetus is infected via the transplacental route, the risk being greatest during the stage of secondary syphilis because of the high load of spirochetes circulating in the mother. Infection after 24 weeks of gestation is also at increased risk.[2,11] Signs of congenital syphilis in an affected child include long bone periostitis, hepatosplenomegaly, jaundice, skin rash, lymphadenopathy, meningitis, and hydrocephalus. Without treatment, late stigmata of the disease can be seen, which includes facial and skin deformities, sensorineural hearing loss, mental retardation, seizures, and hemiplegia.[2] Intracranial involvement results in meningovascular and parenchymal syphilis. Om imaging, there is enhancement of the leptomeninges. The enhancement may extend along the perivascular space into the brain parenchyma and appears as an enhancing parenchymal mass.[1] Inflammatory vasculitis can result in arterial infarctions.[2]

Rubella

Congenital rubella is extremely rare nowadays because of the immunization program and maternal screening during pregnancy. The risk of fetal infection is greater during the first and second trimesters. Affected infants presents with congenital rubella syndrome, which includes growth retardation, ocular abnormalities (cataracts and pigmentory retinopathy), congenital heart defects (patent ductus arteriosus and pulmonary artery stenosis), hepatosplenomegaly, jaundice, and purpuric rash.[3] Neurologic manifestations include hearing loss, microcephaly, meningoencephalitis, psychomotor retardation, speech defects, hypotonia, autism, and bulging fontanelle.[2] Some of these features are present at birth, some develop later. On pathology, affected brain shows microcephaly with ventricular prominence. There are multiple small areas of necrosis and gliosis with calcification in the periventricular white matter, basal ganglia, and brainstem, often as a result of vasculopathy. Myelination is impaired as well.[1] On imaging, there is intracranial calcification in the basal ganglia, periventricular region, and cortex. Multifocal areas of T2/fluid-attenuated inversion recovery (FLAIR) hyperintensity and delayed brain myelination patterns are also seen[12] (**Fig. 3**A, B).

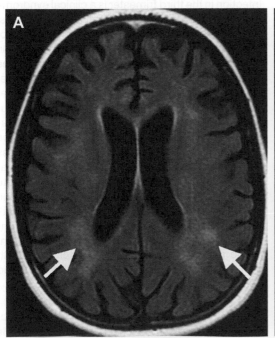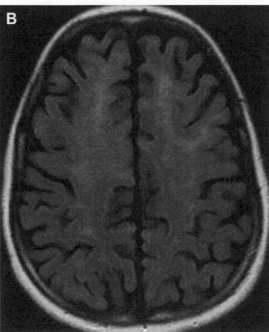

Fig. 2. Congenital HIV. Axial fluid-attenuated inversion recovery (FLAIR)-weighted MR imaging (*A, B*) in a 4-year-old child infected with in utero HIV shows marked brain parenchymal volume loss with ill-defined areas of FLAIR hyperintensities in the white matter of bilateral cerebral hemispheres (*arrows*).

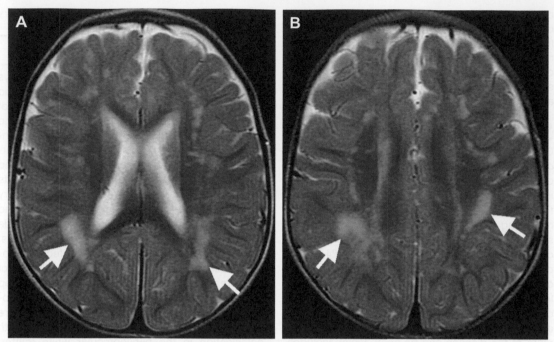

Fig. 3. Congenital rubella. Axial T2-weighted MR imaging (*A, B*) in a 2-year-old patient with congenital rubella infection shows multifocal areas of T2 hyperintensities in the white matter of bilateral cerebral hemispheres (*arrows*).

CT of the temporal bones may show inner ear malformations.[1]

CMV

Cytomegalovirus (CMV) is the commonest viral infection of newborns, with more than 50% of women of childbearing age considered to be sero-positive.[2] Neonatal infection happens when maternal infection or reactivation of infection happens during pregnancy. CMV occurs in approximately 1% of all births, and approximately 10% of these children have hematological, neurologic, and developmental features.[1] Hepatosplenomegaly and skin petechiae are the most commonly seen features. CNS abnormalities are seen in roughly 55% of patients, which includes intracranial calcifications, microcephaly, hearing abnormalities, chorioretinitis, and seizures in order of decreasing frequency.[1,13] Transmission from mother to fetus occurs through the placenta, through direct contact with maternal secretions at the time of birth, or during breast-feeding. Those infected early in gestation have severe disease in which there is multifocal destruction of tissue with associated hemorrhage and dystrophic calcifications. The periventricular subependymal germinal matrix cells are considered most susceptible to early infection. As a result, apart from periventricular calcifications, there are changes of cortical migrational disorders

like lissencephaly, polymicrogyria, heterotopias, and microcephaly. Infection in later gestation produces hydranencephaly and porencephaly. Infection in the third trimester is a clinical syndrome characterized by microcephaly, hearing loss, hyperactivity, ataxia, hypotonia, and behavior problems.[14,15] The imaging features depend on the fetal age at the time of infection and the degree of infection. Patients infected in the first trimester have lissencephaly with thin cortex, cerebellar hypoplasia, delayed myelination, marked ventriculomegaly, and significant periventricular calcifications (**Fig. 4**A, B). Patients with injury later in the second trimester have polymicrogyria and less ventricular dilatation with scattered periventricular calcification or hemorrhage (**Fig. 5**). Infections late in the third trimester or early postnatal period result in mild ventricular prominence. These patients show abnormal white matter signal in the periventricular and subcortical regions, and involvement of the anterior temporal white matter (often with cyst formation[15]; **Fig. 6**A, B), and show scattered periventricular calcifications.

HSV 2

Unlike HSV 1 (discussed later), HSV 2 infection is sexually transmitted and associated with genital lesions. Congenital HSV infection is not a congenital infection; the child acquires the infection during

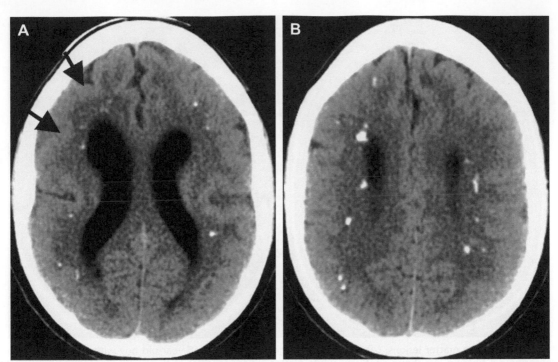

Fig. 4. Congenital CMV; calcification on CT. Axial CT head images (*A, B*) in a 4-month-old patient with congenital CMV infection show multiple foci of dystrophic intraparenchymal calcifications, especially in the periventricular distribution. Cortical migrational abnormalities are also seen in the right frontal cortex (*arrows*).

birth because of contact with genital lesions of the affected mother. Thirty percent of affected infants have brain involvement and, of these, almost 80% do not survive the infection.[2,3] Primary CNS infection by HSV in neonates is diffuse and nonfocal,

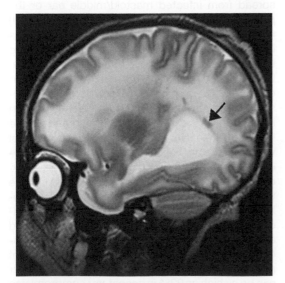

Fig. 5. Congenital CMV; MR imaging. Sagittal T2-weighted MR imaging in a neonate with congenital CMV infection show few punctate areas of T2 hypointensity (*arrow*).

resulting in widespread involvement and brain destruction. In surviving children, severe neurologic sequelae like seizures, microcephaly, multicystic encephalomalacia, and ventriculomegaly are seen.[2] On neuroimaging, findings are nonspecific, especially in the earlier part of the disease. Unlike HSV infection in adults, which tends to localize more in the frontal and temporal lobes, the HSV 2 infection in neonates is diffuse and multifocal, often mimicking changes of diffuse hypoxic-ischemic encephalopathy. These changes are seen as hypoattenuation on CT (**Fig. 7**A, B) and hyperintensity on the T2-weighted images (see **Fig. 7**C). Diffusion-weighted images reveal brain involvement earlier than routine sequences and should be obtained (see **Fig. 7**D). Contrast enhancement is minimal and suggests meningeal involvement. There is eventually severe brain atrophy, encephalomalacia, dystrophic calcification, and ventriculomegaly. Cerebellar involvement is seen in roughly half the patients.[16]

BACTERIAL MENINGITIS

Infectious bacterial meningitis is the most common form of CNS infection in children.[17] It is more common than other forms of infective meningitis like lymphocytic meningitis (usually viral

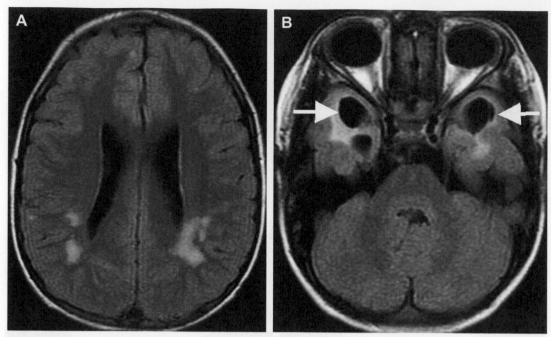

Fig. 6. CMV white matter lesions. (*A*) Axial FLAIR-weighted image in a 5-year-old boy with microcephaly and sensorineural hearing loss shows confluent white matter hyperintensities in the peritrigonal white matter. (*B*) White matter abnormalities with cyst formation are also seen in anterior temporal lobes (*arrows*).

infection) or chronic meningitis (tuberculosis and coccidioidomycosis being common examples).[17] The primary organisms causing infective meningitis in neonates are group B *Streptococcus* and *Escherichia coli*, accounting for nearly 66% of all cases in North America.[18] Ninety percent of neonates with bacterial meningitis of early onset present within the first 24 hours of life. Antenatal chorioamnionitis or premature rupture of membrane, previous newborn with early onset disease, and less than 37 weeks of gestation are some of the risk factors for infective meningitis. Causes of bacterial meningitis in infants include *Streptococcus pneumoniae* or *Neisseria meningitidis*. *Haemophilus influenzae* can also involve this age group but the incidence is decreasing because of vaccinations. The clinical features of infective meningitis in neonates and infants often differ from those of older children, with lethargy, stupor, poor feeding, and irritability being the common symptoms.[19] Seizures are seen in up to 40% of cases.[1,20] Patients can present with bulging fontanelle. Typical signs of infective meningitis, including neck stiffness and Kernig sign, are typically subtle or even absent in these young patients.[20] Cerebrospinal fluid (CSF) evaluation typically shows raised protein and markedly low levels of glucose. The white blood cells are

raised with neutrophilic predominance. Gram stain shows the causative organism.

The infective organisms reach the meninges by any of 5 mechanisms: (1) hematogenous spread from systemic foci of infection, (2) contiguous spread from infected mastoid/middle ear or the paranasal sinuses, (3) via the choroid plexus, (4) rupture of the superficial parenchymal abscess into the subarachnoid space, and (5) penetrating trauma. Previous skull base trauma and dysraphic lesions (mostly dermal tracts and cysts and neuroenteric fistulae) are common in children, often resulting in recurrent meningitis. Once the infection is lodged into the meninges, it can spread via the leptomeningeal sheaths of the penetrating cortical vessels in the perivascular spaces, resulting in cerebritis and brain abscess formation. The thick, creamy leptomeningeal exudates compromise the subarachnoid space and cause extraventricular hydrocephalus. Spread of infection to the ependymal surface with subsequent ventriculitis and aqueductal ependymitis causes obstructive hydrocephalus. Ventriculitis is seen in almost 30% of patients with bacterial meningitis and this number can be as high as 92% in neonates,[1] compromising the secretion of CSF and the washout of the ventricles. Thrombosis of the subependymal veins results in periventricular necrosis. Focal necrosis

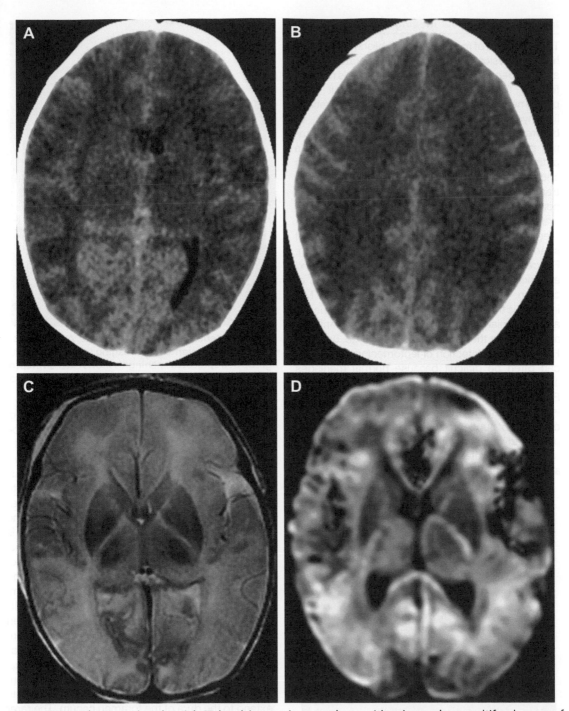

Fig. 7. Neonatal HSV 2. (*A*, *B*) Axial CT head images in a newborn with seizures show multifocal areas of hypoattenuation in the cerebral hemispheres, especially in left frontal and bilateral parietal lobes. (*C*) Axial T2-weighted and (*D*) diffusion-weighted images show multifocal areas of T2 hyperintensity and restricted diffusion in both cerebral hemispheres and involving both the cortex and underlying white matter. This patient had HSV 2 virus on cerebrospinal fluid examination.

within the arterial and venous walls can result in arterial or venous thrombosis, the latter being more common than the former. Overall, cerebral infarctions can be seen in up to 30% of neonates with bacterial meningitis.[1,18] Seepage of inflammatory exudates into the extra-axial space results in subdural hygromas. Secondary infection of these fluid collections results in subdural empyemas.

Imaging of Bacterial Meningitis

The diagnosis of meningitis is established by clinical history, physical examination, and laboratory evaluation, especially CSF evaluation. Imaging is not performed for diagnosis of meningitis, but it is performed to look for associated complications like hydrocephalus, abscess, and empyema, or before lumbar puncture to exclude raised intracranial pressure. Imaging can also be performed in patients with seizures or focal neurologic deficits and in patients in whom there is no treatment response or the response is too slow. A normal CT scan is the most common finding in children with acute bacterial meningitis. Mild ventriculomegaly and enlargement of the subarachnoid spaces are early abnormalities that can be seen. Effacement of the cerebral cortical sulci and enhancing meningitis are seen in less than 50% of children.[1] Contrast-enhanced T1-weighted MR imaging is the standard method of imaging for nearly all intracranial meningitis. Enhancing leptomeninges are seen over the cerebral convexity (Figs. 8 and 9). However, the detection of leptomeningeal disease can often be difficult because normal meninges enhance to some degree. Contrast-enhanced FLAIR imaging increases the specificity compared with contrast-enhanced T1-weighted images for detection of subtle leptomeningeal enhancement,[21] particularly when findings from gadolinium-enhanced weighted images are inconclusive. Evaluation for focal breaches of the osteodural envelopes

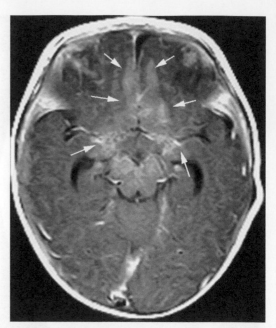

Fig. 9. Bacterial meningitis in a neonate. Axial contrast-enhanced T1-weighted MR imaging in a neonate with group B streptococcal meningitis shows extensive leptomeningeal exudates at the inferior frontal and anterior temporal regions (*arrows*).

of the CNS often requires both CT and MR imaging. For defects along the skull base, high-definition coronal CT is helpful. MR imaging (with high-definition T2-weighted images/constructive interference in steady state/fast imaging employing steady state acquistion (FIESTA) or similar sequences) to show the discontinuity of the bone, fluid accumulation in the adjacent pneumatized structures, and detection of intracranial meningeal enhancement is also good to evaluate these patients. Dorsal dermal sinus tracts are typically found on the dorsal aspect of the spine and in the posterior fossa, and extend into the dorsal aspect of the cord or cerebellum. Diagnosis is best done by sagittal and axial MR imaging, T2-weighted imaging, and T1-weighted imaging, without and with contrast enhancement to show the tract extending across the subcutaneous fat through the posterior wall of the spinal canal and dura toward the cord or cerebellum across the meninges. The nasal dermal tracts extend to the dura of the foramen cecum. The rarer neuroenteric canal is a communication between the respiratory or digestive tract and the anterior aspect of the neural tube posteriorly.

Complications of Bacterial Meningitis

Hydrocephalus

Hydrocephalus in infective meningitis can be communicating or noncommunicating (extraventricular or intraventricular). Obstruction sites may

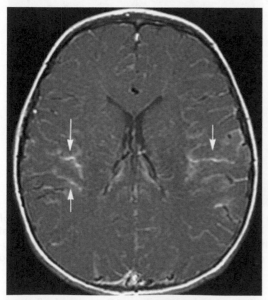

Fig. 8. Bacterial meningitis. Axial contrast-enhanced T1-weighted MR imaging in another child with acute pyogenic meningitis reveals enhancing leptomeningeal exudates over bilateral cerebral convexities (*arrows*).

be multiple and result in complex hydrocephalus with multiple encysted cavities that may or may not communicate, in addition, with parenchymal cavitations. Both CT and MR imaging show the presence of hydrocephalus. MR imaging is superior for localizing the ventricular or the cisternal level(s) of obstruction.

Subdural Effusions and Empyemas

Effusions are simple fluid collections that show CSF like signal on all the pulse sequences and the margins do not enhance. The medial margin of the effusion occasionally shows thin enhancement, presumably because of inflammatory exudate or underlying cortical infarction. Subdural effusions do not need treatment. They typically regress over time with treatment of meningitis. However, they can get infected, resulting in subdural empyemas (SDE). SDE are seen along the cerebral convexities in nearly 50% of cases and along the falx in another 20% of cases.[20,22] SDE typically, but not always, appear crescentic in shape.[22] On CT, SDE appear as extra-axial fluid collections that are isointense to slightly hyperdense to CSF. SDE can be huge, or bilateral. In posterior fossa empyema, bony erosions at the roof of the middle ear cavities can often be observed. On MR imaging, SDE typically appear as crescentic extra-axial fluid collections (Fig. 10A, B), often bilateral, sometimes huge; they are limited by the dural reflections. They show mildly hyperintense signal compared with CSF on T1 and isointensity or hyperintensity compared with CSF on T2-weighted images. There is no water suppression on the FLAIR images, and, because they are made of pus, there is restricted diffusion on diffusion-weighted image and apparent diffusion coefficient (ADC) imaging (see Fig. 10C). This feature is helpful to differentiate them from extra-axial effusions, or from extra-axial hygroma or chronic hematoma. After contrast, there is marked rim enhancement of the limiting membranes caused by inflammatory changes with fibrosis and hypervascularity. There may be internal septations within these collections. The underlying brain may show signal abnormality or enhancement reflecting cerebritis or ischemia because of the involvement of the surface cortical vessels, mostly the veins. There is high propensity for venous thrombosis, especially with SDE, and MR venogram should be performed to evaluate the patency of dural venous sinuses.

Acute parenchymal abscess

Most bacterial abscesses in children are caused by complications of bacterial meningitis. Overall, the most common organisms isolated from the brain abscess include streptococci and staphylococci,

though gram-negative organisms can also be seem. *Citrobacter*, *Proteus*, *Pseudomonas*, and *Serratia* are other common cause of abscesses in neonates. The clinical features of brain abscess include headache, lethargy, obtundation, fever, vomiting, and seizures. Focal neurologic deficits may be seen, depending on the area of brain involved.

Four different stages of evolution of brain abscess from cerebritis are classically known, and these are early cerebritis, late cerebritis, early capsule formation, and late capsule formation.[5] Early cerebritis is the initial stage, lasting for 3 to 5 days, in which the organisms enter the brain parenchyma because of necrotizing vasculitis. Infection is focal and not yet localized. An unencapsulated mass of congested vessels with perivascular neutrophilic infiltrates and edema is seen. In the late cerebritis stage, the necrotic area becomes focal and encapsulation ensues. This stage typically last for between 5 and 14 days. In the early capsule formation stage, collagen and reticulin form a well-defined capsule around the core consisting of liquefied necrotic debris. The capsule is better defined than in the earlier stage. During the late capsule stage, the collagen capsule is complete. It is thicker and better developed than in the previous stage. It is thicker on the cortical side than the ventricular side, probably because of increased vascularity on the cortical surface. The late capsule stage can last for weeks to months. The process of capsule formation from early cerebritis can progress more quickly in neonates than in older children and adults. Brain abscesses in infants and newborns are distinguished by their relatively large sizes, poor capsule formation, and location in the periventricular white matter as opposed to the subcortical white matter seen in adults. Deep location, particularly in the parietooccipital lobes, has a higher propensity of rupture into the ventricular system, resulting in ventriculitis. Intraventricular rupture of brain abscess is associated with poor outcome.[1] Abscesses of the infratentorial structures are uncommon and can be caused by direct extension of disease from the infected middle ear or mastoid air cells. imaging, the early cerebritis stage shows heterogeneous hyperintensity on both T1-weighted and T2-weighted images and shows patchy enhancement with contrast. In late cerebritis and the early capsular stage, the capsule wall appears as a hyperintense rim on T1-weighted images and as a slightly hypointense rim on T2-weighted images. The center of the abscess is heterogeneous on both sequences. The wall shows intense enhancement with contrast. The content of the abscess cavity becomes hypointense on T1-weighted images

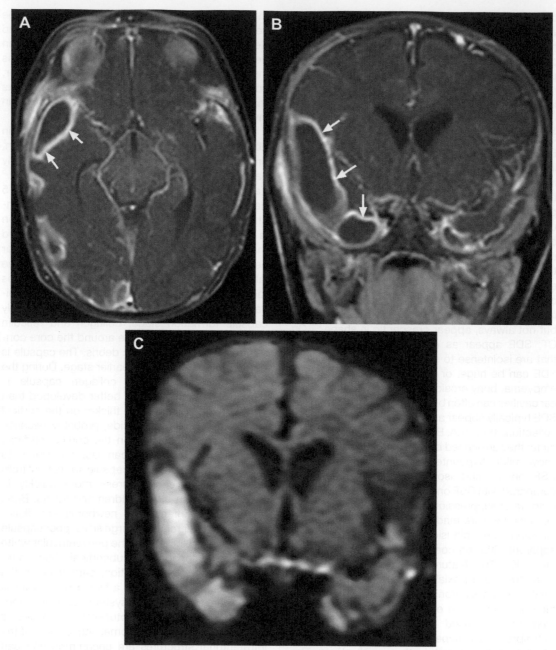

Fig. 10. Subdural empyema. Axial (*A*) and coronal (*B*) contrast-enhanced T1-weighted MR imaging in a neonate with bacterial meningitis show large extra-axial fluid collections, especially over the right temporal convexity. They show thick enhancing peripheral margins (*arrows*). These collection show hyperintensity on the diffusion-weighted images (*C*), which suggests subdural empyema.

and hyperintense on T2-weighted images. The capsule becomes isointense on T1-weighted images and markedly hypointense on T2-weighted images in the late capsular stage (**Fig. 11**A),[17] and it shows smooth and intense enhancement (see **Fig. 11**B). The enhancing rim is thicker toward the cortical surface and thinner as it approaches the ventricles.[17] During the weeks and months after the end of treatment, enhancement may persist where the abscess was, presumably to persistent fibrous tissue. Enhancement therefore is not helpful to assess the response to treatment. Restricted diffusion may have different meanings at different stages. In the cerebritis

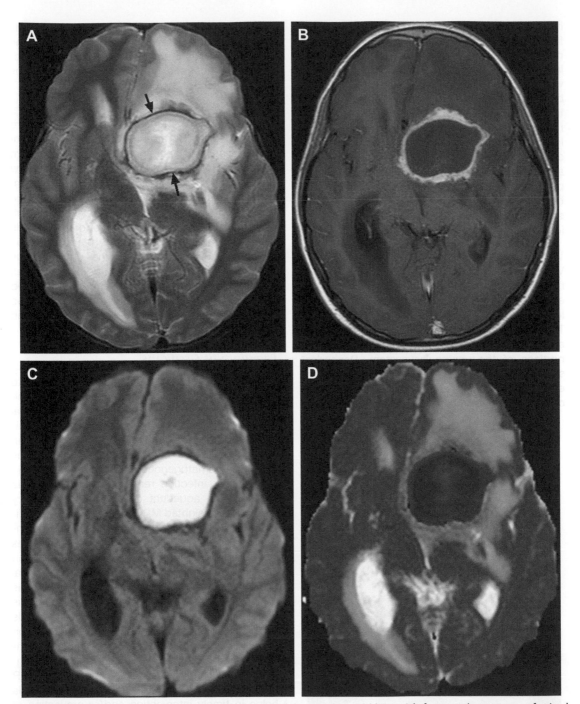

Fig. 11. Brain abscess. Axial T2-weighted MR imaging (*A*) in a 9-year-old boy with fever and symptoms of raised intracranial pressure reveals a large T2 hyperintense lesion in the left frontal lobe with marked surrounding vasogenic edema and mass effect. This lesion has T2 dark rims (*arrows*) that show enhancement with gadolinium (*B*). Diffusion-weighted image (*C*) reveals restricted diffusion within the center of this lesion with dark signal on the corresponding apparent diffusion coefficient map (*D*), which suggests an abscess.

stages, it likely reflects the tissue ischemia with cytotoxic edema that results from the necrotizing vasculitis; the inflammatory hypercellularity may also play a role. In the capsular stage, the restricted diffusion within the abscess cavity is caused by hyperviscosity of the abscess contents and by the hypercellularity that reduces water diffusion (see **Fig. 11**C, D).[23] Diffusion-weighted imaging is thus helpful to differentiate parenchymal abscesses from other cystic lesions and necrotic brain neoplasms. Sequential diffusion imaging correlates well with the response to treatment in children with brain abscesses. MR spectroscopy can also be used to differentiate abscess from necrotic brain tumors. Most tumors show increased choline with reduced N-acetylaspartate on MR spectroscopy. In comparison, brain abscesses show peaks of aliphatic amino acids like alanine, succinate, acetate, leucine, isoleucine, and valine.[24] A lactate peak is seen in all brain abscesses, but it can also be seen in necrotic neoplasms. Based on the specific amino acid peaks, it is even possible to identify the causative organism.[24]

Ventriculitis

Ventriculitis is a common complication of bacterial meningitis. The organism enters the ventricles either caused by direct rupture of the parenchymal lesion or because of spread via the choroid plexus. The classic imaging finding in ventriculitis is presence of proteinaceous debris at the dependent portions of the ventricular system. Dependent secretions show reduced diffusion. Intense enhancement of the ependymal lining is seen after contrast administration (Fig. 12). Because of

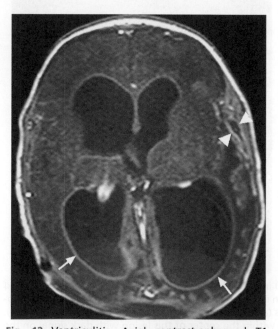

Fig. 12. Ventriculitis. Axial contrast-enhanced T1-weighted MR imaging in a neonate with intraventricular hemorrhage and secondary infection reveals thickening and enhancement of the ventricular lining, suggesting acute ventriculitis (*arrows*). Some debris is noted within the ventricles with ventriculomegaly. Small subdural empyema was also seen over the left temporal convexity (*arrowheads*).

reduced CSF absorption, the ventricles are nearly always dilated. Sometimes there is necrosis of the periventricular white matter, caused by obstruction of the subependymal and periventricular veins or direct effect of the bacterial toxins.[1]

Infarcts

Arterial infarctions in the setting of meningitis are usually caused by arteritis from involvement of the perivascular space and arterial walls from infection. Both CT and MR imaging can show these infarcts, but MR imaging delineates them better. Diffusion-weighted imaging shows the lesions earlier (Fig. 13 A, B). The classic location of arterial infarcts is along the perforator vessels of anterior and middle cerebral arteries. Venous infarcts from thrombosis of the dural venous sinuses can be seen and imaging findings are as per the particular sinus involvement. Compared with arterial infarcts, venous infarcts do not always show restricted diffusion, and these infarcts can often be hemorrhagic.

Labyrinthitis Ossificans

Labyrinthitis ossificans is an end-stage sequela to purulent labyrinthitis characterized by new bone formation in the cochlea and vestibule. Bacterial meningitis is the most common cause of labyrinthitis ossificans, although labyrinthine infection can occur secondary to bacterial middle ear infections or by the hematogenous route. In meningogenic labyrinthitis, infection reaches the inner ear via the cochlear aqueduct or the internal auditory meatus. T2-weighted MR imaging and postgadolinium T1-weighted images can detect early inflammation within the labyrinth before ossification has set in. Early phases of labyrinthine inflammation show a slight reduction in the cochlear fluid signal on T2-weighted MR imaging (Fig. 14A), which is attributed to the presence of intracochlear fibrous tissue.[25] Further evidence of early labyrinthitis ossificans is enhancement of cochlear fluid on gadolinium MR imaging, indicating ongoing inflammation (see Fig. 14B). Early identification of labyrinthine inflammation with gadolinium-enhanced MR imaging along with clinical and audiological criteria helps in timely intervention and/or prevention of labyrinthitis ossificans.[25]

VIRAL ENCEPHALITIS

Encephalitis is a diffuse inflammatory process of the brain and is usually caused by a viral infection. Bacterial causes of meningoencephalitis are unusual, but occur in neonates, most commonly from *E coli* and group B *Streptococci*. Common viruses involving the pediatric age group include

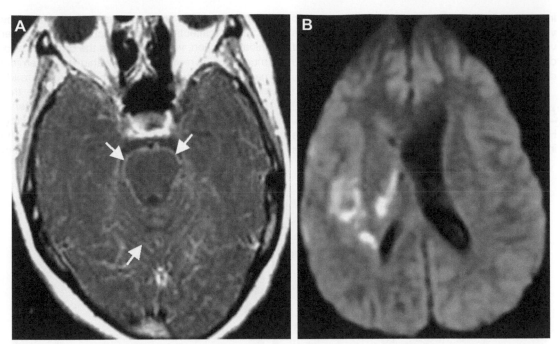

Fig. 13. Postmeningitis vasculitis. (A) Axial contrast-enhanced T1-weighted MR imaging in 6-year-old patient with acute tuberculous meningitis reveals enhancing leptomeningeal exudates over bilateral cerebellar hemispheres and coating the ventral pons (arrows). (B) Axial diffusion-weighted image shows multiple areas of restricted diffusion in right insula, basal ganglia, and thalamus, suggesting postmeningitis vasculitis.

HSV 1, mumps virus, varicella, and arbovirus. Most of the viral involvement of the CNS is via the hematogenous route. Infection by a few viruses, like polio virus and HSV 1, spreads to the CNS via peripheral nerves.[1] Affected brain usually shows neuronal loss and inflammation of the white matter and, at times, of the meninges. The clinical symptoms are often nonspecific and include seizure, delirium, and focal neurologic deficit. Imaging findings are also nonspecific and exhibit considerable overlap, making it , difficult to diagnose the viral cause in many cases. Few viruses have a predilection to involve specific regions of the brain, like involvement of thalami and brainstem, involvement of hippocampi, cingulated gyrus, substantia nigra, or basal nuclei or

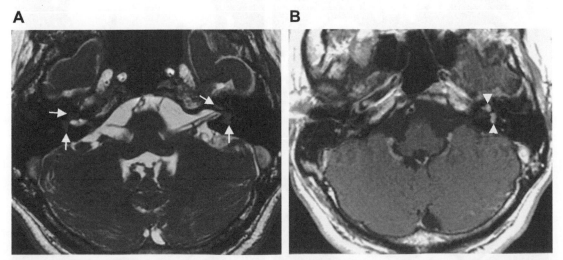

Fig. 14. Postmeningitis labyrinthitis ossificans. Axial FIESTA MR imaging image (A) through the membranous labyrinth shows decrease in the T2 signal within bilateral cochlea and vestibule (arrows). Axial contrast-enhanced T1-weighted image (B) shows enhancement in both the membranous labyrinths (arrowheads). This case was an early stage of postmeningitis labyrinthitis ossificans.

involvement of the cerebellum. A few specific viruses like HSV 1, varicella virus, and measles virus are discussed here, along with a brief discussion on Rasmussen encephalitis and acute disseminated encephalomyelitis (ADEM).

HSV 1

HSV 1 is the common cause of herpes encephalitis in all patients older than 6 month. Patients less than 20 years old comprise nearly 30% of all cases of HSV 1 infection.[26] It is postulated that, after initial infection, virus penetrates the oral and nasal mucosa and remains latent within the trigeminal ganglion. Following reactivation, the virus spreads along the branches of the trigeminal nerve that innervate the meninges, especially in the anterior and middle cranial fossa.[26] The virus probably also has a tropism for the limbic system.[1] The disease begins in the anterior and medial parts of

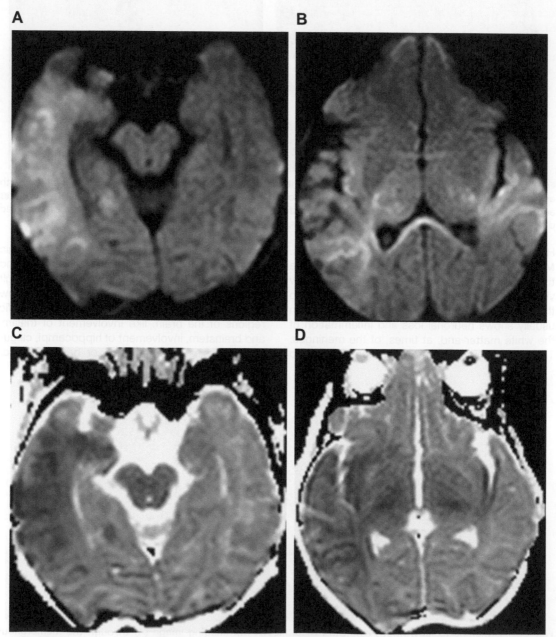

Fig. 15. HSV 1 encephalitis. Axial diffusion-weighted images (*A, B*) in a 4-year-old patient with HSV 1 encephalitis show multifocal areas of restricted diffusion and dark signal on corresponding ADC maps (*C, D*) in the right temporal lobe, right insula, and, to a lesser extent, in the left temporal lobe.

the temporal lobes, spreads to the insular cortex, inferior parts of the frontal lobes, and the cingulated gyri. Basal nuclei are usually spared. Like most viral encephalitis, imaging earlier in the course of the disease is nonspecific and may even be normal. If possible, diffusion-weighted images should be obtained and reviewed in all suspected cases because they show the abnormalities earlier and more extensively than the conventional T2-weighted images, allowing an earlier diagnosis (**Fig. 15**A–D).Hemorrhage can occasionally be seen in the involved regions. Enhancement occurs in the subacute phase of the disease and involves the cortex and overlying meninges. Bilateral involvement is common. In patients who survive the disease, multifocal encephalomalacia, cortical gyriform calcification, and ventriculomegaly is noted.

Varicella Virus

Varicella-zoster infection is common during childhood and results in chickenpox. CNS complication of varicella virus affects less than 0.1% of children.[27] Clinical symptoms usually develop within 10 days of onset of skin rash and include headache, vomiting, dysarthria, hemiparesis, and signs of raised intracranial pressure.[27] Imaging shows lesions in the gray white junction, cerebral cortex, basal ganglia, and in the cerebellum.[1] Sometimes patients present with delayed onset of neurologic deficits often caused by varicella induced

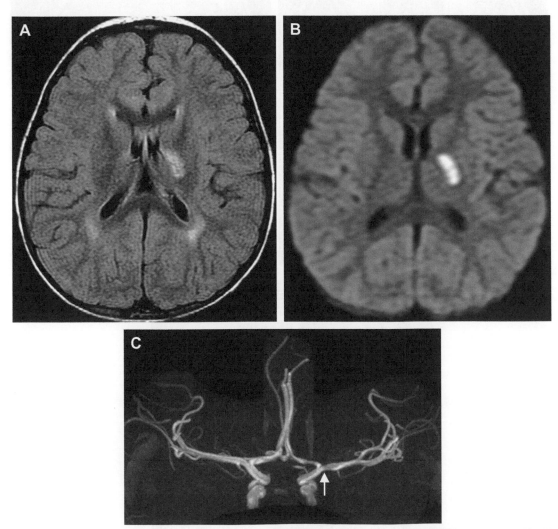

Fig. 16. Postvaricella angiitis. Axial FLAIR-weighted MR imaging (*A*) in a child with right-sided hemiplegia after varicella infection show a focal area of signal abnormality in the posterior limb of the left internal capsule. This area showed restricted diffusion consistent with an acute ischemic lesion (*B*). Time of flight MR angiogram image (*C*) shows focal area of narrowing (*arrow*) in the proximal aspect of the left middle cerebral artery from postvaricella angiitis.

angitis.[28] These patients present 1 to 4 months after initial skin rash and most of them have focal neurologic deficit caused by infarction of basal ganglia (Fig. 16A, B). Narrowing of the distal internal carotid artery and proximal anterior and middle cerebral arteries is seen on angiography (see Fig. 16C).

Measles Virus

Measles virus is known to involve the CNS either as acute postinfectious encephalitis, progressive infectious encephalitis, or as subacute sclerosing panencephalitis.[29] Acute postinfectious encephalitis is thought to be an autoimmune process with perivascular inflammation and demyelination in the affected brain. Imaging reveals areas of T2 hyperintensity in the thalami, basal ganglia, and cortex.[1] Progressive infectious encephalitis is associated with impaired cell immunity. Affected patients show progressive neurologic deterioration including seizures and altered mental status. Subacute sclerosing panencephalitis (SSPE) is thought to be caused by reactivation of the measles

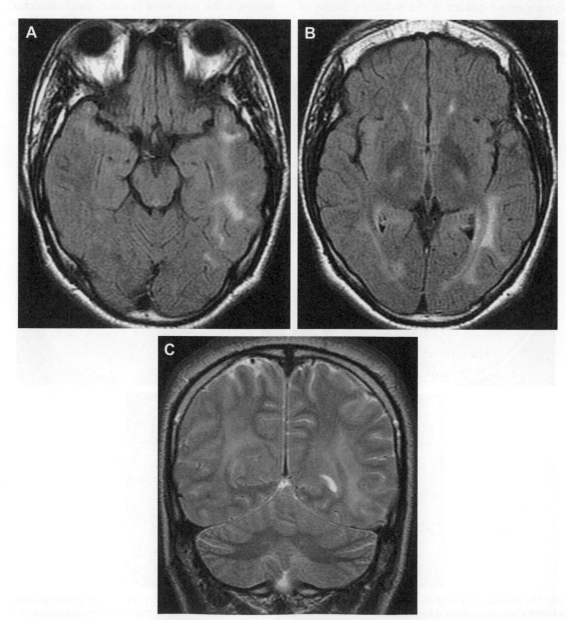

Fig. 17. Postmeasles SSPE. Axial (A, B) FLAIR and coronal T2-weighted (C) MR imaging in a 12-year-old patient with SSPE shows multifocal areas of signal abnormalities in the white matter, especially in left temporal lobe and within bilateral peritrigonal regions.

virus, many years after initial illness.[30] It commonly involves children and presents with behavioral changes, mental deterioration, ataxia, myoclonus, and visual disturbances. Severe dementia, quadriparesis, and autonomic instability eventually follow. Affected patients have a poor prognosis, with most children dying within 1 to 3 years after disease onset.[1] On imaging, there is diffuse atrophy with multifocal areas of signal abnormality (T2 hyperintensity) in periventricular and subcortical white matter (Fig. 17A–C). Contrast enhancement is typically not seen. Involvement is predominantly in the temporal and parietal lobes, often in an asymmetric fashion. Basal ganglia are involved in 20% to 35% of cases,[31] and the brainstem is involved late in the disease.[1]

Rasmussen Encephalitis

Rasmussen encephalitis, or chronic localized encephalitis, was first described by Rasmussen and colleagues[32] in 1958 in series of children with severe progressive focal epilepsy. It is one of the common causes of intractable epilepsy in childhood. Affected patients typically present within the age group of 2 to 14 years, with mean of 7 years.[1] The symptoms include varying degree of hemiparesis, dysphasia, hemianopia, and mental deterioration, along with progressive, refractory seizures. Surgical resection of the affected hemisphere is the only known effective treatment. Although the cause of Rasmussen encephalitis is not known, it is widely

thought to be caused by slow virus infection like Epstein-Barr virus or CMV.[2] Another possibility is an autoimmune process.[33] On imaging, the initial examination is often normal. Subsequent imaging shows areas of T2 prolongation in the cortex, especially in the frontal and temporal lobes. Atrophy of the involved regions (Fig. 18A, B) and involvement of the subcortical white matter is seen later.[34] Basal ganglia involvement is seen in about 65% of cases.[34] Positron emission tomography (PET) imaging using F18-fluorodeoxyglucose shows reduced metabolic uptake in the involved regions of the cerebral hemisphere.[1]

Acute Demyelinating Encephalomyelitis

Acute demyelinating encephalomyelitis (ADEM), or parainfectious encephalomyelitis, is autoimmune postinfectious encephalitis, without or with myelitis, resulting in demyelination. It happens late in the course of a viral illness or after a vaccination. The usual clinical presentation is onset of neurologic signs and symptoms a few days to a few weeks after the viral event. Children present with seizures, ataxia, and altered mental status. Most cases are self-limiting; with most patients making a complete recovery. Between 10% and 30% have some permanent neurologic damage.[35] The disorder rarely shows alternate waxing and waning, leading to the term multiphasic disseminated encephalomyelitis or relapsing disseminated encephalomyelitis.[36] Chances of second attack are

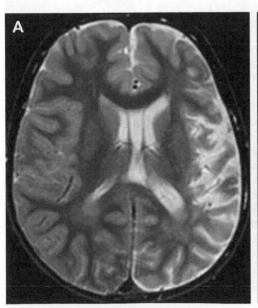
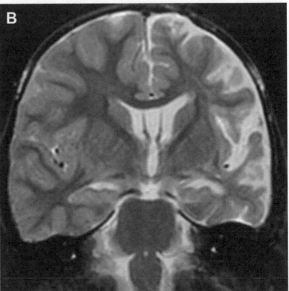

Fig. 18. Rasmussen encephalitis. Axial (A) and coronal (B) T2-weighted MR imaging in a 10-year-old patient with chronic epilepsy shows asymmetric volume loss involving the left cerebral hemisphere, especially in the frontoparietal and temporal lobes.

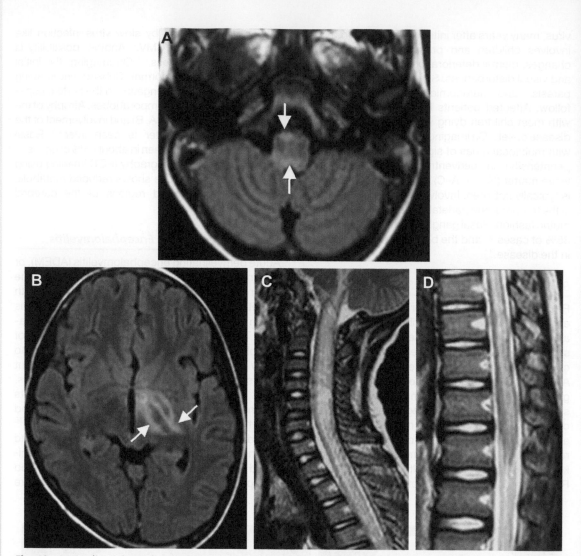

Fig. 19. Acute disseminated encephalomyelitis. Axial FLAIR-weighted MR images show multifocal signal abnormalities within the brainstem (A) and left thalamus/basal nuclei (B) (arrows). Sagittal T2-weighted MR imaging of the spine shows extensive T2 hyperintensity with cord swelling in both cervical (C) and thoracic (D) regions.

greater in patients who are more than 10 years of age at initial presentation.[1] A hemorrhagic variant of ADEM is also described in which the involved regions undergo hemorrhagic necrosis. Affected patients tend to have a grave prognosis, with most dying within days to weeks after onset.[37] On pathology, confluent areas of demyelination are seen both in the brain and spinal cord parenchyma. Cortical and deep gray matter is involved to a lesser extent than the white matter. On imaging, the involved areas are of low attenuation on CT and show increased T2/ FLAIR signal (Fig. 19A, B). The pattern of involvement is bilateral, but often asymmetric. Unlike multiple sclerosis, involvement of periventricular white matter is seen in 50% of cases and corpus callosum is also less involved.[1] Deep cerebral nuclei are involved in almost 50%

of cases and brainstem, cerebellum, and spinal cord are involved in about 30% to 50% of cases.[38] Contrast enhancement is seen in the subacute stage. Diffusion-weighted images show increased water diffusion. Spine imaging should be obtained in suspected cases, which can show varying degrees of spinal cord swelling and increased T2 signal within the cord (see **Fig. 19**C, D). Like the intracranial lesions, spinal cord lesions show contrast enhancement in the subacute stages.

REFERENCES

1. Barkovich AJ. Pediatric neuroradiology. 4th edition. Philadelphia: Lippincott Williams & Wilkins; 2005. p. 801–68.

2. Ressler JA, Nelson M. Central nervous system infections in the pediatric population. Neuroimaging Clin North Am 2000;10:427–43.

3. Bale JF, Murph JR. Congenital infections and the nervous system. Pediatr Clin North Am 1992;39:669–90.

4. Diebler C, Dusser A, Dulac O. Congenital toxoplasmosis: clinical and neuroradiologic evaluation of the cerebral lesions. Neuroradiology 1985;27:125–30.

5. Bale JR. Viral infections. In: Berg BO, editor. Neurologic aspects of pediatrics. Boston: Butterworth-Heinemann; 1992. p. 227–56.

6. Hayward JC, Titelbaum DS, Clancy RR, et al. Lissencephaly-pachygyria associated with congenital cytomegalovirus infection. J Child Neurol 1991;6:109–14.

7. Lindegran M, Byers RJ, Thomas P, et al. Trends in perinatal transmission of HIV/AIDS in the United States. JAMA 1999;282:531–8.

8. Belman AL. Acquired immunodeficiency syndrome and the child's central nervous system. Pediatr Neurol 1992;10:691–714.

9. Barnes PD, Poussaint TY, Burrows PE. Imaging of pediatric central nervous system infections. Neuroimaging Clin North Am 1994;4:367–91.

10. Johann-Liang R, Lin K, Cervia J, et al. Neuroimaging findings in children perinatally infected with the human immunodeficiency virus. Pediatr Infect Dis J 1998;17:753–4.

11. Griffith BP, Booss J. Neurologic infections of the fetus and newborn. Neurol Clin 1994;12:541–64.

12. Lane B, Sullivan EV, Lim KO, et al. White matter MR hyperintensities in adult patients with congenital rubella. AJNR Am J Neuroradiol 1996;17:99–103.

13. Leung A, Sauve R, Davies H. Congenital cytomegalovirus infection. J Natl Med Assoc 2003;95:213–8.

14. Steinlin MI, Nadal D, Eich GE, et al. Late intrauterine cytomegalovirus infection: clinical and neuroimaging findings. Pediatr Neurol 1996;15:249–53.

15. van der Knapp MS, Vermeulen G, Barkhof F, et al. Pattern of white matter abnormalities at MR imaging: use of polymerase chain reaction testing of Guthrie cards to link pattern with congenital cytomegalovirus infection. Radiology 2004;230:529–36.

16. Noorbehesht B, Enzmann DR, Sullinder W, et al. Neonatal herpes simplex encephalitis: correlation of clinical and CT findings. Radiology 1987;162:813–9.

17. Osborn AG. Infections of the brain and its linings. Diagnostic neuroradiology. St Louis (MO): Mosby; 1994. p. 680–2.

18. Shrier LA, Schopps JH, Feigin RD. Bacterial and fungal infections of the central nervous system. In: Berg BO, editor. Principles of child neurology. New York: McGraw-Hill; 1996. p. 766–71.

19. Volpe JJ. Neurology of the newborn. 4th edition. Philadelphia: Saunders; 2001.

20. Lipton JD, Schafermeyer RW. Evolving concepts in pediatric bacterial meningitis: part I: pathophysiology and diagnosis. Ann Emerg Med 1993;22:1602–15.

21. Parmar H, Sitoh YY, Anand P, et al. Contrast enhanced FLAIR imaging in evaluation of infectious leptomeningeal diseases. Eur J Radiol 2006;58:89–95.

22. Wong AM, Zimmerman RA, Simon EM, et al. Diffusion-weighted MR imaging of subdural empyemas in children. AJNR Am J Neuroradiol 2004;25:1016–21.

23. Kim YJ, Chang KH, Song IC, et al. Brain abscess and necrotic or cystic brain tumor: discrimination with signal intensity on diffusion-weighted MR imaging. AJR Am J Roentgenol 1998;171:1487–90.

24. Garg M, Gupta RK, Husain M, et al. Brain abscesses: etiologic categorization with in vivo proton MR spectroscopy. Radiology 2004;230:519–27.

25. Mukerji S, Parmar H, Pynnonen M. Labyrinthitis ossificans. Arch Otolaryngol Head Neck Surg 2007;133: 298–300.

26. Bale JR. Viral infections of the central nervous system. In: Berg BO, editor. Principles of child neurology. New York: McGraw-Hill; 1996. p. 839–58.

27. Johnson R, Milbourn PE. Central nervous system manifestations of chickenpox. Can Med Assoc J 1970;102:831–4.

28. Silverstein FS, Brunberg JA. Postvaricella basal ganglia infarction in children. AJNR Am J Neuroradiol 1995;16:449–52.

29. Norrby E, Kristensson K. Measles virus in the brain. Brain Res Bull 1997;44:213–20.

30. Krawiecki NS, Dyken PR, El Gammal T, et al. CT of the brain in subacute sclerosing panencephalitis. Ann Neurol 1984;15:489–93.

31. Brismar J, Gascon GG, von Steyern KV, et al. Subacute sclerosing panencephalitis: evaluation with CT and MR. AJNR Am J Neuroradiol 1996;17:761–72.

32. Rasmussen T, Olszewski J, Lloydsmith D. Focal seizures due to chronic localized encephalitis. Neurology 1958;8:435–45.

33. Rogers SW, Andrews PI, Gahring L, et al. Autoantibodies to glutamate receptor GluR3 in Rasmussen's encephalitis. Science 1994;265:648–51.

34. Bhatjiwale M, Polkey C, Cox TCS, et al. Rasmussen's encephalitis: neuroimaging findings in 21 patients with a closer look at the basal ganglia. Pediatr Neurosurg 1998;29:142–8.

35. Sriram S, Steinman L. Postinfectious and postvaccinial encephalomyelitis. Neurol Clin 1984;2: 341–53.

36. Stuve O, Zamvil SS. Pathogenesis, diagnosis and treatment of acute disseminated encephalomyelitis. Curr Opin Neurol 1999;12:395–401.

37. Reich H, Lin SR, Goldblatt D. Computerized tomography in acute hemorrhagic leukoencephalopathy: case report. Neurology 1979;29:255–8.

38. Murthy J. Acute disseminated encephalomyelitis. Neurol India 2002;50:238–43.

Imaging in Infections of the Head and Neck

Amogh N. Hegde, MBBS, MD, FRCR[a],*, Suyash Mohan, MD[b],
Amit Pandya, MD[c], Gaurang V. Shah, MD[c]

KEYWORDS

- Head and neck • Infection • Magnetic resonance imaging • Computed tomography
- Complications • Deep neck spaces • Cross sectional imaging • Abscess • Phlegmon

KEY POINTS

- Imaging plays a central role in delineating anatomic extent of infection, detecting complications, assisting in accurate diagnosis, and guiding drainage procedures.
- Computed tomography is the mainstay investigation in the imaging workup for head and neck infections.
- Magnetic resonance imaging is reserved for assessing intracranial extension and intramedullary bone marrow signal, and to monitor response to therapy.
- Ultrasound is preferred for assessment of lymph nodes, salivary glands, and neck abscesses, and plays an important role in imaging the pediatric population.
- Cross-sectional imaging is preferred in presurgical anatomic localization, particularly for deep-seated and locally extensive lesions.

IMAGING IN INFECTIONS OF THE HEAD AND NECK

Infections of the head and neck vary in their clinical course and outcome because of the diversity of organs and anatomic compartments involved. Although the clinical diagnosis is obvious in most cases, some infections may be misleading in their severity and extent owing to limitations of physical examination and complexity of the anatomy involved. Delay in appropriate management increases the risk of life-threatening complications, because of compromise of vital structures like the airway, cervical vessels, optic nerves, intracranial space, and spinal canal.[1] Imaging plays a central role in delineating the anatomic extent of the disease process, identifying the infection source, and detecting complications. The utility of imaging to differentiate between a solid phlegmonous mass and an abscess cannot be overemphasized, the latter being an indication for drainage. This review briefly describes and pictorially illustrates the typical imaging findings of some important head and neck infections, such as malignant otitis externa, otomastoiditis bacterial and fungal sinusitis, orbital cellulitis, sialadenitis, cervical lymphadenitis, and deep neck space infections.

IMAGING MODALITIES

Contrast-enhanced computed tomography (CT) is the mainstay investigation for the infections of the head and neck. The rapid data acquisition of a CT scan nearly completely eliminates motion artifacts from swallowing, respiration, and eye movements and reduces the study duration.[1] Besides high spatial and temporal resolution, multiplanar reformats (MPRs) are made available in a single

[a] Department of Radiology, Singapore General Hospital, Block 4, Level 1, Outram Rd, Singapore 169608;
[b] Department of Radiology, Division of Neuroradiology, University of Pennsylvania School of Medicine, Philadelphia, PA 19104, USA; [c] Department of Radiology, B2 A209, University of Michigan Health System, 1500 E. Medical Center Drive, Ann Arbor, MI 48109-0030, USA
* Corresponding author.
E-mail address: amogh77@yahoo.co.in

Neuroimag Clin N Am 22 (2012) 727–754
doi:10.1016/j.nic.2012.05.007
1052-5149/12/$ – see front matter © 2012 Elsevier Inc. All rights reserved.

acquisition.[2] CT is the modality of choice for imaging temporal bone and paranasal sinuses because of the exquisite bone detail provided. Foreign bodies and salivary duct calculi, which may be the source of infection, are best resolved on this modality. Some deep neck spaces extend into the mediastinum; infections extending into the mediastinum are well resolved on CT scan. A few disadvantages of CT scan are the unavoidable risk of radiation exposure and artifacts from bone, hardware, or dental amalgam.[3] Adverse allergic reactions to iodinated contrast and contrast nephrotoxicity can be a limiting factor in some patients.

Magnetic resonance imaging (MRI) has an inherent advantage of higher soft tissue contrast resolution as compared with CT.[3] Intracranial extension of infections is best assessed with MRI. Although not useful for cortical bone assessment, intramedullary bone marrow signal is best evaluated on this modality.[4,5] The disadvantages of MRI lie in its relatively higher cost, longer scan time, intolerance by claustrophobic patients, the recently discovered risk of nephrogenic systemic fibrosis in renal impairment from some Gadolinium-based agents, and contraindications to usage in patients with implanted devices and metallic foreign bodies near vital structures.[3]

Ultrasound (US) plays an important role in head and neck imaging, especially in the pediatric population, as the relatively superficial nature of the neck structures lends itself readily to ultrasound assessment.[6] US is being widely accepted as the first imaging method for assessment of lymph nodes and major salivary glands in some countries.[7–9] US can help to ascertain the suitability of neck abscesses for drainage and also assist in the same. The limitations include inaccessibility of deep-seated lesions, its inability to penetrate bone or air-filled structures, its operator dependency, and variable reproducibility in serial imaging.[10] Cross-sectional imaging is preferred in presurgical anatomic localization, particularly for more deep-seated and locally extensive lesions.[11]

The role of plain radiographs in head and neck imaging is at best supplementary, limited to confirming a few conditions like acute sinusitis, retropharyngeal swelling, or acute epiglottitis. Dental radiographs, such as the Panorex oral view, are useful in identifying odontogenic sources of infection.[1]

Nuclear medicine studies in head and neck infections are occasionally used to diagnose early osteomyelitis (using 99mTc-labeled methylene diphosphonate [MDP] bone scan). Rarely, gallium and indium may be used for localization of infection.[3]

The imaging features of various head and neck infections are discussed by anatomic region: (1) temporal bone, (2) paranasal sinuses, (3) orbits, (4) salivary glands, (5) cervical lymphadenopathy, (6) deep neck infections and necrotizing fasciitis.

Infections of the Temporal Bone

External auditory canal cholesteatoma

External auditory canal (EAC) cholesteatoma has an estimated incidence of 0.1% to 0.5% of all otologic patients, typically presenting as otorrhoea, dull pain, and conductive hearing loss.[12,13] The exact etiology remains unclear, some cases being spontaneous; postsurgical or posttraumatic etiologies have been implicated. Ear canal stenosis or obstruction may also be a causative factor.[14]

On high-resolution CT (HRCT), the EAC cholesteatoma typically manifests as a soft tissue mass in the EAC with associated bone erosion and intramural bone fragments with a propensity to involve the inferior and/or posterior walls (**Fig. 1**).[13,15] Extension into the middle ear cavity, facial nerve canal, and mastoid air cells may be noted. Imaging differentials include squamous cell carcinoma, severe otitis externa, keratosis obturans, and cerumen.[16] Treatment options range from conservative medical therapy with frequent cleaning

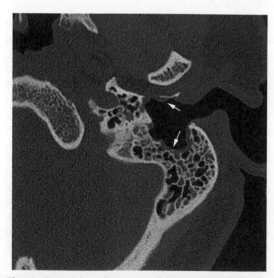

Fig. 1. External auditory canal (EAC) cholesteatoma. Axial high-resolution CT (HRCT) image of the left temporal bone demonstrates widening of the bony portion of the external auditory canal with underlying erosion of the posterior wall, extending into the mastoid air cells. Tiny fragments of bone are seen within the thin rind of soft tissue (*arrows*) that overlies the eroded areas.

and debridement for painless localized EAC cholesteatomas to modified radical mastoidectomy for those with mastoid involvement.[13,17,18]

Malignant otitis externa and skull base osteomyelitis

Skull base osteomyelitis most often is secondary to an infection that has extended beyond the external auditory canal.[19] Diabetes mellitus is the most important associated condition, among other immunocompromised states. *Pseudomonas* and *Aspergillus* (especially in patients seropositive for human immunodeficiency virus [HIV]) are common species of organisms implicated in this condition.[1,20] The typical presentation is that of an elderly diabetic with severe otalgia, otorrhea, hearing loss, and a swollen, tender external auditory canal. Palsies of cranial nerves VII, IX, X, and XI may also be present in severe cases.

The early HRCT findings are characterized by mucosal thickening and enhancement in the external auditory canal with bone erosion, consistent with osteomyelitis (**Fig. 2A, B**). Eventually, the infection spreads to involve the masticator space, middle ear, mastoid and temporomandibular joint well depicted on CT scan. MRI is sensitive to changes in the medullary bone marrow and is better than CT to monitor response to treatment and demonstrate intracranial extension (see **Fig. 2C**).[21,22] Nuclear medicine studies, such as 99mTc- MDP bone scans, [111]Indium-labeled white blood cell scans, or gallium citrate scans, are very sensitive but not specific for detection of skull base osteomyelitis.[22–24] Aggressive intravenous antibiotic therapy, diabetic control, local debridement of granulation tissue/bony sequestrum, and drainage of associated abscess are required for effective management.

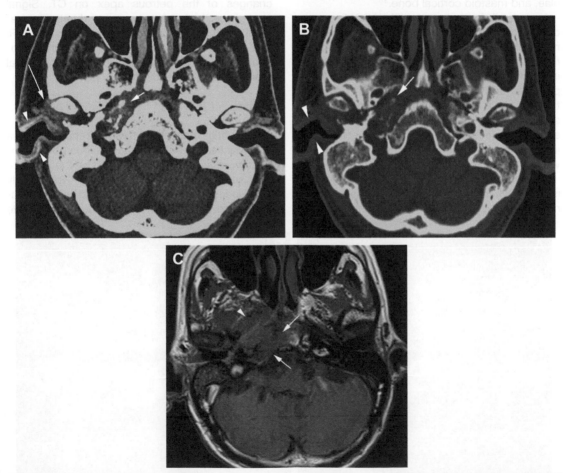

Fig. 2. Right-sided malignant otitis externa. Axial CT image in soft tissue window (*A*) and bone window (*B*) settings reveal soft tissue swelling in the right external auditory canal (*arrowheads*). The soft tissue causes irregular bone destruction at the right petrous apex (*arrow*) and also involves the right temporomandibular joint (*long arrow* in *A*). The clivus appears irregular and sclerotic but T1-weighted MR image (*C*) clearly depicts bone marrow infiltration of the clivus. The soft tissue also extends into the right masticator space (*arrowhead*), obliterating the fat planes between the pterygoid muscles.

Acute infections of the middle ear and mastoids

Acute otitis media (AOM) is inflammation of the middle ear that occurs primarily in children caused by Eustachian tube dysfunction, secondary to hypertrophy of the adenoids. *Streptococcus* (particularly group A beta hemolytic *Streptococcus* and *Streptococcus pneumoniae*) and *Haemophilus influenzae* account for 65% to 80% of bacterial cases.[25] A minority of cases develop acute mastoiditis with symptoms similar to, but longer and recurrent than those of uncomplicated AOM. Patients present acutely, and the diagnosis is based on clinical signs and symptoms of pain, fever, otorrhea, retroauricular swelling, and erythema.[26,27] CT shows nonspecific increased attenuation of the middle ear cavity and mastoid cells, sometimes with fluid levels but with preservation of the ossicular chain, trabeculae, and mastoid cortical bone.[28]

In acute coalescent mastoiditis (ACOM), erosion of the mastoid septa or mastoid walls may be noted on CT scan. Lateral wall erosion may give rise to a subperiosteal abscess, which may extend into the neck as a Bezold abscess (Fig. 3).[29] Apical petrositis and labyrinthitis are known complications (see later in this article). Erosion of the medial sigmoid sinus plate may result in intracranial spread of infection, manifesting as meningitis, or intracranial abscess (Fig. 4) and thrombosis involving the adjacent sigmoid sinus.[25]

On spin-echo MR sequences, loss of signal void is noted, whereas on gradient MR sequences it is represented by a lack of flow-related enhancement.

On contrast-enhanced CT and MRI, sigmoid sinus thrombosis appears as a filling defect in the sinus, surrounded by its enhancing dural lining (Fig. 5). Patients with ACOM require aggressive management with intravenous (IV) antibiotics and/or surgical intervention (myringotomy with or without mastoidectomy).[25]

Petrous apicitis

Medial spread of infection in acute otomastoiditis along a pneumatized petrous apex (exists in 30% population) causes petrositis. However, petrositis may also occur in isolation without otomastoiditis. Patients with petrous apicitis are usually acutely sick with fever and some or all of the symptoms of the Gradenigo triad: ipsilateral cranial nerve VI paralysis, severe facial pain in V distribution, and inflammatory disease of the inner ear or mastoid air cells.[30] Imaging studies demonstrate erosive changes of the petrous apex on CT. Signal changes in the bone marrow and dural enhancement at the petrous apex are noted on MRI (Fig. 6).[25] In most cases, treatment with appropriate intravenous antibiotics suffices and surgical drainage is rarely required.

Chronic infections of the middle ear and mastoids

Chronic otitis media (COM) without cholesteatoma may manifest as noncholesteomatous/postinflammatory ossicular erosion, defined by the absence of a segment of the ossicular chain (commonly distal incus) with or without surrounding inflammatory tissue. Alternatively, it may present as middle

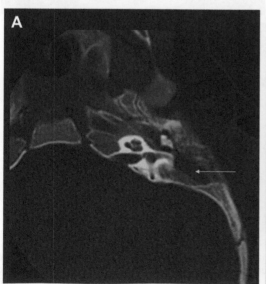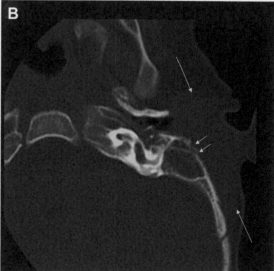

Fig. 3. Coalescent mastoiditis with subperiosteal abscess. Axial CT sections in bone window through the left temporal bone showing opacification of mastoid air cells (*arrow* in *A*) and the middle ear cavity with left post-auricular subperiosteal abscess (*arrows* in *B*). Note subtle erosions in the mastoid cortex (*small arrows* in *B*).

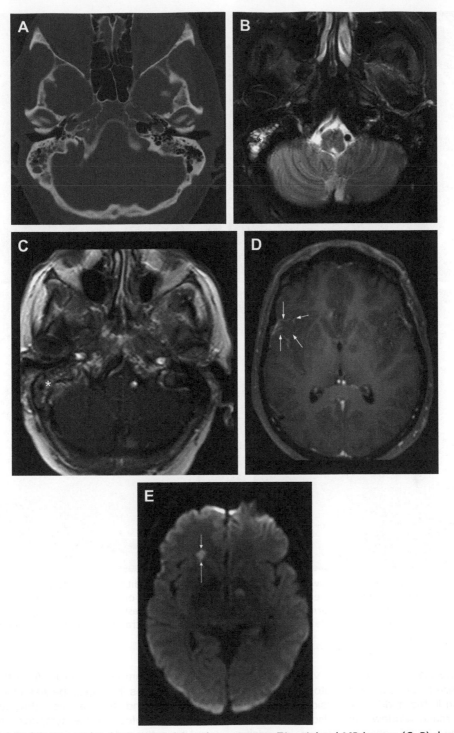

Fig. 4. Axial CT (*A*), T2-weighted MR image (*B*) and postcontrast T1-weighted MR images (*C, D*) showing right mastoiditis (*asterisk*), with focal leptomeningitis in the right sylvian cistern (*white arrows*). Small abscess (*white arrows*) is seen in the right frontal lobe with restricted diffusion on diffusion-weighted image sequence (*E*).

ear granulation tissue, represented by opacification of the middle ear and mastoids. Granulation tissue can be difficult to differentiate from cholesteatoma on CT, with both appearing as soft tissue

densities. However, bony erosion and displacement of ossicles is rare in the former (**Fig. 7**).[31] Sclerosis and opacification of the mastoid air cells is commonly seen.

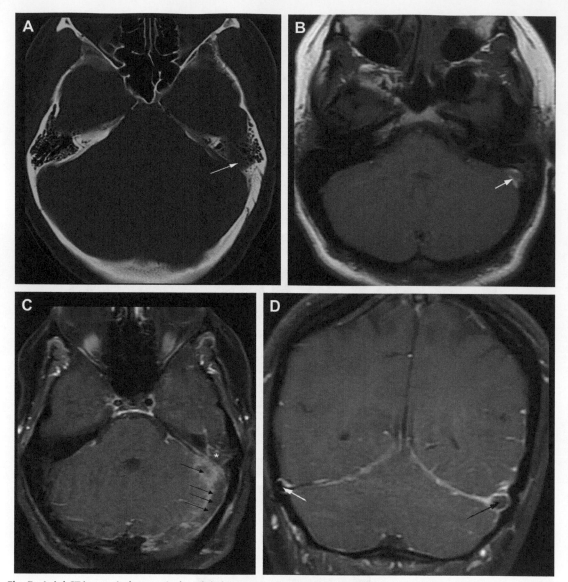

Fig. 5. Axial CT image in bone window (*A*) showing coalescent left mastoiditis (*arrow*). The expected normal flow void of the left sigmoid sinus has been replaced by a hyperintense signal on the T1-weighted MR image (*white arrow*) (*B*). The filling defect (*black arrows*) on axial and coronal postcontrast T1-weighted images (*C, D*) confirms the suspicion of a thrombosis of the left sigmoid sinus, extending into the transverse sinus. Note normal flow void (*white arrow*) in the right transverse sinus.

Tympanosclerosis is a healing variant of COM characterized by postinflammatory new bone deposition in the middle ear, ossicles, mastoids, oval and round windows, and also the tympanic membrane. HRCT shows calcified or ossific foci in the middle ear surrounded by soft tissue, often giving the appearance of extra ossicles (**Fig. 8**).[31–33]

Acquired cholesteatoma

Acquired cholesteatoma may be a complication of repeated or chronic otitis media. The keratinizing stratified squamous epithelium from the external canal accesses the recess between the tympanic membrane and the ossicles (Prussak space) through a defect in the tympanic membrane, usually in the anterosuperior pars flaccida. The radiologic sine qua non of a cholesteatoma is bone erosion, usually involving the long process of incus and scutum, best seen on coronal images (**Fig. 9**). Erosion and medial displacement of the ossicles and extension via aditus ad antrum into the mastoid antrum may occur. Well-recognized complications include facial nerve paralysis,

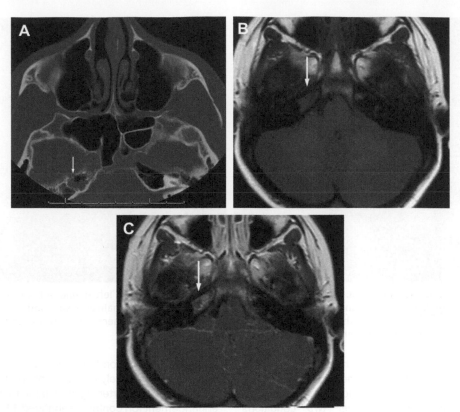

Fig. 6. Petrous apicitis. Axial CT (*A*) image for the paranasal sinuses shows aerated petrous apices bilaterally with fluid in the right petrous apical air cells (*arrow*). Axial T1-weighted (*B*) and postcontrast fat-saturated T1-weighted (*C*) images reveal altered bone marrow signal and abnormal enhancement of the right petrous apex (*arrow*).

labyrinthine fistula, and intracranial extension through the tegmen tympani with sequel of meningitis, dural sinus thrombosis, or abscess (**Fig. 10**).[33] MRI can help to distinguish between fluid, thickened mucosa of COM and cholesteatoma. Fluid, granulation tissue, and cholesteatoma

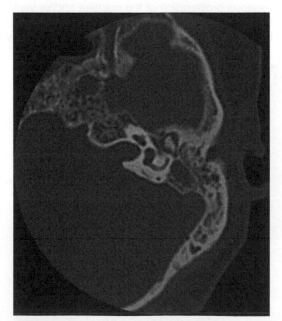

Fig. 7. Chronic otitis media with granulation tissue. Axial HRCT image of the left temporal bone demonstrates opacification of the middle ear and mastoid air cells without ossicular displacement or erosions.

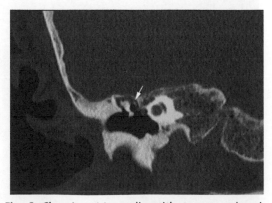

Fig. 8. Chronic otitis media with tympanosclerosis. Axial HRCT image of the right temporal bone depicts opacification of the middle ear with curvilinear calcification medial to the ossicles (*arrow*).

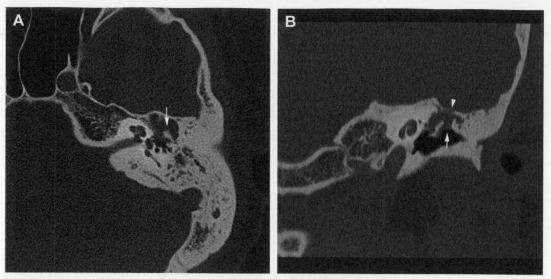

Fig. 9. Acquired cholesteatoma. Axial (*A*) and coronal (*B*) HRCT images of the left temporal bone reveal a soft tissue in the middle ear (*arrow* in *A*) with medial displacement of the ossicular chain and widening of the Prussack space (*arrow* in *B*). Erosions of the scutum and the head of the malleus are evident. Focal erosion of the tegmen tympani (*arrowhead* in *B*) is seen.

appear bright on T2 images; however, cholesteatomas have been found to show increased signal on diffusion-weighted imaging, which can distinguish them from the other two conditions (**Fig. 11**).[34,35] Surgical excision is curative but recurrences are well known.

Labyrinthitis

Labyrinthitis, most commonly caused by a viral infection, presents acutely with sensorineural hearing loss, vertigo, and tinnitus. It may be posttraumatic, secondary to acute otomastoiditis or meningitis or rarely autoimmune in etiology.

On MR, T2 shortening and faint to moderate enhancement (on contrast-enhanced T1-weighted images) within normally fluid-filled spaces of the inner ear is seen (**Fig. 12**).[25] *Labyrinthitis ossificans* often occurs as a response to secondary infection of the endolymph, manifesting as fibrous and/or osseous proliferation of the cochlea and/or vestibules and semicircular canals.[25] On T2-weighted MR images there is a reduction in signal intensity

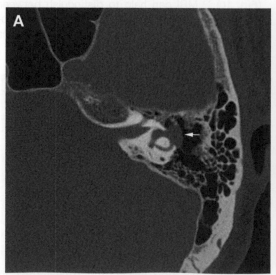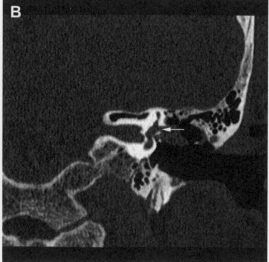

Fig. 10. Acquired cholesteatoma with labyrinthine fistula. Axial (*A*) and coronal (*B*) HRCT images of the left temporal bone show soft tissue in the middle ear (*arrow* in *A*) displacing the ossicles chain anteriorly. There is a defect in the lateral semicircular canal, flush with the soft tissue suggestive of a fistula (*arrow* in *B*).

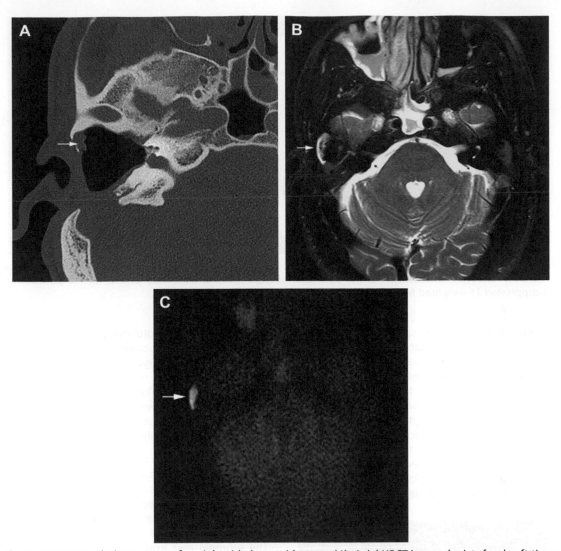

Fig. 11. Recurrent cholesteatoma after right-sided mastoidectomy (*A*). Axial HRCT image depicts focal soft tissue lobulated in the anterior part of the mastoidectomy bowl (*arrow*), appearing hyperintense on axial T2-weighted MR image (*arrow* in *B*). The soft tissue demonstrates restricted diffusion on axial diffusion-weighted image (*arrow* in *C*).

of the usually fluid-filled labyrinth (**Fig. 13**). Ossification is seen well on CT as a hazy increased density within the normally fluid-filled spaces of the membranous labyrinth in mild cases (**Fig. 14**). Severe forms are accompanied by complete obliteration by bone replacement. Evaluation for labyrinthitis ossificans before cochlear implantation can be performed with CT or MRI.[16,36]

Infections of the Sinonasal Cavities

Bacterial sinusitis

Rhinosinusitis is a more accurate term for what is commonly termed sinusitis, because the mucous membranes of the nose and sinuses are contiguous and subject to the same disease processes. Rhinosinusitis may be divided into acute (duration <4 weeks), subacute (duration 4–12 weeks), and chronic (duration >12 weeks).[37] The most common presenting symptoms for acute sinusitis include pain over the involved sinus, fever, and toxicity; chronic sinusitis symptoms include facial pressure, headache, nasal obstruction, postnasal drip, and fatigue. An isolated finding of an air-fluid level is typical of acute sinusitis, although imaging is rarely required for the diagnosis of this condition.[38]

CT is the imaging standard for chronic sinusitis in all age groups.[39,40] With the usage of a lower mA protocol (miniCAT), the radiation dose is similar to

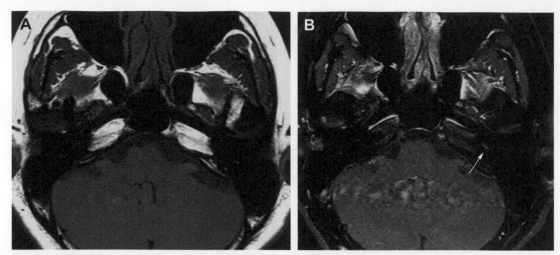

Fig. 12. Left-sided labyrinthitis. Axial T1- weighted MR image (*A*) shows no signal abnormality in the inner ear structures. However, enhancement of the basal turn of the cochlea is illustrated (*arrow*) on the postcontrast fat-suppressed T1-weighted MR image (*B*).

a standard 4-view radiographic series at superior resolution.[41,42] On CT, it appears as diffuse or focal mucosal thickening, with partial or complete sinus opacification; bone remodeling with uniform thickening caused by osteitis from adjacent chronic mucosal inflammation is a feature of chronic rhinosinusitis. These findings often overlap with those of allergic sinusitis, granulomatous inflammation, sinonasal polyposis, and trauma.[43] The pattern of sinus opacification determines if the obstruction is osteomeatal, infundibular, sphenoethmoidal recess, sinonasal polyposis, or unclassifiable and

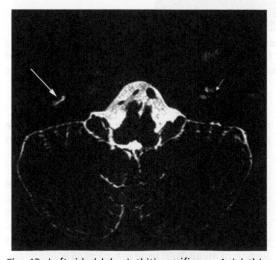

Fig. 13. Left-sided labyrinthitis ossificans. Axial thin-section heavily T2-weighted MR image shows signal drop out in the intralabyrinthine fluid signal within the basal turn of left cochlea (*short arrow*). Notice normal fluid signal in the basal turn of cochlea on the right side (*long arrow*).

is useful to guide the otolaryngologist for planning functional endoscopic sinus surgery (FESS).[44]

MRI may show varying signal of the fluid on T1-weighted images depending on the protein concentration of the fluid. The signal is usually is hyperintense on T2-weighted imaging (**Fig. 15**). MRI is particularly useful for assessing possible intracranial and vascular complications.

Complications of bacterial sinusitis

Persistent obstruction of the sinus drainage and subsequent expansion of the sinus is termed as a mucocele. Mucoceles may occur as a complication of chronic rhinosinusitis among other conditions, such as tumors, polyps, and after surgery. The ethmoid and frontal sinuses are commonly affected; patients present with frontal headache and proptosis.

On CT scan, mucoceles appear as hypodense, nonenhancing masses that fill and expand the sinus cavity. The typical mucocele contents have low density and do not enhance (**Fig. 16**). On MRI, the signal intensity of the mucocele varies with its protein content and the degree of hydration. Postcontrast fat-suppressed T1-weighted images show no/minimal peripheral enhancement of the mucocele. This finding can help rule out solid tumors, which show significant enhancement.[45]

Orbital complications are most often associated with ethmoidal sinusitis, whereas frontal and sphenoid sinusitis is implicated in the intracranial spread of infection. A subgaleal abscess, termed "Pott puffy tumor," may be seen in the frontal region of the scalp as a result of spread of infection in severe frontal sinusitis (**Fig. 17**). Intracranial involvement may lead to meningitis, epidural, subdural,

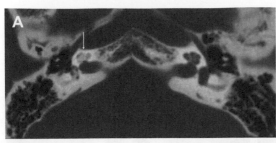
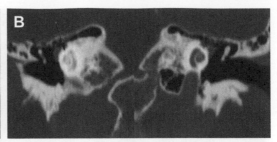

Fig. 14. Right-sided labyrinthitis ossificans. Axial (*A*) and coronal (*B*) HRCT images of the right (abnormal) and left (normal) temporal bones demonstrate near complete ossification of the basal and middle turns of the right cochlea (*arrow*). Foci of calcification/ossification are also seen in the right vestibule. The left-sided cochlea and vestibule show normal intralabyrinthine fluid density.

or intracerebral abscesses and cavernous sinus thrombosis, better resolved by MRI.[45–49]

Fungal sinusitis

The disease is broadly divided into invasive and noninvasive fungal sinusitis depending on the presence or absence of fungal hyphae within the mucosa, submucosa, bone, or blood vessels of the paranasal sinuses. Angioinvasion, intraorbital, intracranial, and maxillofacial involvement and hematogenous dissemination are features of invasive fungal sinusitis.[15] Common organisms implicated in invasive fungal sinusitis include *Rhizopus, Rhizomucor, Mucor, Aspergillus, Bipolaris,* or *Candida.*[50,51] The symptomatology is not useful to distinguish it from other forms of sinusitis. Hence, a high index of suspicion is maintained

in immunocompromised patients with fever of unknown origin after 48 hours of appropriate broad-spectrum intravenous antibiotics or the presence of localizing sinonasal symptoms. In advanced forms, symptoms specific to orbital and intracranial invasion may occur. Acute invasive fungal sinusitis is almost always seen in patients with poorly controlled diabetes or in immunocompromised hosts (patients with hematologic malignancies, solid organ or bone marrow transplantation, chemotherapy-induced neutropenia, or AIDS), and has a fulminant progression. Chronic invasive fungal sinusitis occurs in diabetic, mildly immunocompromised, or immunocompetent individuals and follows a slow but ultimately fatal course over months to years. Chronic granulomatous invasive fungal sinusitis is much rarer,

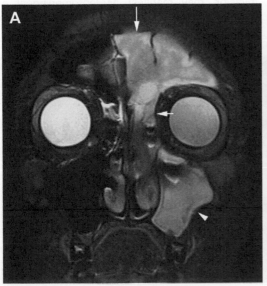
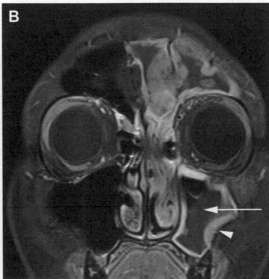

Fig. 15. Coronal T2-weighted (*A*) and postcontrast fat-suppressed T1-weighted (*B*) images reveal involvement of the left frontal (*arrow* in *A*), left ethmoidal (*short arrow*), and left maxillary sinuses (*arrowhead* in *A*), suggesting an osteomeatal pattern of obstruction. Note the intense mucosal enhancement (*arrowhead* in *B*) around the nonenhancing secretions (*long arrow* in *B*), a sign of benign disease.

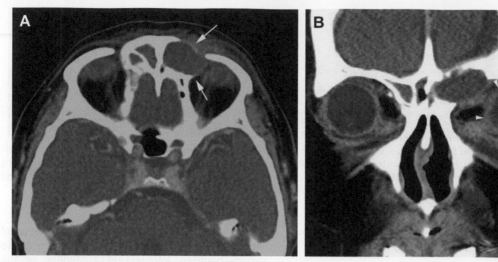

Fig. 16. Left frontal mucocele. Axial (*A*) and coronal (*B*) contrast-enhanced CT images reveal smooth expansion of the left frontal sinus by a soft tissue lesion with no significant enhancement. Marked thinning and dehiscence of the outer and inner tables of the frontal sinus is seen (*arrows* in *A*) with reactive changes in the overlying subcutaneous tissues. Inferolateral displacement of the left eyeball is noted (*arrowheads*).

occurs in immunocompetent individuals, and has similar imaging features as chronic invasive fungal sinusitis. It is not considered to be a different entity by some authors.[52]

On CT scan, severe unilateral nasal cavity soft tissue thickening is the most consistent, although nonspecific, early CT finding of acute invasive fungal sinusitis.[53] Periantral fat obliteration with or without bone erosion, and intraorbital and intracranial invasion are more specific but appear later on in the disease. In chronic fungal sinusitis, besides the nonspecific findings like mucosal

thickening and bony sclerosis (indistinguishable from chronic rhinosinusitis), the sinuses may be opacified with hyperattenuating material, often with foci of central calcifications. Centrally situated intrasinus calcification on CT is characteristic of fungal sinusitis, particularly that caused by *Aspergillus* species (**Fig. 18**). On MRI, decreased signal intensity on T2-weighted images is a characteristic feature of the disease (**Fig. 19**).[51] Variable signal is seen on T1-weighted images. Intracranial invasion may manifest as leptomeningeal enhancement, adjacent cerebritis, granulomas, or

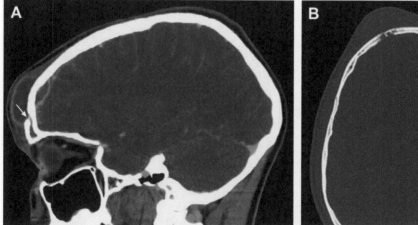
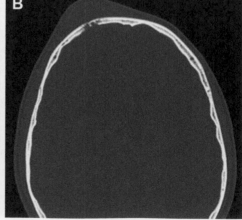

Fig. 17. Pott puffy tumor. Sagittal contrast-enhanced CT scan image (*A*) shows right frontal superficial soft tissue abscess and an underlying epidural abscess. This is secondary to mucosal sinus disease of the frontal sinus where there is cortical destruction of the outer table (*arrow*). Axial CT image in bone window setting (*B*) depicts osseous destruction of the frontal calvarium at the level of the subgaleal and epidural abscesses.

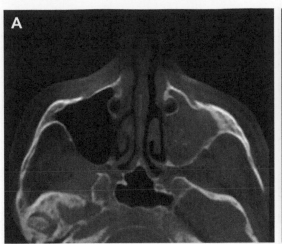
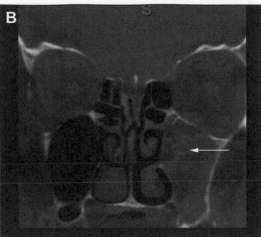

Fig. 18. Chronic fungal sinusitis. Axial (*A*) and coronal (*B*) miniCAT images show complete opacification of the left maxillary sinus and central calcifications (*arrow* in *B*) and marked wall thickening.

cerebral abscess formation. Fungal infections of the sphenoid sinus have a propensity to invade the adjacent cavernous sinus and internal carotid artery. Orbital apex syndrome and related cranial nerve palsies may occur as a result of invasion from the sphenoid sinus (**Fig. 20**). Prompt aggressive surgical debridement of affected tissues and systemic antifungal therapy are the pillars of treatment.

Allergic fungal sinusitis is a noninvasive chronic noninfective rhinosinusitis that manifests in atopic,

immunocompetent individuals. An immunoglobulin E–mediated type of immediate hypersensitivity and type III delayed hypersensitivity to inhaled fungal organisms are thought to be involved.[54] Typically, bilateral rhinosinusitis is seen with complete opacification with expansion, erosion, or remodeling and thinning of the sinuses (**Fig. 21**). The signal intensity on T2-weighted MR sequences is usually low. The treatment involves surgical clearance of the obstructed sinuses followed by topical steroids to prevent recurrence.

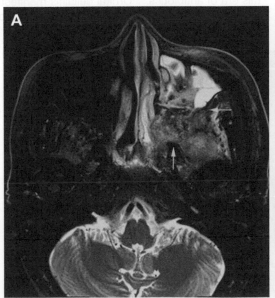
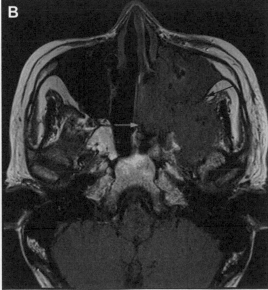

Fig. 19. Invasive maxillofacial fungal sinusitis. Axial T2- weighted (*A*) and T1-weighted (*B*) MR images demonstrate an irregular lesion in the left maxillary antrum with foci of signal drop out. Entrapped secretions are also seen in left antrum. Extrasinus invasion through the posterolateral wall of the left maxillary antrum into the masticator space and pterygopalatine fossa (*arrows*) is seen, with replacement of normal periantral fat (*black arrow* in *B*).

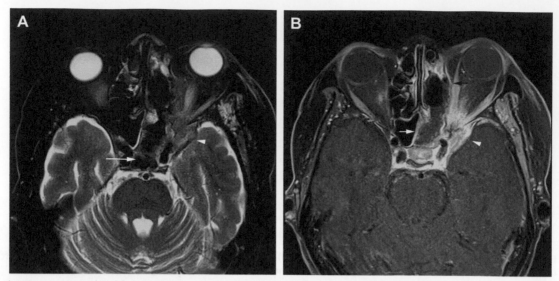

Fig. 20. Invasive orbital fungal sinusitis. Axial T2-weighted (*A*) and postcontrast fat-saturated T1-weighted (*B*) MR images reveal enhancing soft tissue in the sphenoid and left posterior ethmoidal air cells. The signal void in the sphenoid sinus on the T2-weighted image (*arrow in A*) corresponds to soft tissue on T1-weighted image (*arrow in B*). Invasion of the left medial orbital extraconal fat (*black arrow in B*), left cavernous sinus, orbital apex, and left superior orbital fissure (*arrowheads*) is well depicted on the postcontrast T1-weighted MR image.

Infections of the Orbit

Unlike periorbital cellulitis, which is limited to the preseptal soft tissues, orbital cellulitis implies infective postseptal orbital involvement requiring imaging and aggressive treatment. It is most commonly caused by paranasal (usually ethmoidal and frontal) sinusitis, which spreads to the orbit via a perivascular pathway or through natural bony dehiscences.[55–57] Thus, bone destruction is not usually seen. Patients present with swelling and erythema of the eyelids, chemosis, and proptosis.

Orbital cellulitis rarely evolves without prior subperiosteal abscess, typically appearing as a lentiform rim-enhancing collection in the medial orbital wall with adjacent ethmoidal sinusitis (**Fig. 22**). Intraconal orbital abscesses are rare in this era of antibiotics.[58] Orbital cellulitis manifests as inflammatory fat stranding of intraconal and/or

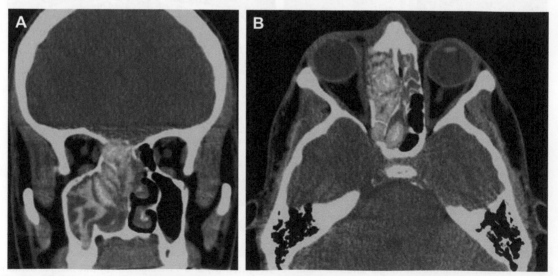

Fig. 21. Allergic fungal rhinosinusitis. Coronal (*A*) and axial (*B*) noncontrast CT images depict complete opacification, bone erosions, and expansion of the right maxillary antrum, ethmoid air cells, and right nasal cavity by a heterogeneous, predominantly hyperdense soft tissue mass. There is a marked expansion of the right maxillary antrum and ethmoidal air cells as a result of bone remodeling.

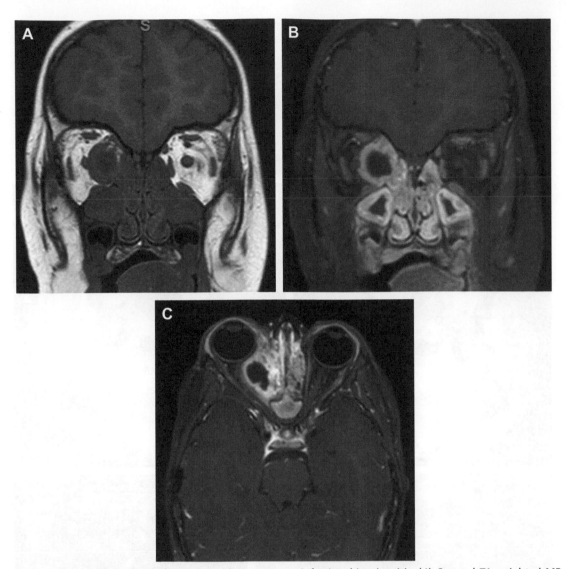

Fig. 22. Subperiosteal orbital abscess secondary to severe infective rhinosinusitis. (*A*) Coronal T1-weighted MR image (*A*) and Coronal (*B*) and axial (*C*) postcontrast fat-suppressed T1-weighted MR images show a rim-enhancing, centrally necrotic, medial extraconal abscess in the right orbit. Marked mucosal thickening and enhancement with complete opacification is seen in bilateral ethmoidal air cells and maxillary sinuses.

extraconal fat and enlargement of the affected structures on CT. Complications of orbital cellulitis include thrombosis of the superior ophthalmic vein, the cavernous sinuses, bacterial meningitis, and intracranial abscesses. Treatment includes intravenous antibiotics and drainage of subperiosteal or orbital abscesses to salvage vision.[54]

Dacryocystitis, an inflammation and dilatation of the lacrimal sac, is diagnosed on clinical signs and symptoms.[59] However, imaging may be requested to exclude orbital cellulitis. The typical imaging finding is a well-circumscribed round lesion that is centered at the lacrimal fossa and that demonstrates peripheral enhancement.

Infections of the Salivary Glands

Acute siloadenitis

Acute siloadenitis usually manifests as painful bilateral swelling of the salivary glands in children, with mumps virus and cytomegalovirus being the commonest viruses implicated.[60] Acute bacterial infections are usually caused by *Staphylococcus aureus* or oral flora and are usually secondary to an obstructive calculus.[61,62]

Ultrasound is well suited for the evaluation of acutely inflamed salivary glands (**Fig. 23**), but extensions into the deep neck spaces are better demonstrated on CT scan (**Fig. 24**). CT is the

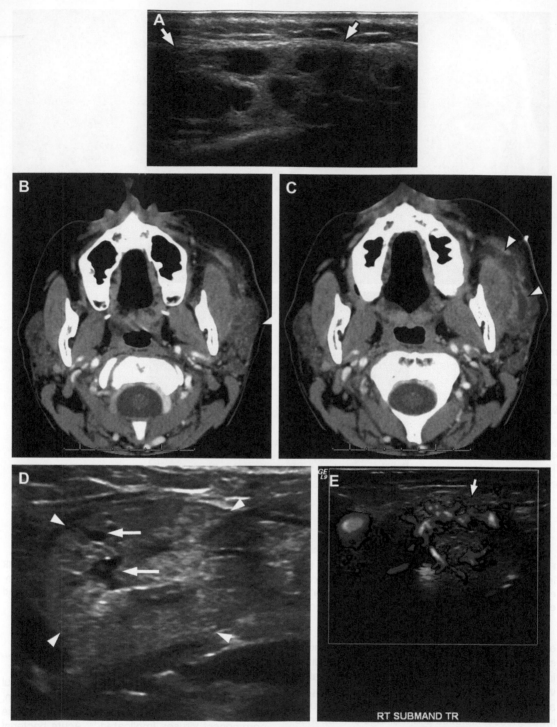

Fig. 23. A 67-year-old woman with left cheek swelling and pain. (*A*) US image of the left parotid gland shows coarse echotexture with multiple hypoechoic and anechoic cystic structures. (*B*) Axial contrast-enhanced CT image shows heterogeneous enhancement with hypodense areas within the left parotid gland with overlying soft tissue stranding. (*C*) The duct was significantly dilated and diffusely enhancing with no definite obstructive stone. (*D*) Grayscale US image of the right submandibular gland in a 68-year-old man who presented with right submandibular swelling and pain showed heterogeneous enlargement of the gland (*arrowheads*) with prominent ducts (*white arrows*). (*E*) Power Doppler US image shows increased vascularity of the gland, indicative of acute sialadenitis.

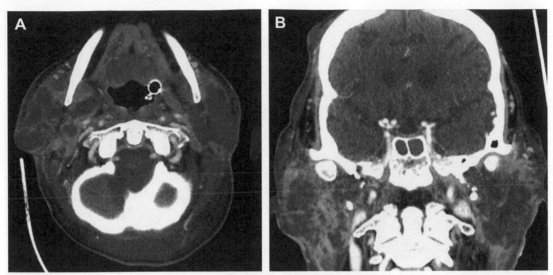

Fig. 24. A 70-year-old woman with type 2 diabetes and methicillin-resistant *Staphylococcus aureus* parotitis. Axial (*A*) and coronal (*B*) contrast-enhanced CT sections showing gross swelling in and around the parotids with multiloculated, edge-enhancing parotid abscesses.

most sensitive imaging modality for detecting calculi within the duct system or the glandular parenchyma.[63] On US, suppurative siloadenitis manifests as an enlarged, heterogeneous gland with hypoechoic foci representing lymph nodes or small abscesses (see **Fig. 23**).[64] On cross-sectional studies, the inflamed gland is enlarged and hypodense (on CT) or hyperintense (on T2-weighted MRI) (see **Fig. 24**). Avid contrast enhancement is noted, especially in bacterial siloadenitis. Inflammatory stranding of the adjacent soft tissues and intraglandular and locoregional adenopathy are accompanying features (**Fig. 25**). A search for an obstructing sialolith in the path of the Stenson or Wharton ducts is often rewarding in cases of unilateral siloadenitis.[63]

Lymphoepithelial cysts in HIV
The characteristic parotid lesion in HIV infection is a benign lymphoepithelial cyst (BLEC), generally

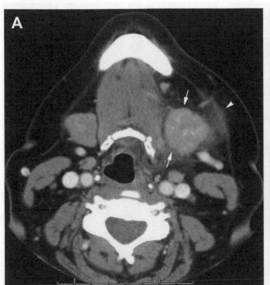
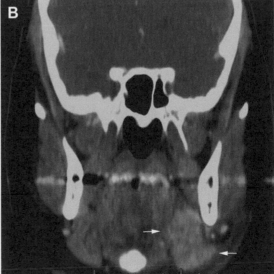

Fig. 25. Left submandibular siloadenitis. Axial (*A*) and coronal (*B*) contrast-enhanced CT images reveal marked enlargement and enhancement of the left submandibular gland (*arrows*). Significant stranding and fluid is seen in the periglandular soft tissues (*arrowhead* in *A*).

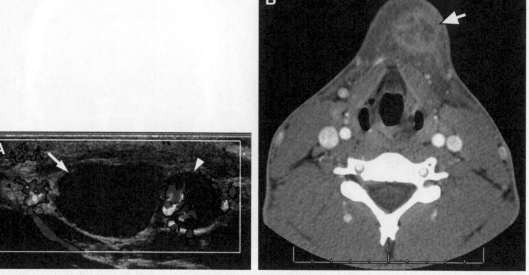

Fig. 26. Suppurative lymphadenitis. (*A*) Color Doppler US image of the left submandibular space showing a hypo-echoic necrotic avascularized enlarged lymph node (*arrow*) and an adjacent enlarged lymph node with increased vascularity (*arrowhead*). (*B*) Corresponding axial contrast-enhanced CT image showing a necrotic rim-enhancing left submandibular lymph node with significant surrounding soft tissue thickening (*arrow*).

presenting as bilateral multiple painless swellings and cervical adenopathy.[65–68] Although the presence of BLEC is considered an indicator of HIV infection, the pathogenesis is not related to direct HIV infection of the gland per se.[65–68]

Infections of the Cervical Lymph Nodes

Cervical lymphadenitis denotes an inflammation of the lymph nodes of the neck caused by an infectious process, often secondary to viral respiratory infections in the pediatric age group.[69,70]

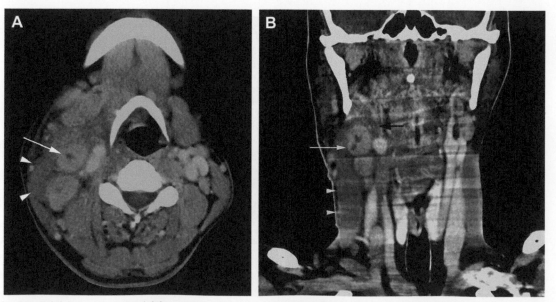

Fig. 27. Axial (*A*) and coronal (*B*) contrast-enhanced CT images demonstrate enlarged, round, enhancing right side upper cervical lymph nodes with central necrosis (*arrow*). Fat stranding is seen adjacent to the nodes (*black arrow* in *B*) and right sternocleidomastoid muscle is edematous (*arrowheads*).

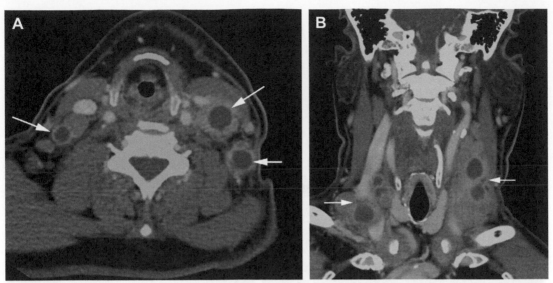

Fig. 28. Tuberculous lymphadenitis. Axial (*A*) and coronal (*B*) contrast-enhanced CT images demonstrate enlarged, enhancing bilateral cervical lymph nodes with central necrosis (*arrows* in *A*). No fat stranding is seen adjacent to the nodes. The matting of the necrotic nodes (*arrows* in *B*) is better seen on the coronal image.

Suppurative adenitis indicates a lymph node that has undergone liquefactive necrosis, usually attributable to acute bacterial infections like *Staphylococcus aureus* or Group A *Streptococcus*.[71] The symptomatology is acute with fever and painful, erythematous lumps over the neck. Tuberculous cervical lymphadenitis (also known as scrofula) is caused by *Mycobacterium tuberculosis* and presents with malaise, weight loss, and nontender neck lumps. Three typical features of tuberculous lymphadenitis are multiplicity, matting, and caseation.[72] Nontuberculous mycobacterial adenitis is commoner in the pediatric age group, *Mycobacterium avium* and *Mycobacterium intracellulare*

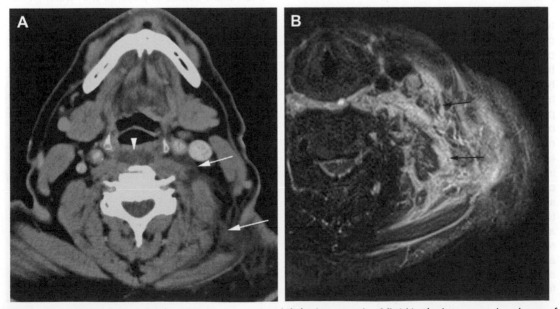

Fig. 29. Necrotising fasciitis. Axial contrast-enhanced CT (*A*) depicts strands of fluid in the intermuscular planes of the left side of the neck (*arrows*). Note is made of the nonabscess fluid in the retropharyngeal space (*arrowhead*). Axial fat-suppressed T2-weighted MR image (*B*) confirms the presence of fluid in the intermuscular planes (*black arrows*) along with increased signal from the muscles.

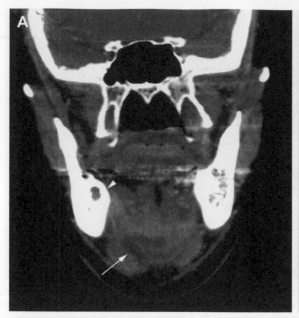

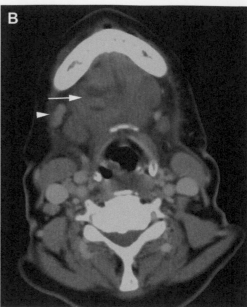

Fig. 30. Ludwig angina. Coronal (*A*) and axial (*B*) CT images depict linear fluid collections in the right sublingual and submandibular spaces, crossing the midline (*arrows*), suggestive of abscesses. Fat stranding and fluid is seen in the right submandibular space with submandibular adenopathy (*arrowhead* in *B*). The probable source of infection is dental caries, as shown by the well-defined periapical cyst at the level of the second mandibular molar tooth (*arrowhead* in *A*).

accounting for most cases. The typical clinical manifestation is that of slowly enlarging and unilateral submandibular or preauricular mass of nodes. Constitutional symptoms, such as fever, fatigue, and failure to thrive may be present in 50% of patients.[73,74]

On gray-scale sonography, the inflamed nodes tend to be enlarged, rounded, and hypoechoic compared with the adjacent muscles.[75] Central cystic changes appear in suppurative and in tuberculous lymphadenitis with loss of echogenic hilum (Fig. 26A).[76,77] On CT scan, cervical adenitis manifests as enlarged enhancing nodes, with a preserved oval shape, usually accompanied by mild perinodal fat stranding. Suppurative lymph nodes display central nonenhancing foci with thick enhancing rims and marked perinodal fat stranding (see Fig. 26B). Extensive edema of subcutaneous tissues and adjacent muscles may be seen (Fig. 27). Suppurative adenitis may progress to abscess formation. Tuberculous lymphadenitis also appears as rim-enhancing nodes with central necrosis; however, matting of the adjacent nodes and a relative lack of fat stranding and effacement are typical imaging features that differentiate it from suppurative adenitis (Fig. 28).[77–79]

Infections of the Deep Neck Spaces

Deep neck space infections are usually polymicrobial, commonly seen in patients with recent

illnesses like tonsillitis/pharyngitis, dental caries or procedures, trauma, or intravenous drug use. The usual clinical presentations include pain, fever, swelling, dysphagia, trismus, dysphonia, otalgia, and dyspnea. These infections may follow a fulminant course in patients with weak immune mechanisms.[80–82]

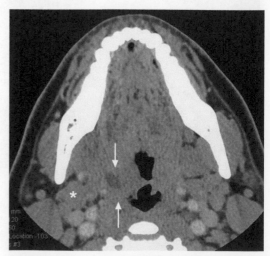

Fig. 31. Right peritonsillar abscess. Contrast-enhanced axial CT image showing right peritonsillar nonenhancing collection with no overt rim (*arrows*). Enlarged right level II lymph nodes (*asterisk*) are also noted.

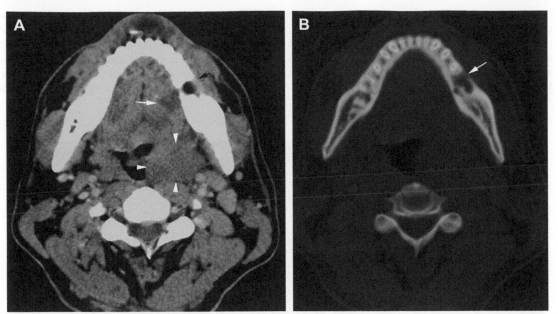

Fig. 32. Sublingual abscess with parapharyngeal phlegmon. Axial contrast-enhanced CT image in soft tissue (*A*) demonstrates an irregular fluid collection in the left sublingual space (*arrow*) suggestive of an abscess. A phlegmon is demonstrated in the left parapharyngeal space (*arrowheads*). Periapical lucency in the bone window setting (*arrow* in *B*) in relation to the left mandibular premolar tooth suggests an odontogenic source of infection.

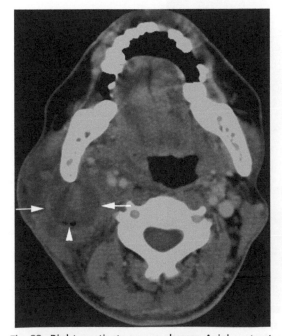

Fig. 33. Right masticator space abscess. Axial contrast-enhanced CT image shows a right-sided masticator space abscess (*arrows*) with pockets of gas within (*arrowhead*). Perilesional fat stranding is seen with edema of the right sternocleidomastoid muscle.

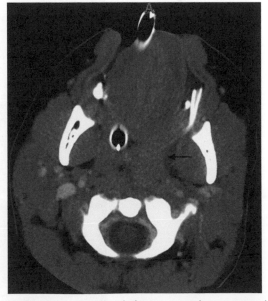

Fig. 34. Retropharyngeal abscess secondary to spread from left parapharyngeal abscess: axial contrast-enhanced CT image shows soft tissue swelling in the retropharyngeal space with irregular peripherally enhancing fluid collection (*asterisk*). Also note poorly marginated small fluid collection in the left parapharyngeal space (*black arrow*).

CT is the modality of choice for evaluation of deep neck space infection.[81] As the visceral, retropharyngeal, danger and perivertebral spaces extend into the mediastinum, it is imperative to include the upper sections of the mediastinum in the CT scan coverage.

US is useful to evaluate if the abscess is liquefied enough to be drained and may also assist in the drainage.[83] On CT, fluid and fat stranding in the subcutaneous tissues and along fascial planes may be representative of cellulitis. Myositis appears as enlargement and hyperenhancement

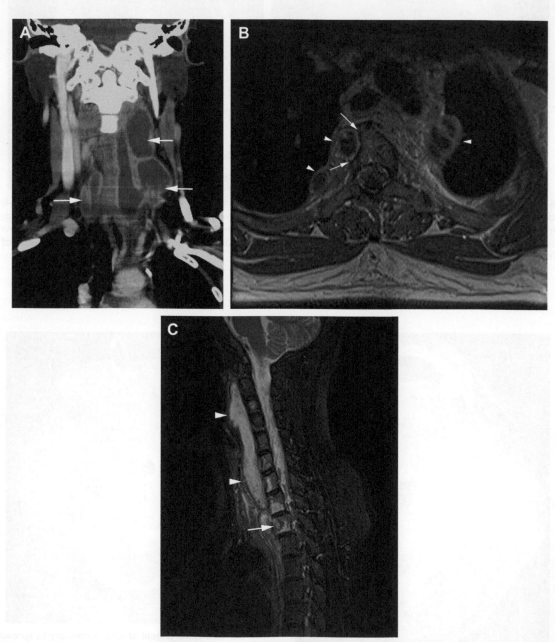

Fig. 35. Prevertebral abscess secondary to tuberculous spondylodiscitis at the T3/4 vertebral level. Coronal contrast-enhanced CT image (A) illustrates multiple loculated rim-enhancing collections in the perivertebral space on either side of the midline, suggestive of perivertebral abscesses (arrows in A). Axial contrast-enhanced T1-weighted MR image (B) and sagittal fat-suppressed contrast-enhanced T1- weighted MR image (C) depict the extensive perivertebral abscesses on either side of the midline (arrowheads) and reveal a destructive lesion in the right half of the T3 vertebral body (arrows in B and C).

of the muscles.[84] Aggressive monitoring and management of the airway is the most urgent and critical aspect of care, followed by appropriate antibiotic coverage and surgical drainage, when needed.

Necrotizing fasciitis

Necrotizing fasciitis is a rapidly progressive and often fatal infection of subcutaneous tissues and deep fasciae arising from an odontogenic or oropharyngeal source. The infection may follow surgical procedures or trauma. Necrotizing fasciitis generally is characterized by extensive collections of subcutaneous and subfascial gas and fluid. Marked cellulitis or myositis involving the deep fascial planes and neck spaces is seen (**Fig. 29**).[84-86] Broad-spectrum antibiotics, aggressive surgical treatment, and supportive therapy are the cornerstones of successful treatment.

Oral cavity

The deep neck spaces around the oral cavity are composed of midline submental and laterally situated sublingual and submandibular spaces, communicating freely with one another and with the parapharyngeal and anterior visceral spaces.[80,84] The major source of infection is odontogenic. The spread of dental infection depends on the insertion of the dental roots in relation to the mylohyoid. Infections involving second and third mandibular molars spread into the submandibular space, whereas those involving the first molar/premolars spread into the sublingual space.[84] Other sources of infection include siloadenitis, suppurative lymphadenitis, oral trauma, and upper respiratory infections.

Ludwig angina is an infective cellulitis of bilateral sublingual, submental, and submandibular spaces, usually seen in patients with diabetes or individuals with other forms of immunocompromise. Progression into fasciitis and frank abscess formation occurs if not treated adequately.[87,88] Contrast-enhanced CT depicts these changes well (**Fig. 30**). Submental or submandibular lymphadenopathy is also seen. There is a potential risk of rapidly progressive airway obstruction and asphyxiation if airway compromise is not urgently addressed.

Peritonsillar and parapharyngeal space

Peritonsillar abscess results from tonsillitis and is often a clinical diagnosis. CT is reserved for complicated cases with deep involvement and failing to respond to antibiotics; it helps to differentiate cellulitis from a drainable abscess (**Fig. 31**). Parapharyngeal space is an inverted pyramid-shaped space, which extends from the base of the skull down to the hyoid bone. This space is secondarily involved by infections like pharyngitis, tonsillitis, otitis, mastoiditis, parotitis, and odontogenic infections (**Fig. 32**).[80,89,90] Spread of infection to the carotid sheath results in complications such as Lemierre syndrome, an infective internal jugular vein thrombosis, mycotic carotid artery aneurysm, ipsilateral Horner syndrome, and cranial nerve palsies (IX to XII). Direct inoculation into the neck results in carotid space infections, as is seen in intravenous drug abusers and following central venous catheter placement.

Masticator space

Most masticator space infections originate from the posterior mandibular molars; less common sources include trauma and surgery. CT is invaluable in the assessment of masticator space infections as it can often influence the surgical (intraoral versus external) approach and distinguish abscess from cellulitis (**Fig. 33**).[89]

Retropharyngeal, danger, and prevertebral spaces

The retropharyngeal and danger spaces extend from the base of the skull into to the mediastinum (up to T2 thoracic vertebral level) and diaphragm respectively, separated from one another by the alar fascia. The prevertebral space lies posterior to the danger space with an intervening

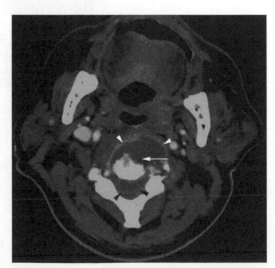

Fig. 36. Prevertebral abscess secondary to infective spondylodiscitis at the C2/3 vertebral level. Axial contrast-enhanced CT image depicts the rim-enhancing collection in the prevertebral space (*arrowheads*) along with the erosion in the anterior part of the C3 vertebra (*arrow*). Note a large epidural component of the abscess (*black arrowheads*) causing severe compromise of the spinal canal. (*Courtesy of* Dr Lim Teh Aun, Singapore General Hospital, Singapore.)

prevertebral fascia between them and extends down to the coccyx.[80] Infections of the retropharyngeal space originate from the retropharyngeal lymph nodes (in the pediatric age group), from the parapharyngeal space, or may be posttraumatic.[83] Life-threatening complications, such as airway obstruction and aspiration, may occur following rupture of an abscess into the airway. Prevertebral phlegmon/abscess results from bacterial or tuberculous spondylodiscitis, penetrating injuries to the posterior pharyngeal wall, and secondary spread from retropharyngeal and danger space infections. The infections of the danger space are secondary to spread from

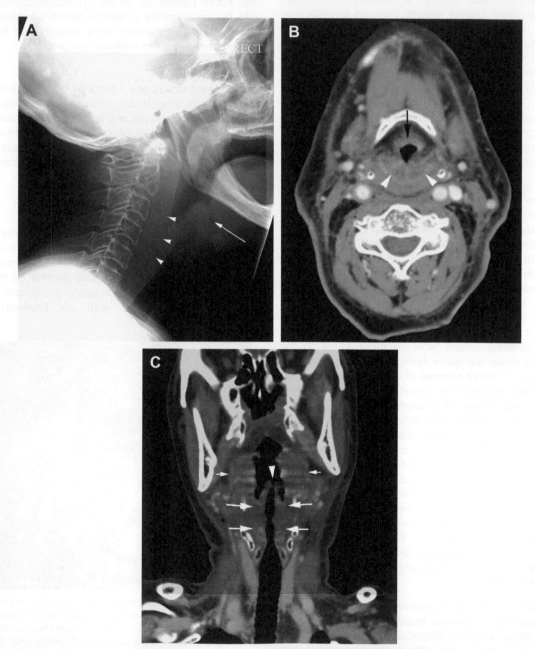

Fig. 37. Supraglottitis. A lateral radiograph of the neck of (*A*) shows a swollen epiglottis (*arrow*) and thickened prevertebral soft tissues (*arrowheads*) in keeping with supraglottitis. Axial (*B*) and coronal (*C*) contrast-enhanced CT images depict edema of the preglottic (*black arrow* in *B*), posterior hypopharyngeal wall (*arrowheads* in *B*). Edema of the epiglottis (*arrowhead* in *C*) and supraglottic fat (*arrows* in *C*) is well seen on the coronal image. (*Courtesy of* Dr Lim Eng Hoe Winston, Singapore General Hospital, Singapore.)

retropharyngeal and prevertebral spaces and are difficult to distinguish from those of the retropharyngeal space on imaging.[91]

Retropharyngeal suppurative adenitis is heralded by appearance of enlarged paramedian retropharyngeal lymph nodes that contain low-attenuation centers. A retropharyngeal abscess commonly results from a rupture of a suppurated retropharyngeal node. It appears as a low-attenuation fluid collection with a thin enhancing rim in some cases, distending the retropharyngeal space and flattening the prevertebral muscles (**Fig. 34**). MRI may help to delineate the abscess better and differentiate it from cellulitis.[22] Symmetric and smooth expansion of the retropharyngeal space by fluid density without an enhancing rim (termed retropharyngeal edema or nonabscess fluid) may be seen in early infection, internal jugular vein thrombus, postradiation states, and in prevertebral calcific tendonitis (see **Fig. 29A**). No surgical drainage is necessary.[22,92] In patients with prevertebral abscesses, changes of spondylodiscitis may be sought on plain radiographs or cross-sectional imaging modalities. MRI, including fat-saturated, contrast-enhanced T1 sequences, best delineates epidural phlegmon or drainable empyema (**Figs. 35 and 36**).

Anterior visceral space

Infections of the anterior visceral space often originate from traumatic perforation of the anterior esophageal wall and, less commonly, from neck trauma or thyroiditis. Infections of this space are associated with laryngeal and pharyngeal edema and are prone to life-threatening complications like mediastinitis.[81]

Epiglottitis, more appropriately referred to as supraglottitis, is classically seen in children and is uncommon after the development of *H influenzae type b* vaccines. Adults may also be affected, and the organisms implicated include group A and group F β-hemolytic *Streptococcus pyogenes* and *Staphylococcus aureus*.[93] The clinical presentation is acute, often with muffled voice, fever, drooling, and stridor in the pediatric age group.

A plain radiograph of the neck is sufficient to make the diagnosis, the findings being an enlargement of the epiglottis, enlarged aryepiglottic folds and arytenoids, prevertebral soft tissue swelling, and ballooning of the hypopharynx (**Fig. 37**).[94] CT is recommended to exclude complications such as abscesses. CT findings include swelling of the supraglottis with obliteration of surrounding fat planes, and thickening of the platysma muscle (see **Fig. 37B, C**).[95] Treatment centers on airway maintenance and intravenous antibiotics.

SUMMARY

Infections of the head and neck may be misleading in terms of their severity and anatomic extent and are prone to serious complications secondary to involvement of vital structures, such as the orbits, cranium, and airway. The role of imaging is to delineate the extent of anatomic involvement, detect complications, and to assist in the diagnosis and drainage of abscesses.

REFERENCES

1. Hurley MC, Heran MK. Imaging studies for head and neck infections. Infect Dis Clin North Am 2007;21(2):305–53.
2. Lewis MA. Multislice CT: opportunities and challenges. Br J Radiol 2001;74(885):779–81.
3. Ouyang T, Branstetter BF. Advances in head and neck imaging. Oral Maxillofac Surg Clin North Am 2010;22:107–15.
4. Kaneda T, Minami M, Ozawa K, et al. Magnetic resonance imaging of osteomyelitis in the mandible. Comparative study with other radiologic modalities. Oral Surg Oral Med Oral Pathol Oral Radiol Endod 1995;79:634–40.
5. Lee K, Kaneda T, Mori S, et al. Magnetic resonance imaging of normal and osteomyelitis in the mandible: assessment of short inversion time inversion recovery sequence. Oral Surg Oral Med Oral Pathol Oral Radiol Endod 2003;96:499–507.
6. Evans RM, Ying M, Ahuja AT. Ultrasound. In: Ahuja AT, Evans RM, King AD, et al, editors. Imaging in head and neck cancer: a practical approach. London: Greenwich Medical Media Limited; 2003. p. 3–16.
7. Alyas F, Lewis K, Williams M, et al. Diseases of the submandibular gland as demonstrated using high resolution ultrasound. Br J Radiol 2005;78:362–9.
8. Ridder GJ, Richter B, Disko U, et al. Grayscale sonographic evaluation of cervical lymphadenopathy in cat-scratch disease. J Clin Ultrasound 2001;29:140–5.
9. Ying M, Ahuja A, Metreweli C. Diagnostic accuracy of sonographic criteria for evaluation of cervical lymphadenopathy. J Ultrasound Med 1998;17:437–45.
10. Douglas SA, Jennings S, Owen VM, et al. Is ultrasound useful for evaluating paediatric inflammatory neck masses? Clin Otolaryngol 2005;30:526–9.
11. Smith J, Hsu J, Chang J. Predicting deep neck space abscess using computed tomography. Am J Otolaryngol 2006;27(4):244–7.
12. Anthony PF, Anthony WP. Surgical treatment of external auditory canal cholesteatoma. Laryngoscope 1982;92:70–5.

13. Piepergerdes MC, Kramer BM, Behnke EE. Keratosis obturans and external auditory canal cholesteatoma. Laryngoscope 1980;90:383–91.

14. Holt JJ. Ear canal cholesteatoma. Laryngoscope 1992;102:608–13.

15. Garin P, Degols JC, Delos M. External auditory canal cholesteatoma. Arch Otolaryngol Head Neck Surg 1997;123:62–5.

16. Martin B, Hirsch BE. Imaging in hearing loss. Otolaryngol Clin North Am 2008;41:157–78.

17. Shire JR, Donegan JO. Cholesteatoma of the external auditory canal and keratosis obturans. Am J Otol 1986;7:361–4.

18. Heilbrun ME, Salzman KL, Glastonbury CM, et al. External auditory canal cholesteatoma: clinical and imaging spectrum. AJNR Am J Neuroradiol 2003; 24:751–6.

19. Nadol JB. Histopathology of pseudomonas osteomyelitis of the temporal bone starting as malignant external otitis. Am J Otolaryngol 1980;1:359–71.

20. Ress BD, Luntz M, Telischi FF, et al. Necrotizing external otitis in patients with AIDS. Laryngoscope 1997;107:456–60.

21. Grandis JR, Curtin HD, Yu VL. Necrotizing (malignant) external otitis: prospective comparison of CT and MR imaging in diagnosis and follow-up. Radiology 1995;196:499–504.

22. Wiggins RH. Necrotising external otitis. In: Harnsberger HR, Wiggins RH, Hudgins PA, et al, editors. Diagnostic imaging head and neck. 1st edition. Salt Lake City (UT): Amirsys Inc; 2004. p. 10–3 I(2).

23. Mendelson DS, Som PM, Mendelson MH, et al. Malignant external otitis: the role of computed tomography and radionuclides in evaluation. Radiology 1983;149:745–9.

24. Stokkel MP, Takes RP, van Eck-Smit BL, et al. The value of quantitative gallium-67 single-photon emission tomography in the clinical management of malignant external otitis. Eur J Nucl Med 1997;24: 1429–32.

25. Vazquez E, Castellote A, Piqueras J, et al. Imaging of complications of acute mastoiditis in children. Radiographics 2003;23:359–72.

26. Valvassori GE, Buckingham RA. Imaging of the temporal bone. In: Valvassori GE, Mafee MF, Carter BL, editors. Imaging of the head and neck. New York: Thieme; 1995. p. 1–156.

27. Veillon F, Riehm S, Roedlich MN, et al. Imaging of middle ear pathology. Semin Roentgenol 2000;35: 2–11.

28. Dhooge IJ, Vandenbussche T, Lemmerling M. Value of computed tomography of the temporal bone in acute otomastoiditis. Rev Laryngol Otol Rhinol 1998;119:91–4.

29. Antonelli PJ, Garside JA, Mancuso AA. Computed tomography and the diagnosis of coalescent mastoiditis. Otolaryngol Head Neck Surg 1999; 120:350–4.

30. Motamed M, Kalan A. Gardenigo's syndrome. Postgrad Med J 2000;76:559–60.

31. Schwartz J. Chronic otitis media with tempanosclerosis. In: Harnsberger HR, Wiggins RH, Hudgins PA, et al, editors. Diagnostic imaging head and neck. 1st edition. Salt Lake City (UT): Amirsys Inc; 2004. p. 56–9 I(2).

32. Weissman J. Hearing loss. Radiology 1996;199: 593–611.

33. Shah L, Wiggins RH. Imaging of hearing loss. Neuroimaging Clin N Am 2009;19:287–306.

34. Stasolla A, Magliulo G, Parrotto D, et al. Detection of postoperative relapsing/residual cholesteatomas with diffusion-weighted echo-planar magnetic resonance imaging. Otol Neurotol 2004;25(6):879–84.

35. Vercruysse JP, De Foer B, Pouillon M, et al. The value of diffusion-weighted MR imaging in the diagnosis of primary acquired and residual cholesteatoma: a surgical verified study of 100 patients. Eur Radiol 2006;16(7):1461–7.

36. Harnsberger HR, Dart DJ, Parkin JL, et al. Cochlear implant candidates: assessment with CT and MR imaging. Radiology 1987;164(1):53–7.

37. Hahnel S, Ertl-Wagner B, Tasman AJ, et al. Relative value of MR imaging as compared with CT in the diagnosis of inflammatory paranasal sinus disease. Radiology 1999;210:171–6.

38. Zinreich SJ, Abayram S, Benson ML, et al. The ostiomeatal complex and functional endoscopic surgery. In: Som PM, Curtin HD, editors. Head and neck imaging. 4th edition. St Louis (MO): Mosby; 2003. p. 149–74.

39. Benninger MS, Ferguson BJ, Hadley JA, et al. Adult chronic rhinosinusitis: definitions, diagnosis, epidemiology, and pathophysiology. Otolaryngol Head Neck Surg 2003;129:S1–32.

40. Kronemer KA, McAlister WH. Sinusitis and its imaging in the pediatric population. Pediatr Radiol 1997;27:837–46.

41. Rao VM, el-Noueam KI. Sinonasal imaging: anatomy and pathology. Radiol Clin North Am 1998;36:921–39.

42. Tack D, Widelec J, De Maertelaer V, et al. Comparison between low-dose and standard-dose multidetector CT in patients with suspected chronic sinusitis. AJR Am J Roentgenol 2003;181:939–44.

43. Campbell PD, Zinreich SJ, Aygun N. Imaging of the paranasal sinuses and in-office CT. Otolaryngol Clin North Am 2009;42:753–64.

44. Epstein VA, Kern RC. Invasive fungal sinusitis and complications of rhinosinusitis. Otolaryngol Clin North Am 2008;41:497–524.

45. Younis RT, Lazar RH, Anand VK. Intracranial complications of sinusitis: a 15-year review of 39 cases. Ear Nose Throat J 2002;81:636–44.

46. Kraus M, Tovi F. Central nervous system complications secondary to oto-rhinologic infections. An analysis of 39 pediatric cases. Int J Pediatr Otorhinolaryngol 1992;24:217–26.
47. Yousem DM. Imaging of sinonasal inflammatory disease. Radiology 1993;188:303–14.
48. Eustis HS, Mafee MF, Walton C, et al. MR imaging and CT of orbital infections and complications in acute rhinosinusitis. Radiol Clin North Am 1998;36(6):1165–83.
49. Sonkens JW, Harnsberger HR, Blanch GM, et al. The impact of screening sinus CT on the planning of functional endoscopic sinus surgery. Otolaryngol Head Neck Surg 1991;105:802–13.
50. Gillespie MB, O'Malley BW Jr, Francis HW. An approach to fulminant invasive fungal rhinosinusitis in the immunocompromised host. Arch Otolaryngol Head Neck Surg 1998;124(5):520–6.
51. Aribandi M, McCoy V, Bazan C. Imaging features of invasive and noninvasive fungal sinusitis: a review. Radiographics 2007;27:1283–96.
52. Stringer SP, Ryan MW. Chronic invasive fungal rhinosinusitis. Otolaryngol Clin North Am 2000;33(2):375–87.
53. DelGaudio JM, Swain RE Jr, Kingdom TT, et al. Computed tomographic findings in patients with invasive fungal sinusitis. Arch Otolaryngol Head Neck Surg 2003;129(2):236–40.
54. Schubert MS. Allergic fungal sinusitis. Otolaryngol Clin North Am 2004;37(2):301–26.
55. Mafee MF. Orbit: embryology, anatomy, and pathology. In: Som PM, Curtin HD, editors. Head and neck imaging. 4th edition. St Louis (MO): Mosby; 2003. p. 529–654.
56. Zimmerman RA, Bilaniuk LT. CT of orbital infection and its cerebral complications. Am J Roentgenol 1980;134:45–50.
57. Wald ER. Periorbital and orbital infections. Pediatr Rev 2004;25:312–20.
58. Jain A, Rubin PA. Orbital cellulitis in children. Int Ophthalmol Clin 2001;41:71–86.
59. Kassel EE, Schatz CJ. Lacrimal apparatus. In: Som PM, Curtin HD, editors. Head and neck imaging. 4th edition. St Louis (MO): Mosby; 2003. p. 655–733.
60. Sikorowa L, Meyza JW, Ackerman LW. Salivary gland tumors. New York: Pergamon; 1982.
61. Brook I. Acute bacterial suppurative parotitis: microbiology and management. J Craniofac Surg 2003;14:37–40.
62. Howlett DC, Kesse KW, Hughes DV, et al. The role of imaging in the evaluation of parotid disease. Clin Radiol 2007;57:692–701.
63. Zenk J, Iro H, Klintworth N, et al. Diagnostic imaging in sialadenitis. Oral Maxillofac Surg Clin North Am 2009;21:275–92.
64. Garcia CJ, Flores PA, Arce JD, et al. Ultrasonography in the study of salivary gland lesions in children. Pediatr Radiol 1998;28:418–25.
65. Litzau D, Harnsberger HR. Benign lymphoepithelial lesions—HIV. In: Harnsberger HR, Wiggins RH, Hudgins PA, et al, editors. Diagnostic imaging head and neck. 1st edition. Salt Lake City (UT): Amirsys Inc; 2004. p. 8–11 III(7).
66. Elliott JN, Oertel YC. Lymphoepithelial cysts of the salivary glands. Histologic and cytologic features. Am J Clin Pathol 1990;93:39–43.
67. Kirshenbaum KJ, Nadimpalli SR, Friedman M, et al. Benign lymphoepithelial parotid tumors in AIDS patients: CT and MRI findings in nine cases. AJNR Am J Neuroradiol 1991;12:271–4.
68. Soberman N, Leonidas JC, Berdon WE, et al. Parotid enlargement in children seropositive for human immunodeficiency virus: imaging findings. Am J Roentgenol 1991;157:553–6.
69. Peters TR, Edwards KM. Cervical lymphadenopathy and adenitis. Pediatr Rev 2000;21:399–405.
70. Rudolph CD, Rudolph AM, Hostetter MK, et al, editors. Rudolph's pediatrics. 21st edition. New York: McGraw Hill Medica; 2003.
71. Baker CJ. Group B streptococcal cellulitis-adenitis in infants. Am J Dis Child 1982;136:631–3.
72. Desa AE. Tuberculosis of lymph glands. In: Rao KN, editor. Text book of tuberculosis. New Delhi (India): Vikas Publishing House; 1981. p. 476–81.
73. Polesky A, Grove W, Bhatia G. Peripheral tuberculous lymphadenopathy: epidemiology, diagnosis, treatment, and outcome. Medicine 2005;84:350–62.
74. Marais BJ, Wright CA, Schaaf HS, et al. Tuberculous lymphadenitis as a cause of persistent cervical lymphadenopathy in children from a tuberculosis-endemic area. Pediatr Infect Dis J 2006;25:142–6.
75. Ying M, Ahuja A. Sonography of neck lymph nodes. I. Normal lymph nodes. Clin Radiol 2003;58:351–8.
76. Ahuja A, Ying M. Sonography of neck lymph nodes. II. Abnormal lymph nodes. Clin Radiol 2003;58:359–66.
77. Ahuja A, Ying M, Yuen YH, et al. Power Doppler sonography to differentiate tuberculous cervical lymphadenopathy from nasopharyngeal carcinoma. AJNR Am J Neuroradiol 2001;22:735–40.
78. Hanck C, Fleisch F, Katz G. Imaging appearance of nontuberculous mycobacterial infection of the neck. AJNR Am J Neuroradiol 2004;25(2):349–50.
79. Burrill J, Williams CJ, Bain G, et al. Tuberculosis: a radiologic review. Radiographics 2007;27(5):1255–73.
80. Vieira F, Allen SM, Stocks RS, et al. Deep neck infection. Otolaryngol Clin North Am 2008;41:459–83.
81. Boscolo-Rizzo P, Marchiori C, Zanetti F, et al. Conservative management of deep neck abscesses in adults: the importance of CECT findings. Otolaryngol Head Neck Surg 2006;135(6):894–9.

82. Lee J, Kim H, Lim S. Predisposing factors of complicated deep neck infection: an analysis of 158 cases. Yonsei Med J 2007;48(1):55–62.

83. Yellon RF. Head and neck space infections. In: Bluestone CD, Casselbrant ML, Stool SE, et al, editors. Pediatric otolaryngology, vol. 2, 4th edition. Philadelphia: Saunders; 2003. p. 1681–701.

84. Mosier KM. Nononcologic imaging of the oral cavity and jaws. Otolaryngol Clin North Am 2008; 41:103–37.

85. Becker M, Zbaren P, Hermans R, et al. Necrotizing fasciitis of the head and neck: role of CT in diagnosis and management. Radiology 1997;202:471–6.

86. Fugitt B, Puckett ML, Quigley MM, et al. Necrotizing fasciitis. Radiographics 2004;24(5):1472–6.

87. Bross-Soriano D, Arrieta-Gomez J, Prado-Calleros H, et al. Management of Ludwig's angina with small neck incisions: 18 years experience. Otolaryngol Head Neck Surg 2004;130(6):712–7.

88. Wasson J, Hopkins C, Bowdler D. Did Ludwig's angina kill Ludwig? J Laryngol Otol 2006;120(5): 363–5.

89. Weed HG, Forest LA. Deep neck infection. In: Cummings CW, Flint PW, Harker LA, et al, editors.

Otolaryngology: head and neck surgery, vol. 3, 4th edition. Philadelphia: Elsevier Mosby; 2005. p. 2515–24.

90. Oh J, Kim Y, Kim C. Parapharyngeal abscess: comprehensive management protocol. ORL J Otorhinolaryngol Relat Spec 2007;69(1):37–42.

91. Castellote A, Vazquez E, Vera J, et al. Cervicothoracic lesions in infants and children. Radiographics 1999;19(3):583–600.

92. Eastwood JD, Hudgins PA, Malone D. Retropharyngeal effusion in acute calcific prevertebral tendinitis: diagnosis with CT and MR imaging. AJNR Am J Neuroradiol 1998;19:1789–92.

93. Shih L, Hawkins DB, Stanley RB. Acute epiglottitis in adults: a review of 48 cases. Ann Otol Rhinol Laryngol 1988;97:527–9.

94. Nemzek WR, Katzberg RW, Van Slyke MA, et al. A reappraisal of the radiologic findings of acute inflammation of the epiglottis and supraglottic structures in adults. AJNR Am J Neuroradiol 1995;16: 495–502.

95. Smith MM, Mukherji SK, Thompson JE, et al. CT in adult supraglottitis. Am J Neuroradiol 1996;17: 1355–8.

Spine Infections

John L. Go, MD[a],*, Stephen Rothman, MD[b],
Ashley Prosper, MD[c], Richard Silbergleit, MD[d],
Alexander Lerner, MD[e]

KEYWORDS

- Spinal infections • Fungal • Tuberculosis

KEY POINTS

- Infections of the spine represent a rare but potentially debilitating and neurologically devastating condition for patients.
- Early diagnosis, imaging, and intervention may prevent some of the more critical complications that may ensue from this disease process, including alignment abnormalities, central canal compromise, nerve root impingement, vascular complications, and spinal cord injury.
- A variety of imaging modalities are used to diagnose infections of the spine and spinal cord.

INTRODUCTION

Infection of the vertebral column without (spondylitis) or with involvement of the disk space (spondylodiscitis) constitute fewer than 2% to 4% of all cases of osteomyelitis.[1,2] A progressive increase has been seen in the number of vertebral infections in the setting of tuberculosis in HIV-positive patients and the homeless, and in hematogenous seeding in intravenous drug abusers and immunocompromised patients. The relative incidence of infectious spondylitis is more common in men than women, with a relative ratio of 1.5 of 3:1. It has a relative peak incidence in the sixth decade of life, although infections have been reported at all age ranges.[3] Risk factors for the possibility of spinal infection include recent surgery, immunocompromised state, diabetes, recent genitourinary surgery in male patients, and older age.[4,5]

CLINICAL PRESENTATION

Patients typically present with back pain, tenderness, and rigidity at the site of involvement.[6]

Accompanying fever should alert clinicians to the possibility of infection. Paravertebral involvement and involvement of the neural foramina and exiting nerve roots may present as a radiculopathy or polyradiculopathy. Additional involvement of the thecal sac and contents may lead to worsening neurologic deficits. Delay in diagnosis may be the result of a nonfocal neurologic examination.[4,7] Patients may also present with nonrelating symptoms, such as pleural effusion, which may delay diagnosis.[8,9]

SPONDYLITIS AND SPONDYLODISCITIS
Pathogenesis

Infection to the spinal column may occur through several routes. The most common manifestation is through hematogenous seeding directly to the vertebral bodies, usually resulting from septicemia. The segmental arteries providing the blood supply to the vertebral bodies provide the vascular blood supply to the peripheral third of the end plates. At each motion segment, the segmental

[a] Division of Neuroradiology, Department of Radiology, Keck School of Medicine, University of Southern California, Room 3740F, 1200 North State Street, Los Angeles, CA 90033, USA; [b] Department of Radiology, Keck School of Medicine, University of Southern California, Room 3740A, 1200 North State Street, Los Angeles, CA 90033, USA; [c] Diagnostic Radiology Residency Program, Keck School of Medicine, University of Southern California, Room 3D321, 1200 North State Street, Los Angeles, CA 90033, USA; [d] Diagnostic Radiology, William Beaumont Hospital, Oakland University William Beaumont School of Medicine, 3601 West 13 Mile Road, Royal Oak, MI 48073, USA; [e] Division of Neuroradiology, Department of Radiology, Keck School of Medicine, University of Southern California, Room 3750E, 1200 North State Street, Los Angeles, CA 90033, USA
* Corresponding author.
E-mail addresses: jlgomd@me.com; jlgo@usc.edu

Neuroimag Clin N Am 22 (2012) 755–772
http://dx.doi.org/10.1016/j.nic.2012.06.002

artery supplying the subjacent end plates provides nutrients to the disk space through simple diffusion. In adults, no vessels service the intervening disk space, although bridging arteries exist in children between the segmental arteries, servicing the superior and inferior end plates at the motion segment. These vessels enter the disk space through the ossification center of the end plates and from the longitudinal ligaments. By 13 years of age, this network of vessels within the disk space is no longer present.[10,11] Hematogenous spread occurs at the end arterioles at the site adjacent to the end plates posterior to the anterior longitudinal ligament both superiorly and inferiorly, with inoculation of organism within the vertebral bodies. In the setting of pyogenic infection, the infection then spreads from the vertebral body into the disk space and to the adjacent end plate. In children, the organisms may inoculate the bridging arteries within the disk space, and thus children may initially present with only discitis. With stretching of the anterior longitudinal ligament from traction, children may present with abdominal pain as their initial presenting symptom (**Fig. 1**).

Organisms that lack the proteolytic enzymes to digest the disk (tuberculosis) may initially present with spondylitis, and disk space involvement is spared in the early course of disease. Eventual collapse of the vertebral body may lead to secondary collapse and destruction of the disk space late in the disease process (**Fig. 2**).

Another mode of hematogenous spread is through a transvenous route. Batson plexus, which forms the epidural venous plexus within the central canal, represents a series of valveless veins that extend the length of the spinal canal. Cases have been described of transvenous hematogenous seeding in patients with inflammatory bowel disease, urinary tract infections, and septic abortions.[3]

Direct inoculation of the spine may occur in penetrating trauma or direct exposure related to skin breakdown or open wounds. Nosocomial infections may also occur as a rare complication of spine surgery or secondary to inadvertent exposure related to nonspinal surgery. Interventional or diagnostic procedures such as lumbar puncture; pain management procedures such as epidural block, nerve block, facet block, vertebroplasty, and kyphoplasty; and the use of indwelling catheters may result in infection.[12,13]

The lumbar spine is the most common location for spondylodiscitis in 50% of cases, followed by

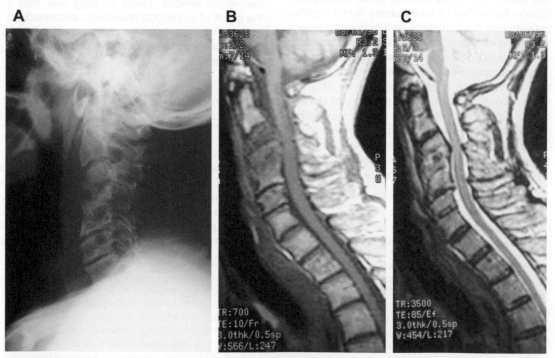

Fig. 1. *Staphylococcus aureus* spondylodiscitis. (*A*) Lateral plain film shows disk space narrowing with erosion of the end plates at the C3-4 level. Also note C4-5 severe disk space narrowing and fusion related to prior infection. (*B*) T1 sagittal image shows decreased signal of C3 and C4 vertebral bodies with loss of the hypointense band of the adjacent end plates. Note obliteration of the C4-5 disk space. (*C*) T2 sagittal image shows increased signal intensity of the C3-4 disk space.

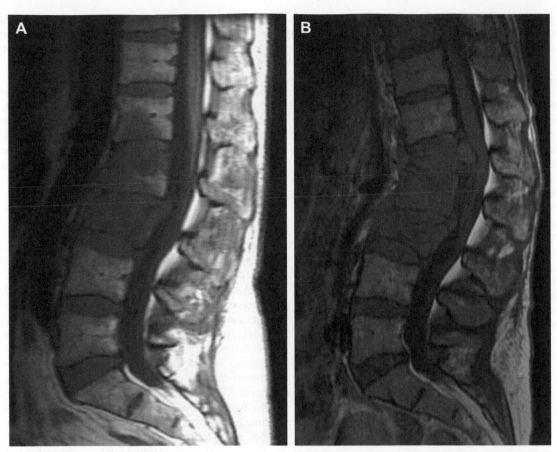

Fig. 2. Tuberculous spondylitis with progressive deformity. (*A*) T1 sagittal image of abnormal hypointense signal within L1-3 showing mild height loss of the L2 and L3 vertebral bodies with mild height loss of the L2-3 disk space. (*B*) Nineteen months later, image shows progressive height loss of L3 and progressive erosion and height loss of L1 with worsening kyphosis and compression of the thecal sac.

the thoracic spine in 33%, with cervical spine involvement the least common (3%–10%).[14–17]

ORGANISMS
Bacterial

A host of organisms have been reported as causing vertebral osteomyelitis, although the most common organism in more than 50% of cases is *Staphylococcus aureus*.[18–21] An increased incidence of *Pseudomonas* infection may be seen in intravenous drug abusers and *Salmonella* infection in patients with sickle cell anemia. *Haemophilus influenzae* can be a cause of spine infection in patients with meningitis.[18]

Tuberculous

Tuberculous infection was more prevalent in the eighteenth and nineteenth centuries but with the development of antibiotics had decreased in the twentieth century. A resurgence of tuberculosis

has been seen within the third world and in immunocompromised patients, those with HIV disease, and the homeless. Patients may present with low-grade fever and mild elevation of erythrocyte sedimentation rate (ESR) and C-reactive protein (CRP). Tuberculous spondylitis is most common within the thoracic spine, followed by the lumbar and cervical regions. The infection begins within the vertebral bodies, with the anterior superior aspect of the vertebral body the most common location. The mycobacterium lack the proteolytic enzymes to digest the disk, and sparing of the disk space distinguishes tuberculous spondylitis from pyogenic infection. Subligamentous spread is typically seen, with adjacent vertebral bodies involved. Skip lesions may also occur within the spine. Involvement of the posterior elements is much more common with tuberculous spondylitis, because pyogenic infection usually does not involve this area. The development of paravertebral abscesses is much more common than in pyogenic infection. Fistulous tracts may also involve the pleural space and occur within the pelvis and groin (**Fig. 3**).[22–26]

Fungal

Fungal infections of the spine are most commonly seen in patients with diabetes or who are immuno-compromised, including those with HIV, those who have undergone transplantation, and those undergoing chemotherapy that leads to immuno-suppression. Exposure to endemic areas with high levels of fungal particles may also lead to fungal spondylitis/spondylodiscitis. Coccidiomy-cosis is endemic in the San Joaquin Valley in California and in Central and South America[27,28]; histoplasmosis is endemic in the Ohio River Valley; and blastomycosis is endemic in areas bordering the Mississippi and Ohio Rivers, the Great Lakes, and the St. Lawrence River, and in Central and South America, Africa, and the Middle East.[29,30] Fungal infections such as mucormycosis and aspergillosis may be more prevalent in patients with diabetes. *Candida* infection may also be

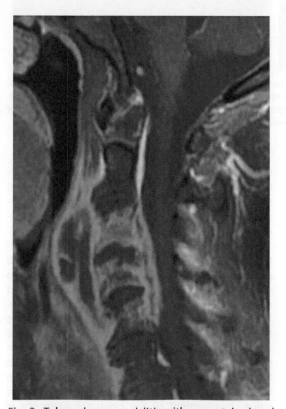

Fig. 3. Tuberculous spondylitis with prevertebral and epidural abscess. Postcontrast T1 sagittal image shows enhancement of the C4, C5, and C6 vertebral bodies with extensive prevertebral abscess and epidural component compressing the thecal sac.

seen in immunocompromised hosts. *Candida* may gain access via intravenous lines, monitoring devices, or implantable devices. Intravenous drug abusers are also at risk (**Figs. 4** and **5**).[31–33]

The imaging of fungal spinal infection is fairly nonspecific and may mimic either tuberculous or pyogenic infection. Coccidiomycosis frequently involves the spine and is characterized by disk space narrowing and the presence of paraspinal masses with little bony erosion, although lytic lesions may be seen, and may also involve the ribs.[34]

Parasitic

Parasitic infection in the spine may affect the thecal sac and its contents. This involvement is usually the result of direct hematogenous seeding of the subarachnoid space from meningitis or implantation of the offending organism with involvement of the spinal cord. Neurocysticerco-sis, the most common parasitic infection in the world, is caused by hematogenous spread of the immature form of *Taenia solium* and may result in spread within the subarachnoid space to the thecal sac or direct implantation of the spinal cord. A full discussion of neurocysticercosis may be found elsewhere in this issue. Echinococcal infection has a similar route of spread, and may be seen more commonly in sheepherders in Australia and in the Middle East.[35,36] Schistosomi-asis, related to ingestion of parasitic trematodes, may occasionally involve the spine and include *Schistosoma mansoni*, *S japonica*, and *S haema-tobium*. Infection after ingestion of the flukes occurs through vascular venous channel from the pelvic veins to the paramedullary veins, and thus involvement of the lower thoracic and lumbar region is the most common location. Schistosomal infection may present as a myelitis of the cord with irregular enhancement and edema, or may present as masses within the thecal sac that may repre-sent the eggs with a surrounding inflammatory reaction. These lesions may be mistaken for an in-tramedullary neoplasm or multiple masses within the thecal sac, such as neurofibromatosis type I or II or metastatic disease (**Figs. 6** and **7**).[37,38]

Laboratory Assessment

Initial workup should include blood cultures and Gram stain, white blood cell count, ESR, and CRP level. In conjunction with blood cultures and Gram stain, ESR has been shown to be most useful as a marker of infection, with elevation seen in 70% to 100% of infections, although its use for following disease progression and response should be cautioned because of its

A   B   C

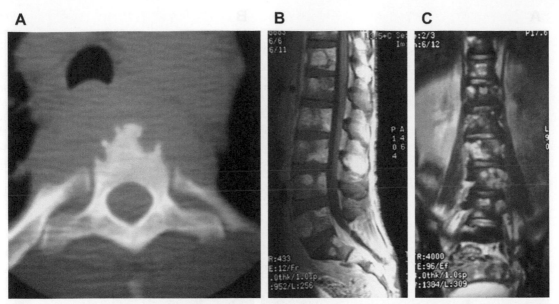

Fig. 4. Coccidiomycosis. (A) CT axial image in the midthoracic spine shows extensive prevertebral soft tissue mass and multiple lytic lesions associated with the vertebral body. (B) T1 sagittal and (C) T1 coronal images show numerous areas of signal abnormality involving the vertebral bodies with sparing of the disk spaces.

nonspecificity.[39–41] Leukocytosis has also been shown to be a good marker for infection, with elevation seen in 13% to 60% of cases.[14,42,43] CRP, an acute phase reactant, is also used in conjunction with ESR.

The clinical presentation and laboratory values may help differentiate between pyogenic and granulomatous infection. Pyogenic spondylodiscitis presents with sharp point tenderness at the site of infection, whereas granulomatous infection presents with dull achy pain. In addition, patients with pyogenic infection may present with markedly elevated spiking fevers, whereas those with granulomatous infection present with low-grade fevers. The white count in pyogenic spondylodiscitis may be markedly elevated, with a shift of polymorphonuclear neutrophils to the left. Patients with granulomatous infectious may have normal or even decreased white counts, especially those who are immunocompromised. The ESR and CRP level may help determine whether the infection may be pyogenic or granulomatous in nature. Although both may be elevated in spondylitis/spondylodiscitis, a marked elevation of ESR and CRP is seen in the setting of pyogenic infection compared with granulomatous disease.

The efficacy of biopsy is somewhat controversial, because 30% of needle biopsies and 14% of open biopsies in the setting of infection may show negative cultures.[41,44] The technique used may determine yield, because soft tissue paravertebral biopsies and disk aspirations may provide lower yields. Higher yield may be achieved with direct bone biopsy or sampling from the end plate.

IMAGING FEATURES
Plain Films

Detection of spondylitis/spondylodiscitis may be difficult or impossible during early infection. Because of replacement of the normal bony matrix as a result of infection, a relative decreased density of the vertebral body with lysis of bone may be seen. Detection of bone loss requires a 30% to 40% loss of the bony matrix, which may occur at approximately 2 weeks during an acute spine infection.[45,46] Thus, plain film radiography is insensitive in the detection of early disease. As disease progresses, lytic lesions of bone may be seen, with eventual involvement of the disk space, and erosive changes of the end plates with or without disk height loss may be apparent (see **Fig. 1**). End plate erosion is often subtle, but is the most reliable sign that can be detected on plain films and is the single most important observation to be made in evaluating any radiograph of the lumbar spine. Prevertebral or paravertebral soft tissue densities may also be detected on plain film radiography in the setting of early infection. In the setting of chronic infection after 4 months, spinal deformity such as kyphosis, scoliosis, or both may be seen (see **Fig. 1**).[3,47]

A   **B**

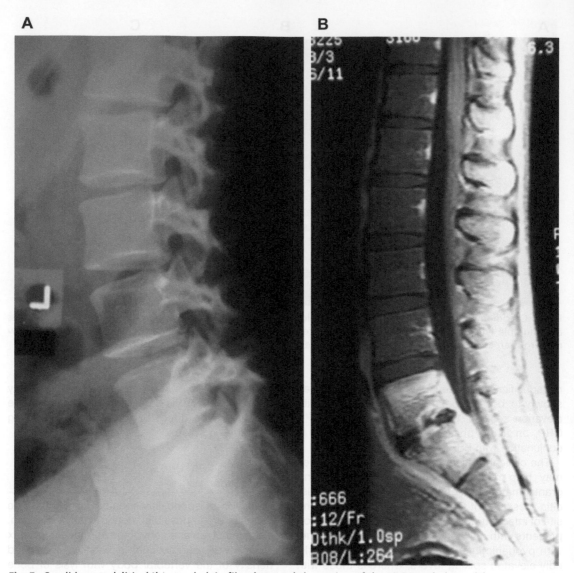

Fig. 5. Candida spondylitis. (*A*) Lateral plain film shows subtle erosion of the L5-S1 end plates. (*B*) Postcontrast T1 sagittal image shows enhancement of the L5 and S1 vertebral bodies with disk space narrowing.

A   **B**   **C**

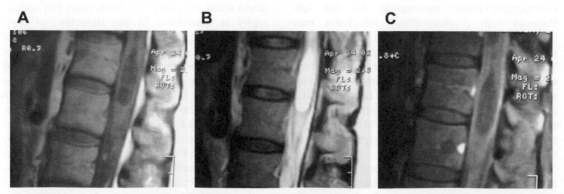

Fig. 6. Neurocysticercosis. (*A*) T1 sagittal image shows a well-circumscribed hypointense lesion within the distal thoracic cord, which is hyperintense on the T2-weighted image (*B*, *C*) Postcontrast image shows no enhancement. Surgical removal showed the vesicular stage of neurocysticercosis.

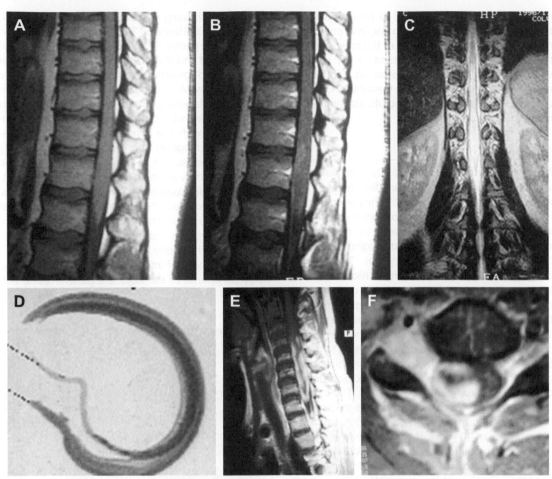

Fig. 7. Schistosomiasis. Precontrast (*A*) and postcontrast (*B*) sagittal images show an enhancing lesion within the distal thoracic cord. Coronal T2-weighted image (*C*) shows increased signal intensity within the thoracic cord. (*D*) Cerebrospinal fluid analysis showed presence of *Schistosomiasis mansoni* on hematoxylin-eosin–stained slide. (*E*) Postcontrast T1 sagittal image and axial image (*F*) shows enhancing intramedullary and extramedullary masses within the thecal sac in a different patient who, after swimming in Lake Victoria in Nigeria, developed progressive upper and lower extremity weakness.

CT

Because this modality is more readily available than MR imaging, a review of CT findings of infection is relevant. At the authors' institution, CT imaging is performed to determine the extent of bony involvement, whereas MR imaging is performed to determine the involvement of the central canal and spinal cord. Intravenous contrast is typically not administered except in the presence of a contraindication to MR imaging. Intravenous contrast may be administered to opacify the epidural venous plexus, which may help determine the degree of mass effect on the thecal sac. If the thecal sac is still not well seen, myelography and postmyelography CT imaging are performed.

Because of the direct involvement of bone, deossification of bone with loss of the normal architecture of the trabecular bone may be seen. As the infection spreads, soft tissue replacement of the bone may be seen. Involvement of the bone may lead to erosive changes of the end plates. Direct inoculation of the disk space may also occur, with involvement of the subjacent end plate, which may lead to collapse of the disk space.[48–50] Abscess formation may also occur within the disk space. As phlebitis or thrombophlebitis of the paravertebral veins occurs, the infection may then spread in a prevertebral and paravertebral location. This spread may be seen as surrounding soft tissue masses with extension into the paravertebral musculature and may lead to impingement of the nerve roots at the neural foramen. In many cases, however, this soft tissue mass represents an aggressive inflammatory response to the infection, and biopsies of this soft tissue component may lead to negative cultures in most cases. Direct extension of the infection posteriorly may lead to involvement of the epidural venous plexus, which may present as a soft tissue mass with compression of the thecal sac. For evaluation of the thecal sac and its contents, MR imaging is needed (Fig. 8).

MR Imaging

MR imaging has shown superiority in the detection and assessment of inflammatory disorders.[1,19,51–53] In the setting of early spondylitis, the earliest finding is the presence of bone marrow edema within the vertebral bodies, which is seen as hypointense signal intensity on T1-weighted imaging (T1WI) and hyperintense signal intensity on T2-weighted imaging (T2WI)/short-tau inversion recovery (STIR) images. After the administration of contrast, this may show enhancement. Infection begins subjacent to the end plates and, as the disease progresses, involvement of the end plates and the intervening disk is seen. Early discitis may be difficult to detect but should be seen as hyperintense signal intensity on T2WI. A fairly reliable sign of early discitis is loss of the internuclear cleft on T2WI.[54–56] The internuclear cleft, seen as part of the normal appearance of the degenerative disk in up to 94% of patients after the age of 40 years, is typically seen as a linear transverse hypointense band on T2WI within the central portion of the disk on sagittal or coronal images.[56] Erosion of the end plates may be seen

as marked thinning or absence of the hypointense band of cortical bone on T1WI and T2WI associated with the end plates (Fig. 9). Bone marrow edema of the adjacent end plates may also be seen as part of the normal degenerative course of the disk, and is described by Modic as a type I reactive end plate change.[57] However, signal abnormality of the end plates and erosion of the end plates with edema associated with the disk space are usually indicative of a pyogenic spondylodiscitis. In severely degenerative spines, edema or fluid within the disk space may be seen as hyperintense in signal intensity, with associated signal changes of the end plate. However, close inspection of the cortical hypointense band of the end plate and its presence without erosion should suggest a sterile spondyloarthropathy.

Development of inflammation around the spine may be edema of the adjacent paravertebral soft

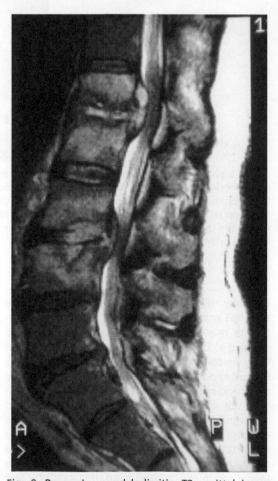

Fig. 9. Pyogenic spondylodiscitis. T2 sagittal image shows loss of the internuclear cleft of the L1-2 and L3-4 disk spaces. Also note subtle loss of the hypointense band of the end plates at the L3-4 level.

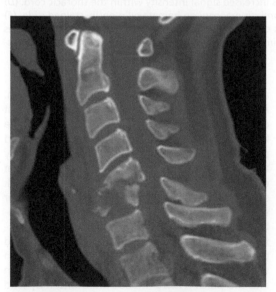

Fig. 8. Tuberculous spondylitis. CT sagittal image shows pathologic fractures of C5 and C6 vertebral bodies with associated bony and end plate erosions and joint space narrowing.

tissues seen as hyperintense signal intensity on the T2WI or as an enhancing inflammatory soft tissue mass. This mass/phlegmon is isointense to hypointense to muscle on T1WI and hyperintense on T2WI/STIR. After administration of contrast, heterogenous moderate to avid enhancement of the soft tissue is seen. Abscesses of the paravertebral soft tissues should show the presence of ring-enhancing fluid collections with thick irregular walls. The fluid material may be heterogenous in nature and have signal intensity higher than cerebrospinal fluid on T1WI, and be

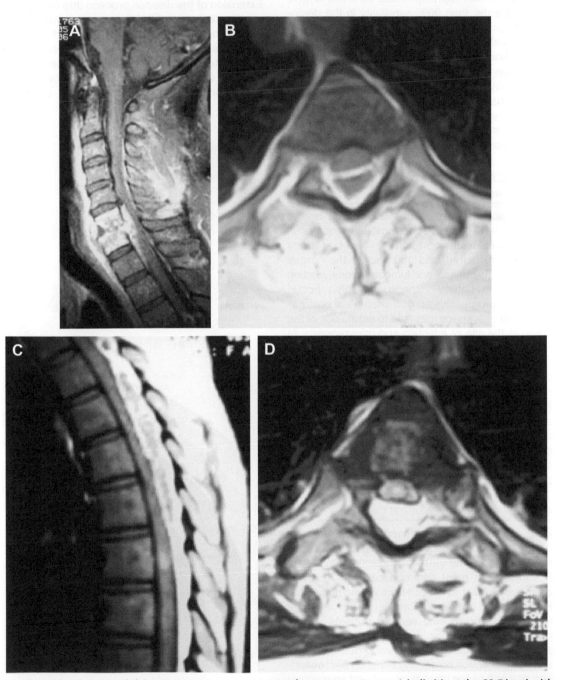

Fig. 10. Epidural abscess. (*A*) Postcontrast T1 sagittal image shows pyogenic spondylodiscitis at the C6-7 level with enhancing epidural process from the C5-6 to the T1-2 level. Note enhancing prevertebral mass. In a different patient with posterior epidural fluid collection in the midthoracic spine, postcontrast axial (*B*) and sagittal images (*C*) show ring enhancing epidural abscess. T2-weighted image shows the collection to be hyperintense in signal intensity (*D*).

hyperintense on T2WI without enhancement. Diffusion of the spine may show diffusion abnormality of these collections, as is true for abscesses in other parts of the body.

Nuclear Medicine

Technetium-99m diphosphonate bone scans have shown greater than 90% sensitivity in the depiction of spondylitis and spondylodiscitis. Gallium scan has also shown 90% sensitivity in the setting of infection. Combined technetium and gallium scans have shown sensitivity of greater than 94%. During the healing phase of infection, gallium imaging has been negative, whereas technetium imaging remains positive, and gallium imaging alone is sufficient for follow-up in determining progression or response to therapy.[19,47,58]

COMPLICATIONS OF SPONDYLODISCITIS
Alignment Abnormalities

Erosion and destruction of the vertebral bodies may lead to alignment abnormalities of the spine. Progressive destruction of the vertebral body may lead to height loss and loss of the normal lordosis in the cervical and lumbar regions, leading to kyphosis. Lateral listhesis may also occur, leading to progressive scoliosis. Eventual obliteration of the disk space may lead to autofusion of the spine at the site of infection and may progress to accelerated degenerative changes to adjacent motion segments of the spine. These alignment abnormalities may lead to progressive compromise of the central canal and neural foramina. Pott disease, the sequel of chronic tuberculous spondylitis with collapse of the vertebral body causing a gibbus deformity of the spine, was described by Percivall Pott[59] (1714–1788) based on clinical observations in severely scoliotic patients.

Epidural Abscess and Spinal Cord Injury

Prior studies have determined the relative incidence of epidural abscess to be 0.2 to 1.96 cases per 10,000.[60] By far the most common pathogen is S aureus. The most common cause of epidural abscess is direct extension from spondylodiscitis. However, an increasing incidence of epidural infections is now being seen in patients undergoing epidural block.[61] Epidural abscess is a misnomer, because an epidural process associated with infection presenting either as fluid collection or a soft tissue mass is considered an epidural abscess. Epidural abscess should be distinguished from subligamentous infection, which is contained by the posterior longitudinal ligament

(PLL). Spondylodiscitis may posteriorly displace the PLL, but the disease process is not in the epidural space and is contained. These types of lesions do not necessitate surgical intervention. The subligamentous component may displace the thecal sac posteriorly, but is contained by the PLL and does not extend around the thecal sac. Extension of the disease process into the epidural space will show a soft tissue mass or fluid extending around the anterior and lateral portions of the thecal sac. Once the disease process involves the epidural space, direct involvement of the epidural venous plexus may occur. Compression and thrombophlebitis of the epidural veins may

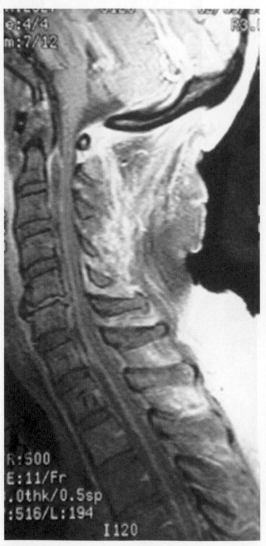

Fig. 11. Postcontrast T1 sagittal image shows extensive ring-enhancing lesion anterior to the cervicothoracic cord, proven to be a subdural abscess at surgery.

cause venous congestion within the spinal cord and will eventually lead to venous ischemia or venous infarct of the spinal cord. Arterial infarction of the spinal cord may also occur, with associated vasculitis of the radiculopial and radiculomedullary branches feeding the spinal cord. The detection of an epidural abscess necessitates emergent surgical intervention to prevent the devastating neurologic complications of spinal cord injury. Once vascular injury to the spinal cord occurs, the consequences may be irreversible (**Fig. 10**).[62-64]

Subdural Abscess

The subdural space is a potential space within the thecal sac with the arachnoid membrane directly deep to the dura. Separation of the arachnoid from the dura may lead to the presence of a subdural collection. Infections associated with the dura may lead to separation of the arachnoid from the dura, leading to presence of effusions or infected fluid. Subdural abscess may form and is seen as a crescentic fluid collection with irregular thick-walled enhancement. Subdural abscess

may be differentiated from epidural abscess, because the normal configuration of the thecal sac is maintained. However the crescentic fluid collection may decrease the overall size of the subarachnoid collection, with apparent compression of the nerve roots within the sac or the spinal cord (**Fig. 11**).[65,66]

Paravertebral Abscess

Prevertebral and paravertebral abscesses result from the contiguous spread of the infection from the spine to adjacent soft tissues. In addition, involvement of the paravertebral veins provides a way for the infection to access the adjacent soft tissues from resulting phlebitis or thrombophlebitis. Abscess formation may occur as previously described. The incidence of abscess formation is greater in granulomatous spondylitis, especially tuberculosis spondylitis, which may necessitate aspiration and drainage. In extensive paravertebral inflammation, secondary involvement of the adjacent vascular structures, such as the aorta, is seen, which may lead to vasculitis and mycotic aneurysm formation (see **Fig. 3**).[67-70]

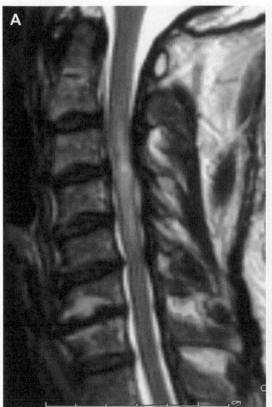 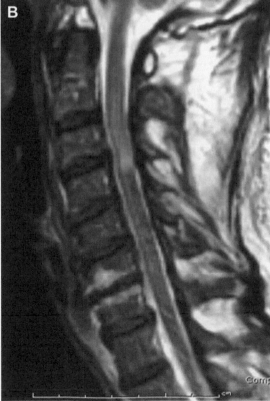

Fig. 12. *Staphylococcus myelitis* with improvement on antibiotics. (*A*) T2 sagittal image shows signal abnormality within the cord from the C3 to C5 levels. After a 2-week course on vancomycin, follow-up T2 sagittal image (*B*) shows marked improvement of cord signal abnormality.

DIRECT SPINAL CORD INFECTION
Myelitis

Direct infection of the spinal cord may result in infectious myelitis. Although myelitis more commonly results from vascular complications in the setting of spondylitis/spondylodiscitis, direct inoculation of the spinal cord may occur. This inoculation classically occurs from a hematogenous route, with viral myelitis by far more common than pyogenic or granulomatous myelitis. Clinical manifestations may vary and may result in progressive neurologic decline, with signs and symptoms of upper motor neuron disease. MR is the mainstay form of imaging of the spinal cord. Myelitis typically shows increased signal of the spinal cord on T2WI in a nonvascular distribution most commonly seen as central cord signal abnormality with cord expansion. The abnormal signal intensity is isointense to hypointense to the spinal cord on T2WI. After the administration of contrast, the areas of signal intensity may or may not enhance. The pattern of enhancement typically is indistinct. Hemorrhage may be seen in viral myelitis, and is not commonly seen in pyogenic or granulomatous myelitis. In HIV myelitis, direct invasion of the spinal cord leads to vacuolar myelopathy, with imaging features typical of apparent volume loss. T2 hyperintensity may also be seen within the spinal cord (**Figs. 12–14**).[71–82]

Spinal Cord Abscess

Spinal cord abscess is a rare occurrence in the antibiotic era, but its presence portends a high morbidity and mortality rate. Spinal cord abscess in children may be the result of hematogenous spread through a congenital defect, urogenital or lung infection, or endocarditis, although in more than 50% of cases it is the result of a dermal sinus

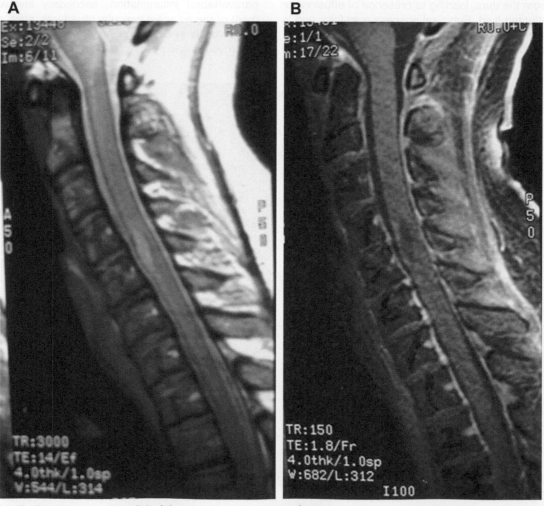

Fig. 13. Coccidiomycosis myelitis. (*A*) T2 sagittal image shows focal area of hyperintense signal abnormality from the C4 to C5 levels and cord expansion. (*B*) Postcontrast image shows no enhancement.

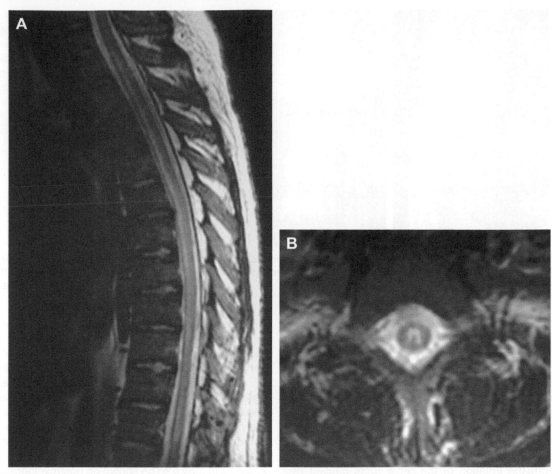

Fig. 14. HIV vacuolar myelopathy. (*A*) T2 sagittal image shows extensive abnormal hyperintense signal intensity within the thoracic cord located within the central aspect of the cord (*B*).

tract. In adults, its origin may also be from a hematogenous source or complication of pyogenic myelitis. *S aureus* is often the offending organism, although tuberculosis, *Streptococcal spp*, *Listeria monocytogenes*, *Candida albicans*, and *Brucella spp* have been described.[83–87] The features of the spinal cord abscess are similar to those seen in other parts of the body, showing a fluid collection within the cord with irregular thick walled rim enhancement. On diffusion-weighted images, diffusion abnormality is seen within the fluid component, as is typical with these types of lesions (**Fig. 15**).[88,89]

Facet Infection

Facet infection may result from involvement of the middle column related to the infection associated with the vertebral column, or as an isolated event. Direct contiguous spread, hematogenous spread, or direct inoculation from an interventional procedure, such as adjacent surgery or facet block,

may lead to infection. The presence of fluid alone does not suggest facet infection. Fluid may be seen within the facet related to acute inflammation or noninfectious spondyloarthropathy. However, erosive changes associated with the subchondral surface of the facet joint and associated enhancing soft tissue mass may suggest the presence of infection. Extension of the infection may occur around the facet, with inflammation of the surrounding soft tissues and possible presence of abscess formation. Because of the relationship of the facet to the central canal, extension of infection into the central canal may lead to an epidural process within the posterior aspect of the epidural space initially, different from the anterior location of epidural spread seen in the setting of spondylodiscitis (**Fig. 16**).[90–96]

Arachnoiditis

Arachnoiditis, which represents infection or inflammation within the thecal sac, is more typically

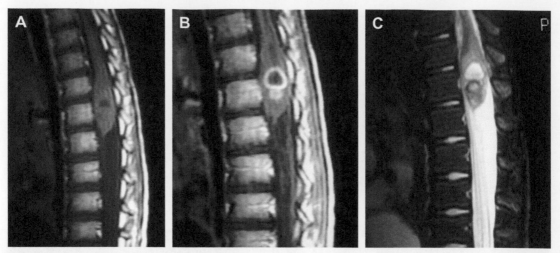

Fig. 15. *Staphylococcus aureus* spinal cord abscess. Precontrast (*A*), postcontrast (*B*), and T2-weighted (*C*) images show a ring enhancing fluid collections in the distal thoracic cord. Note the hypointense capsule of the fluid collection on the T2-weighted image in (*C*).

caused by irritation from older contrast media introduced into the thecal sac, or irritation from the presence of blood products. Infectious seeding of the subarachnoid space may lead to infectious arachnoiditis. Infection is usually caused by secondary spread of infection related to meningitis. Contamination may also occur related to prior surgery, trauma, or hematogenous spread with inoculation of the cerebrospinal fluid space. Clinical manifestations, such as pain, may result from the irritation of the nerve roots caused by involvement of the arachnoid membrane. Involvement of multiple nerve roots results in

a polyradicular distribution. On MR imaging, this may be seen initially as enhancement of the nerve roots, which may be smooth or nodular. Isolated nerve root enhancement may be seen as a result of contrast-related enhancement of the veins associated with a nerve root.[97,98] Multiple enhancing nerve roots, however, should suggest the possibility of arachnoiditis. As the inflammation/infection spreads, clumping of the nerve roots may occur; this is best seen on T2-weighted axial images but may also be shown on postmyelogram CT images. Stranding or synechiae may form, with the presence of loculated fluid collections within

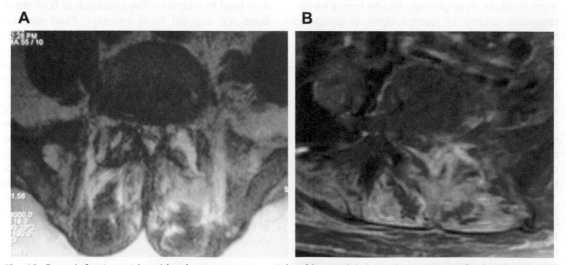

Fig. 16. Facet infection with epidural extension. T2-weighted image (*A*) shows hyperintense fluid within the left L5-S1 joint space. Note loss of the hypointense subchondral signal intensity of bone along the joint space. Postcontrast axial image (*B*) shows enhancement of the facet joint and the adjacent epidural space within the central canal.

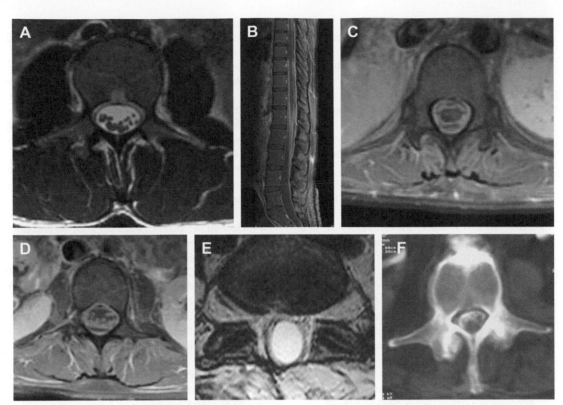

Fig. 17. Examples of arachnoiditis. (*A*) T2-weighted axial image shows clumping of the nerve roots within the thecal sac. Tuberculous arachnoiditis showing enhancing material within the thecal sac on the postcontrast sagittal (*B*) and axial (*C*) images. (*D*) Postcontrast images show enhancement of the cauda equina. (*E*) T2-weighted axial image shows the empty sac sign. (*F*) Noncontrast CT demonstrates calcifications within the thecal sac in this example of arachnoiditis ossificans.

the thecal sac, which may represent intradural arachnoid cysts. Because inflammatory tissue may be associated with the nerve roots, the nerve roots may be adherent to the thecal sac, with the presence of a faceless thecal sac on MR imaging or postmyelogram CT images. In the setting of infection, the subarachnoid fluid may not be homogenous in signal because of the presence of exudate, and may be heterogeneously hypointense on T1WI and heterogeneously hyperintense on T2WI. Late-stage arachnoiditis may lead to the presence of heterotopic calcifications within the thecal sac, appropriately named *arachnoiditis ossificans* (**Fig. 17**).[99–106]

SUMMARY

Infections of the spine, although rare, may have far-reaching consequences for patients. Early detection and management require astute correlation of the clinical history, physical examination, and imaging features to prevent the potential for significant bony and neurologic complications. This article provides a summary of the imaging features that may be seen in spine infections.

REFERENCES

1. Maiuri F, Laconetta G, Gallicchio B, et al. Spondylodiscitis: clinical and magnetic resonance diagnosis. Spine 1997;22:1741–6.
2. Stefanovski N, Van Voris LP. Pyogenic vertebral osteomyelitis: report of a series of 23 patients. Contemp Orthop 1995;31:159–64.
3. Stabler A, Reiser M. Imaging of spinal infection. Radiol Clin 2001;39(1):115–35.
4. Cahill DW, Love LC, Rechtine GR. Pyogenic osteomyelitis of the spine in the elderly. J Neurosurg 1991;74:878–86.
5. Honan M, White GW, Eisenberg GM. Spontaneous infectious discitis in adults. Am J Med 1996;100:85–9.
6. Elghazawi AK. Clinical syndromes and differential diagnosis of spinal disorders. Radiol Clin North Am 1991;29:651–63.
7. Carragee EJ. The clinical use of magnetic resonance imaging in pyogenic vertebral osteomyelitis. Spine 1997;22:780–5.
8. Bass SN, Ailani RK, Shekar R, et al. Pyogenic vertebral osteomyelitis presenting as exudative pleural effusion: a series of five cases. Chest 1998;114:642–7.

9. Liesker KR, Taconis WK, Plasmans CM. Vertebral osteomyelitis caused by thoracic empyema or vice versa? Eur Respir J 1996;9:2426–8.

10. Hassler O. The human intervertebral disc. Acta Orthop Scand 1970;40:765–72.

11. Hirsch C, Schajkowicz F. Studies on structural changes in the lumbar annulus fibrosus. Acta Orthop Scand 1952;22:184–231.

12. Dullerud R, Nakstad PH. Side effects and complications of automated percutaneous lumber nucleotomy. Neuroradiology 1997;39:282–5.

13. Guyer RD, Ohnmeiss DD, Mason SL, et al. Complications of cervical discography: findings in a large series. J Spinal Disord 1997;10:95–101.

14. Hadjipavlou AG, Mader JT, Necessary JT, et al. Hematogenous pyogenic spinal infections and their surgical management. Spine 2000;25:1668–79.

15. Malawski SK, Lukawski S. Pyogenic infection of the spine. Clin Orthop 1991;272:58–66.

16. Schimmer RC, Jeanneret C, Nunley PD, et al. Osteomyelitis of the cervical spine: a potentially dramatic disease. J Spinal Disord Tech 2002;15:110–7.

17. Spies EH, Stucker R, Reichelt A. Conservative management of pyogenic osteomyelitis of the occipitocervical junction. Spine 1999;24:818–22.

18. Sapico FL, Montgomerie JA. Vertebral osteomyelitis. Infect Dis Clin North Am 1990;4:539–50.

19. Modic MT, Feiglin DH, Piraino DW, et al. Vertebral osteomyelitis: assessment using MR. Radiology 1985;157:157–66.

20. Resnick D, Niwayama G. Osteomyelitis, septic arthritis, and soft tissue infection: axial skeleton. In: Resnick D, editor. Diagnosis of bone and joint disorders. 3rd edition. Philadelphia: WB Saunders; 1995. p. 2419–47.

21. Resnick D. Diagnosis of bone and joint disorders. 3rd edition. Philadelphia: WB Saunders; 1995.

22. Shanley DJ. Tuberculosis of the spine: imaging features. AJR Am J Roentgenol 1995;164:659–64.

23. Villoria MF, Fortea F, Moreno S, et al. MR imaging and CT of central nervous system tuberculosis in the patient with AIDS. Radiol Clin North Am 1995;33:805–20.

24. Al-Mulhim FA, Ibrahim EM, El-Hassan AY, et al. Magnetic resonance imaging of tuberculous spondylitis. Spine 1995;20:2287–92.

25. Ridley N, Shaikh MI, Remedios D, et al. Radiology of skeletal tuberculosis. Orthopedics 1998;21:1213–20.

26. Smith AS, Weinstein MA, Mizushima A, et al. MR imaging characteristics of tuberculous spondylitis vs vertebral osteomyelitis. AJR Am J Roentgenol 1989;153:399–405.

27. Pritchard DJ. Granulomatous infection of bones and joints. Orthop Clin North Am 1975;6:1029–47.

28. Winter WG, Larson RK, Zettas JP, et al. Coccidioidal spondylitis. J Bone Joint Surg Am 1978;60:240–4.

29. Chapman SW. Blastomyces dermatitidis. In: Mandell GL, Bennett JE, Dolin R, editors. Principles and practice of infectious diseases. New York: Churchill Livingstone; 1995. p. 2353–65.

30. Goldman AB, Freiberger RH. Localized infectious and neuropathic diseases. Semin Roentgenol 1979;14:19–32.

31. Friedman BC, Simon GL. Candida vertebral osteomyelitis. Report of three cases and a review of the literature. Diagn Microbiol Infect Dis 1987;8:31–6.

32. Edwards JE. Candida species. In: Mandell GL, Gennett JE, Dolin R, editors. Principles and practice of infectious diseases. New York:: Churchill Livingstone; 1995. p. 2289–306.

33. O'Connell CJ, Cherry AV, Zoll JG. osteomyelitis of cervical spine: candida guilliermondii. Ann Intern Med 1973;79:748.

34. Olson EM, Duberg AC, Herron LD, et al. Coccidioidal spondylitis: MR findings in 15 patients. AJR Am J Roentgenol 1998;171:785–9.

35. Gunecs M, Akdemir H, Tuğcu B, et al. Multiple intradural spinal hydatid disease: a case report and review of the literature. Spine (Phila Pa 1976) 2009;34(9):E346–50.

36. Viljoen H, Crane J. Hydatid disease of the spine. Spine (Phila Pa 1976) 2008;33(22):2479–80.

37. Junker J, Eckardt L, Husstedt I. Cervical intramedullary schistosomiasis as a rare cause of acute tetraparesis. Clin Neurol Neurosurg 2001;103:39–42.

38. Jiang Y, Zhang M, Xiang J. Spinal cord schistosomiasis japonica: a report of 4 cases. Surg Neurol 2008;69:392–7.

39. Garcia A Jr, Gratham SA. Hematogenous pyogenic vertebral osteomyelitis. J Bone Joint Surg Am 1960;42:429.

40. Carragee EJ, Kim D, VanDer Vlugt T, et al. The clinical use of erythrocyte sedimentation rate in pyogenic vertebral osteomyelitis. Spine 1997;15:2089–93.

41. Sapico FL, Montgomerie JA. Pyogenic vertebral osteomyelitis. Report of nine cases and review of literature. Rev Infect Dis 1979;1:754–76.

42. Emery SE, Chan DP, Woodward HR. Treatment of hematogenous pyogenic vertebral osteomyelitis with anterior debridement and primary bone grafting. Spine 1989;14:284–91.

43. Jensen AG, Espersen F, Skinhoj P, et al. Increasing frequency of vertebral osteomyelitis following staphylococcus aureus bacteraemia in Denmark 1980-1990. J Infect 1997;34:113–8.

44. Sapico FL. Microbiology and antimicrobial therapy of spinal infections. Orthop Clin North Am 1996;27:9–13.

45. Bonakdar-pour A, Baines VD. The radiology of osteomyelitis. Orthop Clin North Am 1983;14: 21–37.

46. Hovi I, Lamminen A, Salonen O, et al. MR imaging of the lower spine. Acta Radiol 1994;35:532–40.

47. Ozuna RM, Delamarter RB. Pyogenic vertebral osteomyelitis and postsurgical disc space infections. Orthop Clin North Am 1996;27:87–94.

48. Brant-Zawadzki M, Burke VD, Jeffrey RB. CT in the evaluation of spine infection. Spine 1983;8:358–64.

49. Raininko RK, Aho AJ, Laine MO. Computed tomography in spondylitis: CT versus other radiographic methods. Acta Orthop Scand 1985;56:372–7.

50. McGahan JP, Dublin AB. Evaluation of spinal infections by plain radiographs, computed tomography, intrathecal metrizamide, and CT-guided biopsy. Diagn Imaging Clin Med 1985;54:11–20.

51. Post MJ, Quencer RM, Montalvo BM, et al. Spinal infection: evaluation with MR imaging and intraoperative US. Radiology 1988;169:765–71.

52. Sharif HS. Role of MR imaging in the management of spinal infections. AJR Am J Roentgenol 1992; 158:1333–45.

53. Thrush A, Enzmann D. MR imaging of infections spondylitis. AJNR Am J Neuroradiol 1990;11: 1171–80.

54. Varma R, Lander P, Assaf A. Imaging of pyogenic infectious spondylodiskitis. Radiol Clin North Am 2001;39(2):203–13.

55. Naul LG, Peet GJ, Maupin WB. A vascular necrosis of the vertebral body: MR imaging. Radiology 1989;172:219–22.

56. Aguila LA, Piraino DW, Modic MT, et al. The intranuclear cleft of the intervertebral disc: magnetic resonance imaging. Radiology 1985;155:155–8.

57. Modic MT, Steinberg PM, Ross JS, et al. Degenerative Disk Disease: Assessment of Changes in Vertebral Body Marrow with MR Imaging. Radiology 1988;166(1):193–9.

58. Onofrio BM. Intervertebral discitis: incidence, diagnosis and management. Clin Neurosurg 1980;27: 481–516.

59. Pott P. The chirurgical works of Percivall Pott, F.R.S., surgeon to St. Bartholomew's Hospital, a new edition, with his last corrections, 1808. Clin Orthop Relat Res 2002;(398):4–10.

60. Hlavin ML, Kaminski HJ, Ganz E. Spinal epidural abscess: a ten-year perspective. Neurosurgery 1990;27(2):177–84.

61. Khan SH, Hussain MS, Griebel RW, et al. Comparison of primary and secondary spinal epidural abscesses: a retrospective analysis of 29 cases. Surg Neurol 2003;59:28–33.

62. Browder J, Meyers R. Pyogenic infections of the spinal epidural space: a consideration of the anatomic and physiologic pathology. Surgery 1941;10:296–308.

63. Feldenzer JA, McKeever PE, Schaberg DR, et al. The pathogenesis of spinal epidural abscess: microangiopathic studies in an experimental model. J Neurosurg 1988;69:110–4.

64. Darouiche R. Current concepts: epidural abscess. N Engl J Med 2006;355:2012–20.

65. Darouiche RO. Spinal epidural abscess and subdural empyema. Handb Clin Neurol 2010;96C:91–9.

66. Velissaris DE, Aretha D, Fligou F, et al. Spinal subdural staphylococcus aureus abscess: case report and review of the literature. World J Emerg Surg 2009;4:31.

67. Learch TJ, Sakamoto B, Ling AC, et al. Salmonella spondylodiscitis associated with a mycotic abdominal aortic aneurysm and paravertebral abscess. Emerg Radiol 2009;16(2): 147–50.

68. Chen SH, Lin WC, Lee CH, et al. Spontaneous infective spondylitis and mycotic aneurysm: incidence, risk factors, outcome and management experience. Eur Spine J 2008;17(3):439–44.

69. Dahl T, Lange C, Odegard A, et al. Ruptured abdominal aortic aneurysm secondary to tuberculous spondylitis. Int Angiol 2005;24(1):98–101.

70. Englert C, Aebert H, Lenhart M, et al. Thoracics spondylitis from a mycotic (Streptococcus pneumonia) aortic aneurysm: a case report. Spine (Phila Pa 1976) 2004;29(17):E373–5.

71. Thurnher MM, Post MJ, Jinkins JR. MRI of infections and neoplasms of the spine and spinal cord in 55 patients with AIDS. Neuroradiology 2000; 42(8):551–63.

72. Quencer RM, Post MJ. Spinal cord lesions in patients with AIDS. Neuroimaging Clin N Am 1997;7(2):359–73.

73. Hosaka A, Nakamagoe K, Watanabe M, et al. Magnetic resonance images of herpes zoster myelitis presenting with Brown-Séquard syndrome. Arch Neurol 2010;67(4):506.

74. Portolani M, Pecorari M, Gennari W, et al. Case report: primary infection by human herpes virus 6 variant a with the onset of myelitis. Herpes 2006; 13(3):72–4.

75. Mewasingh LD, Christians FJ, Dachy B, et al. Cervical myelitis from herpes simplex virus type 1 [Erratum appears in: Pediatr Neurol 2004;31(3):234]. Pediatr Neurol 2004;30(1):54–6.

76. Marriage SC, Booy R, Hermione Lyall EG, et al. Cytomegalovirus myelitis in a child infected with human immunodeficiency virus type 1. Pediatr Infect Dis J 1996;15(6):549–51.

77. Petereit HF, Bamborschke S, Lanfermann H. Acute transverse myelitis caused by herpes simplex virus. Eur Neurol 1996;36(1):52–3.

78. Cumming WJ. Myelitis and toxic, inflammatory and infectious disorders. Curr Opin Neurol Neurosurg 1992;5(4):549–53.

79. Lesca G, Deschamps R, Lubetzki C, et al. Acute myelitis in early Borreliaburgdorferi infection. J Neurol 2002;249(10):1472–4.

80. Huisman TA, Wohlrab G, Nadal D, et al. Unusual presentations of Neuroborreliosis (Lyme disease) in childhood. J Comput Assist Tomogr 1999;23(1): 39–42.

81. Puvabanditsin S, Wojdylo EW, Garrow E, et al. Group B streptococcal meningitis: a case of transverse myelitis with spinal cord and posterior fossa cysts. Pediatr Radiol 1997;27(4):317–8.

82. Friess HM, Wasenko JJ. MR of staphylococcal myelitis of the cervical spinal cord. AJNR Am J Neuroradiol 1997;18(3):455–8.

83. Citow JS, Ammirati M. Intramedullary tuberculoma of the spinal cord: case report. Neurosurgery 1994;35:327–30.

84. Cokca F, Meco O, Arasil E, et al. An intramedullary dermoid cyst abscess due to Brucella abortus biotype3 at T11-12 spinal levels. Infection 1994; 22:359–60.

85. King SJ, Jeffree MA. MRI of an abscess of the cervical spinal cord in a case of Listeria meningoencephalomyelitis. Neuroradiology 1993; 35:495–6.

86. Lindner A, Becker G, Warmuth-Metz M, et al. Magnetic resonance image findings of spinal intramedullary abscess caused by candida albicans: case report. Neurosurgery 1995;36: 411–2.

87. Menezes AH, Graf CJ, Perret GE. Spinal cord abscess: a review. Surg Neurol 1977;8:461–7.

88. Morandi X, Mercier P, Fournier HD, et al. Dermal sinus and intramedullary spinal cord abscess. Report of two cases and review of the literature. Childs Nerv Syst 1999;15:202–8.

89. Al Barbarawi M, Khriesat W, Qudsieh S, et al. Management of intramedullary spinal cord abscess: experience with four cases, pathophysiology and outcomes. Eur Spine J 2009;18(5):710–7.

90. Ehara S, Khurana JS, Kattapuram SV. Pyogenic vertebral osteomyelitis of the posterior elements. Skeletal Radiol 1989;18:175–8.

91. Roberts WA. Pyogenic vertebral osteomyelitis of a lumbar facet joint with associated epidural abscess. Spine 1988;13:948–52.

92. Swayne LC, Dorsky S, Caruana V, et al. Septic arthritis of a lumbar facet joint: detection with bone SPECT imaging. J Nucl Med 1989;30:1408–11.

93. Heenan SD, Britton J. Septic arthritis in a lumbar facet joint: a rare cause of an epidural abscess. Neuroradiology 1995;37:462–4.

94. Angtuaco EJ, McConnell JR, Chadduck WM, et al. MR imaging of spinal epidural sepsis. Am J Roentgenol 1987;149:1249–53.

95. Halpin DS, Gibson RD. Septic arthritis of a lumbar facet joint. J Bone Joint Surg 1987;67:457–9.

96. Hickey NA, White PG. Septic arthritis of a lumbar facet joint causing multiple abscesses. Clin Radiol 2000;55(6):481–3.

97. Jinkins JR, Roeder MB. MRI of benign lumbosacral nerve root enhancement. Semin Ultrasound CT MR 1993;14(6):446–54.

98. Alatorre-Fernández CP, Venzor-Castellanos JP, Contreras-Cabrera JA, et al. Arachnoiditis and tuberculous cortical encephalitis in an HIV+ patient. Gac Med Mex 2009;145(3):239–40.

99. Belahsen MF, Maaroufi M, Messouak O, et al. Spinal tuberculous arachnoiditis with intradural extramedullary tuberculomas. J Neuroradiol 2006;33(2): 140–3.

100. Agrawal A, Agrawal A, Agrawal C, et al. An unusual spinal arachnoiditis. Clin Neurol Neurosurg 2006; 108(8):775–9.

101. Sarrazin JL. Imaging of postoperative lumbar spine. J Radiol 2003;84(2):241–50.

102. Ross JS. Magnetic resonance imaging of the postoperative spine. Semin Musculoskelet Radiol 2000; 4(3):281–91.

103. Gundry CR, Fritts HM. Magnetic resonance imaging of the musculoskeletal system. Part 8, The spine, Section 1. Clin Orthop Relat Res 1997;338:275–87.

104. Kumar A, Montanera W, Willinsky R, et al. MR features of tuberculous arachnoiditis. J Comput Assist Tomogr 1993;17(1):127–30.

105. Smith AS, Blaser SI. Infectious and inflammatory processes of the spine. Radiol Clin North Am 1991;29(4):809–27.

106. Chang KH, Han MH, Choi YW, et al. Tuberculous arachnoiditis of the spine: findings on myelography, CT and MR imaging. AJNR Am J Neuroradiol 1989;10(6):1255–62.

Pathologic Basis of Central Nervous System Infections

Paul E. McKeever, MD, PhD

KEYWORDS

- Central nervous system • Infection • Pathology • Biopsy

KEY POINTS

- If an infectious cause is suggested at or before the time of biopsy, the surgeon should be notified to send cultures.
- Radiology provides valuable gross pathologic information about central nervous system (CNS) infections, and major categories of infectious lesions of the brain and spinal cord are recognized by imaging such as diffuse, focal, or multifocal.
- This article further discusses cellular responses to infections including meningitis, encephalitis, gliosis, and demyelination; and histologic features of CNS infections.
- Key features of viral, bacterial, fungal, treponemal, prion, and parasitic diseases are illustrated.

BIOPSIES OF INFECTIOUS DISEASES

If imaging and clinical findings to suggest infectious central nervous system (CNS) disease and cerebrospinal fluid (CSF) are unrevealing, biopsy may be undertaken to search for a definitive diagnosis. Because infections involve CNS and its coverings, the biopsy should (1) include dura, arachnoid, and gray and white matter; and (2) be performed in the site of a recently radiologically enhancing lesion, when feasible.

Microbial Culture

If an infectious cause is suggested at or before the time of biopsy, the surgeon should be notified to send cultures.

Special Stains

A combination of histochemical microbial stains is used in the setting of inflammation to evaluate for organisms and assess for specific cell types. Immunohistochemistry or in situ hybridization may help to identify organisms, particularly *Toxoplasma*, viruses (including Herpes, cytomegalovirus [CMV], and JC viruses), fungi, spirochetes, and rickettsia.[1,2] Available molecular biologic approaches for identification of microorganisms vary among institutions. Some require frozen section, but polymerase chain reaction (PCR) usually can be performed on DNA extracted from paraffin-embedded sections of tissue following deparaffinization steps. Most useful is the ability to detect and classify the strain of mycobacteria in the setting of necrotizing granulomatous inflammation. Detection with in vitro cultures are more sensitive than PCR, but they take longer.

Electron microscopy has a role in the identification of microorganisms that do not grow in culture and are hard to stain, including viruses, Whipple bacillus, and amoebae.

GROSS FEATURES OF CNS INFECTIONS

Radiology provides valuable gross pathologic information about CNS infections. Major categories of infectious lesions of the brain and spinal cord are recognized by imaging such as diffuse, focal, or multifocal. Regardless of category, specimens to culture for suspected microorganisms should be sent in sterile containers directly from

Department of Pathology, University of Michigan Medical Center, Med. Science I Bldg., Rm 4207/Box 5602, 1301 Catherine Road, Ann Arbor, MI 48109-5602, USA
E-mail address: paulmcke@umich.edu

Neuroimag Clin N Am 22 (2012) 773–790
http://dx.doi.org/10.1016/j.nic.2012.06.001
1052-5149/12/$ – see front matter © 2012 Elsevier Inc. All rights reserved.

the operating room to microbiology. The pathologic basis of infectious lesions in these categories is discussed in this article.

One problem is the multifocal lesion. If multifocal lesions are encountered, the surgeon should target a radiographic lesion. In my experience, biopsy of a normal region or a so-called unguided or undirected (blind) biopsy in this setting unnecessarily risks a waste of effort. To optimize the probability of a pathologic diagnosis, the biopsy should be directed at a region of recent radiologic abnormality. If feasible, it should include (1) dura, (2) arachnoid, (3) gray matter, and (4) white matter.

CELLULAR RESPONSES TO INFECTIONS
Polymorphonuclear Leukocytes

Polymorphonuclear (PMN) leukocytes or neutrophils are the first-responder cells to move into the injured CNS (Fig. 1). PMN can be found sticking to vascular endothelium hours after injury, as shown by tissue from long neurosurgical procedures. In less than 24 hours, PMN are found in damaged CNS tissue, such as cerebral infarcts. PMN are particularly attracted to rapidly growing bacteria, bacteria that may directly enter the brain from a penetrating wound, from a bacteremia or shower of septic emboli, or from a meningeal infection. Acute bacterial encephalitis, often called cerebritis, is brain with acute inflammation caused by bacteria. At first, the inflammation is primarily composed of PMN. After 2 days, macrophages enter the inflammation and, later, lymphocytes are evident.

In chronic situations, bacteria are walled off from the CNS, either by the pia (bacterial meningitis), by the arachnoid membrane (dural meningitis), or by fibroblast growth from vessels in CNS tissue (abscess). In the CNS or elsewhere, suppurative bacteria shed chemicals that continue to attract PMN, and PMN continue to ingest and kill bacteria, destroying themselves in the process. The product of this battle is a collection of PMN and their debris called pus.

Macrophages and Microglial Cells

Macrophage means big eater, a name that reflects their common role in phagocytosis, but does not address their role in antigen presentation.[3] Macrophages are the most common cells reacting to most subacute infections, and are often seen in chronic infections. They take 2 or 3 days to find the infection, and remain there long after inflammation and CNS injury have subsided.

There are (1) rod-shaped microglial cells with little cytoplasm and thin nuclei, (2) round macrophages with abundant granular or foamy cytoplasm (gitter cells), and (3) epithelioid macrophages with or without multinucleated giant cells. The pathologic basis of these different forms reflects how much they have eaten and their state of activation. Microglial cells are located in brain tissue, and they are often called resident macrophages. When they took up residence in brain tissue is a matter of debate. Terms that better address what is known about their structure and pathophysiology might be nonphagocytic or prephagocytic macrophages. They are thin because they are not engorged with brain tissue fragments (Fig. 2). Some of them are perivascular, participate in inflammation, present antigens to lymphocytes, and express the marker of activated macrophages, CD163.[3]

Gitter cells are macrophages engorged with tissue fragments (Fig. 3). Their lysosomes are loaded with cellular debris, and may contain fungi,

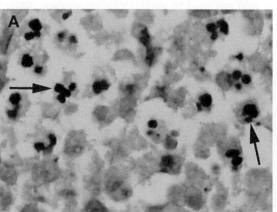
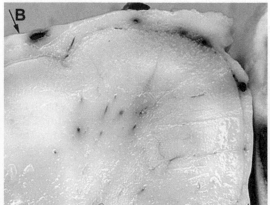

Fig. 1. (A) PMN leukocytes usually have 3 to 5 segments of nuclei per cell (*arrows*) and granular cytoplasm that disintegrates as the cell consumes and kills microbes and tissue. (B) Acute *Streptococcus pneumoniae* bacterial meningitis in a 1-year-old child has filled the space below the arachnoid membrane (*arrow*) with PMN leukocytes. The leptomeningeal vessels are congested.

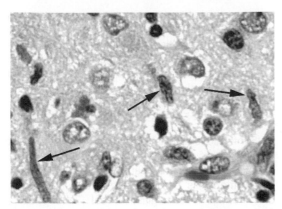

Fig. 2. Microglial cells are thin macrophages with long, thin nuclei (*arrows*). Some microglial cells are residents in the brain but, when they are seen in numbers, they are usually activated macrophages part of an inflammation such as encephalitis.

bacteria, parasites, and other organisms. They are seen in a wide variety of infections that injure CNS tissue.[4,5] The origin of many of these cells is bone marrow via the bloodstream. Blood monocytes enter the brain parenchyma in response to damage.[6] Resident macrophages also participate in phagocytosis, and, if engorged with tissue fragments, they transform into gitter cells.[7] Distinguishing their origins is experimentally possible but not practical.

Epithelioid macrophages are long, wide, and flat cells that superficially resemble squamous epithelial cells. They are seen in granulomas and chronic active inflammation mixed with fibroblasts. Granulomatous inflammation is seen in chronic fungal, treponemal and mycobacterial infectious diseases of the CNS and sarcoid.[8]

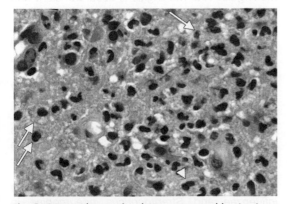

Fig. 3. Macrophages that have consumed brain tissue with or without microorganisms are usually round with bubbly cytoplasm (*arrows*). Most have a single whole nucleus, but they can fuse to end up with more than 1 nucleus (*arrowhead*).

In the CNS and elsewhere, a useful diagnostic immunohistochemical marker for all macrophages is CD68 (KP-1). CD68 frequently identifies considerably more macrophages than anticipated by hematoxylin-eosin (H&E) evaluation. A special stain for myelin, such as, Luxol fast blue-hematoxylin and eosin, identifies engulfed myelin debris. A stain for axons helps to distinguish between CNS necrosis (axons disintegrate and leave axonal debris in macrophages) and demyelination (axons are intact, and foamy macrophages contain only myelin). CNS necrosis occurs in various infections, most prominently in toxoplasmosis. Postinfectious encephalomyelitis and progressive multifocal leukoencephalopathy produce demyelination.

Glial fibrillary acidic protein (GFAP) immunostain is helpful to discern gemistocytic reactive astrocytes from macrophages. Reactive macrophages must be distinguished from the histiocytoses.

Foamy macrophages are common in necrosis and demyelination; macrophages swollen plump by phagocytosis within the CNS are called granular or gitter cells (see **Fig. 3**). Hemosiderin-laden macrophages can be noted around organizing hemorrhages, including mycotic aneurysms and septic emboli. Lipid-laden macrophages can be distinguished from amoebae in amoebic brain abscess by their larger and more distinct nuclei and less chromatin clumping than amoebae, and by their CD68 positivity (discussed later).

Epithelioid macrophages are activated, thin, and nonfoamy macrophages identified in granulomas.

Microglial cells are macrophages that closely resemble antigen-presenting dendritic cells seen elsewhere in the body and play a key role in response to a variety of causal insults.[6,7] They have a spindle-shaped nucleus and no discernible cytoplasm, and must be distinguished from infiltrating glial cells and endothelial cell nuclei. They are CD68 positive. A few microglial cells are scattered diffusely in normal CNS tissue. They increase in infections. Microglial cells are particularly common in viral, spirochetal, and rickettsial diseases, and around dying neurons. In encephalitis, microglial cells accompany small inflammatory aggregates, so-called microglial nodules. When a microglial nodule is accompanied by multinucleated giant cells in brain tissue, human immunodeficiency virus (HIV) encephalitis is a strong possibility.

Giant cell macrophages are produced by the coalescence of macrophages. They are frequently found associated with large material that a single macrophage cannot get around, such as parasites, fungi, and material foreign to the CNS. Nondigestible organisms like mycobacteria and substances like hair also elicit a giant cell macrophage reaction.

Lymphocytes

Lymphocytes are small cells with a dark nucleus and a thin rim of cytoplasm (Fig. 4). Lymphocytes direct the inflammatory response to infections. Cluster designation (CD) immunohistochemical markers distinguish lymphocytes from other cells, and subclassify T-cell and B-cell lymphocytes. Most brain infections elicit more of a cellular than a humoral immune response, and T-cell lymphocytes are often more common in the brain than B-cell lymphocytes and plasma cells.

Gliosis

Gliosis is a reaction of the CNS to any injury, including injury from infection. Gliosis is defined as either (1) increased number of astrocytes, (2) increased number and length of astrocytic processes, or (3) increased cytoplasmic synthesis of GFAP representing a swollen reactive or gemistocytic astrocyte. These 3 features frequently occur in combination. Anti-GFAP immunostain highlights the increased production of GFAP in astrocytes and their cellular processes, which makes gliosis easier to recognize and distinguish from other reactive changes.

Gliosis takes more time to develop than macrophage reaction. In adults, gliosis is usually evident by 2 weeks after an injury. In children, gliosis may be evident earlier. Because nearly any injury of the CNS can cause gliosis, it is not diagnostic of infection, or of any other specific pathologic entity. Subtle astrocytic changes in reaction to injury occur earlier than gliosis, such as astrocyte swelling with fluid.

Gliosis is itself a contracting reaction in the CNS, although this distinction is unclear in infections

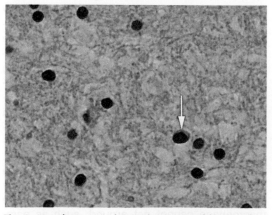

Fig. 4. Lymphocytes in brain tissue resemble oligodendroglial cells. Distinguishing features of lymphocytes include lack of a perinuclear halo seen around oligodendroglia, and a thin rim of cytoplasm around the lymphocyte nucleus (arrow).

that disrupt the blood brain barrier and cause brain swelling.

Gliosis in brain tissue often surrounds an expanding abscess. Excessive fibrillarity and even Rosenthal fibers may occur with gliosis associated with CNS infection.

HISTOLOGIC FEATURES OF CNS INFECTIONS

CNS infections are difficult to classify with respect to the type of disease they cause because some infectious organisms cause several diseases. This difficulty is particularly true of fungi, which can cause meningitis, focal encephalitis, abscesses, and hemorrhage. Variable inflammatory infiltrates are elicited by fungi, most often chronic and granulomatous. Despite such variability, the physician sees the disease first, and must deal with possible infectious agents from that perspective, which creates a need to know the agents most often associated with a specific disease. These agents and associated diseases are discussed below.

Meningitis

The term meningitis literally means inflammation of the meninges. Pachymeningitis means thick meningitis and dural meningitis. Leptomeningitis means inflammation of the thin meninges (ie, inflammation of the leptomeninges: the arachnoid and pial membranes).

Leptomeningitis matures like most inflammatory diseases. Acute inflammation is characterized by neutrophils (see Fig. 1). Subacute and chronic inflammation is characterized by lymphocytes and macrophages.

Most microorganisms, particularly bacteria but also viruses, fungi, and mycobacteria, can cause meningitis. Viral meningitis is usual transient and self-limited. Biopsy specimens are seldom taken. Bacterial and fungal meningitides are serious. Mycobacterial, spirochetal, and some fungal meningitides become granulomatous, relentless, and dangerous.

In neonates, bacterial meningitis is commonly caused by *Escherichia coli*, group B β streptococci, and *Listeria monocytogenes* in neonates. *E coli* is the leading cause, and the k1 antigen is associated with invasive *E coli*. Clinical recognition and prophylaxis has decreased cases of postpartum group B β streptococci.

Meningitis is commonly caused by *Haemophilus influenzae* and *Streptococcus pneumoniae* in children (see Fig. 1). Recent incidence of *S pneumoniae* has been reduced by vaccination. Complications of *H influenzae* include vascular ischemic disease and subdural hygroma.

In young adults and adolescents, *Neisseria meningitidis* causes meningitis. Septicemia precedes the meningitis, and may cause hemorrhages including conspicuous cutaneous petechiae. Perivascular hemorrhage may precede neutrophil reaction and show a ring of hemorrhage around an affected vessel.

In older adults, meningitis is commonly caused by streptococci or staphylococci. *S pneumoniae* used to be common, but its recent incidence has been reduced by vaccination. Properly preserved, it shows a green meningeal exudate.

Cryptococcal meningitis is a common form of fungal meningitis. Cryptococcus has a thick, nonantigenic capsule that delays the inflammatory response to the organism (**Fig. 5**). Mucicarmine stains this capsule of *Cryptococcus*, and helps to identify the organism. As with many organisms, microbiologic culture is best for confirmation and speciation. *Cryptococcus* occurs as an opportunistic infection in immunocompromised patients in whom it may not elicit much inflammation. Depending on variable inflammatory responses, some chronic infections produce granulomatous inflammation.

Granulomatous Meningitis

Granulomatous inflammation is characterized by meningeal thickening (**Fig. 6**). The meninges may be studded with round firm nodules. The nodules are composed of round clusters of lymphocytes, activated epithelioid macrophages, fibroblasts, and collagen (**Fig. 7**). Giant cells formed by the fusion of macrophages are often present (see **Fig. 7**; **Figs. 8** and **9**). Macrophages are abundant and flat. They circle around other constituents producing a multilayered whorled pattern (see **Fig. 9**).

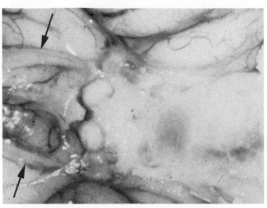

Fig. 6. Base of the brain shows mesial portions of frontal and temporal lobes with arrows pointing at olfactory nerves in the rostral portion of the picture. The leptomeninges are thickened by granulomatous inflammation of chronic meningeal tuberculosis, obscuring the midline structures.

Organisms that cause granulomatous meningitis include bacteria, fungi, and parasites: mycobacteria, *Nocardia*, *Treponema pallidum*, *Aspergillus*, *Candida*, and *Strongyloides stercoralis*. Both Grocott methenamine silver (GMS) and periodic acid Schiff (PAS) should be used on suspected fungi because some forms stain better with one than the other stain.

Atypical mycobacteria and tuberculosis and can involve the CNS or its coverings, principally causing meningitis and meningoencephalitis (**Fig. 10**). Fite and similar stains for acid-fast bacilli (AFB) are useful and rapid when enough organisms are present to find them (**Fig. 11**). Microbial

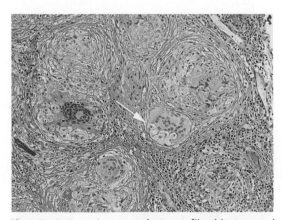

Fig. 7. Activated macrophages, fibroblasts, and collagen form multiple whorls of tissue with lymphocytes predominating between each whorl in this granulomatous inflammation. One of 3 giant cells appears to be growing by coalescing with additional macrophages (*arrow*).

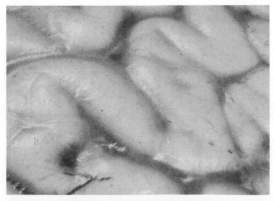

Fig. 5. Leptomeninges over cerebral gyri and sulci show the paucity of inflammation often found with acute cryptococcal meningitis.

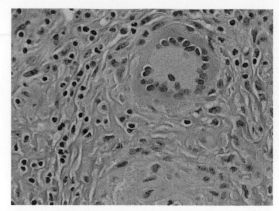

Fig. 8. Langhans giant cell is typically seen in tuberculous meningitis and tuberculomas. However, Langhans giant cells can also be seen in association with other microorganisms and with sarcoidosis.

cultures are more sensitive than AFB stains, but slower. A role for PCR in identifying and speciating mycobacteria has been established.[9] In patients with HIV–acquired immune deficiency syndrome (AIDS), newly acquired tuberculosis can spread and progress rapidly to active disease. In heavily immunodeficient patients, the inflammatory reaction is weak, macrophages are indolent, and there is little or no granulomatous reaction (**Fig. 12**). Tuberculosis may be the first clinical manifestation of immunodeficiency in some patients.

Fungi tend to cause granulomatous meningitis following an acute phase of infection. Yeast forms including *Cryptococcus neoformans*, *Coccidioides immitis*, *Histoplasma*, and, rarely, *Blastomyces* cause meningitis (**Fig. 13**). Hyphal fungi may also

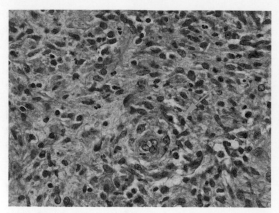

Fig. 10. A patient immunocompromised by anti-inflammatory medications. Epithelioid macrophages cluster around each other forming whorls in this granulomatous meningitis (*arrow*).

cause meningitis, but vascular disease is often more prominent.

Infection of the CNS often spreads via the bloodstream from an initial pulmonary infection, and it can extend directly from a nearby wound, otitis, osteomyelitis, or an infected cranial sinus. Zygomycetes extension from a nasal sinus infection is a particular risk in diabetic patients.[10] As with other organisms, fungal organisms may spread from the subarachnoid space along communicating perivascular spaces to involve parenchyma. Many fungi including *Cryptococcus*, *Aspergillus*, *Zygomycetes*, and *Candida* are more opportunistic than pathogenic, and do not usually infect immune-competent patients. *Histoplasma* and *Blastomyces* are both pathogenic and opportunistic.

Part of understanding fungal infections is knowing their habitats and geographic distribution. The natural habitat of most fungi is the soil,

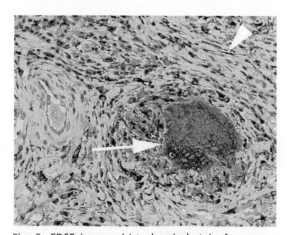

Fig. 9. CD68 immunohistochemical stain for macrophages shows that giant cells in a granuloma are macrophages (*arrow*). Other activated macrophages are elongated (*arrowhead*), and are often are called epithelioid macrophages.

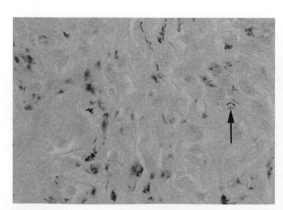

Fig. 11. A patient immunocompromised by anti-inflammatory medications. Fite stain for AFB reveals rosy red rods of mycobacteria (*arrow*).

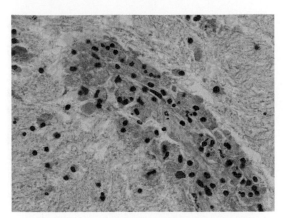

Fig. 12. This patient with HIV-AIDS has perivascular macrophages and lymphocytes. However, there is no granulomatous response to the organism. Mycobacterial brain infection was proved by culture.

so it is easiest to remember that and the exceptions, like *Candida*, that live in the human digestive track. *C neoformans* is worldwide, but cases are most often reported from Australia and the southern United States. *Histoplasma* is common around large rivers of the midwestern United States. *Blastomyces* is common in all of the aforementioned regions of the United States, but it rarely infects the CNS.

Immunodeficiency states including HIV-AIDS have been associated with an increase in syphilis.[11] Syphilis causes a wide variety of diseases, the most frequently encountered now being syphilitic meningitis, which usually manifests as a chronic inflammation with fibrosis and vascular wall thickening. Focal lymphoplasmacytic inflammatory infiltrates are often perivascular. Gummas or syphilitic granulomas may be part of the inflammation. Silver stains for spirochetes do not work well in brain because of background staining, and immunohistochemical stains for *T pallidum* are recommended (Fig. 14).

Encephalitis and Myelitis

The terms encephalitis and myelitis literally mean inflammation of the brain parenchyma and inflammation of the spinal cord parenchyma, respectively.[12] Acute inflammation is characterized by neutrophils and subacute and chronic inflammation characterized by lymphocytes and macrophages. These forms of inflammation can be seen in infectious processes and also in autoimmune inflammatory processes.

Viruses usually cause inflammation of brain tissue that is more diffuse than that caused by larger microorganisms. By convention, this diffuse viral brain inflammation is usually called viral encephalitis or just encephalitis. The brain may show little change (Fig. 15), and thus require careful sampling to find histologic abnormalities. The triad of histologic features of viral encephalitis is perivascular cuffs of inflammation (Fig. 16), microglial nodules (Fig. 17), and neuronophagia (see Fig. 17; Figs. 18 and 19). The presence of all 3 features is strong evidence for a viral encephalitis. If the viral encephalitis is acute, PMN leukocytes (neutrophils) predominate in the inflammatory response. Subacute and chronic encephalitis brings more lymphocytes and macrophages, and eventually substantial gliosis.

Perivascular cuffs of inflammation are composed of macrophages and T-cell and B-cell lymphocytes, usually in that order of abundance. Perivascular cuffs are not specific indicators of viral inflammation. They can be seen in bacterial (see Fig. 12), fungal, and parasitic diseases. The

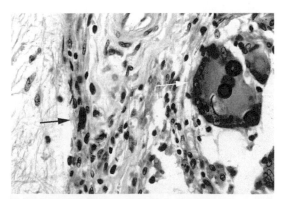

Fig. 13. Fungal spherules with diameters between 20 and 35 μm have been engulfed by a giant cell macrophage (*white arrow*) in this granulomatous meningitis (*black arrow*). *C immitis* stained with cresyl violet and eosin.

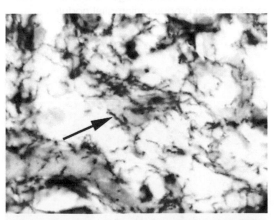

Fig. 14. Immunohistochemical stain for *T pallidum* shows numerous long microorganisms with a dotted or undulated appearance to their true spiral structure (*arrow*).

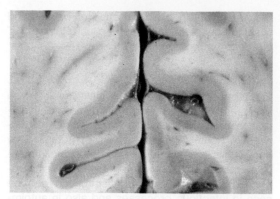

Fig. 15. Prominent gray patches present in gray and white matter are better seen in white matter where they stand out against the white myelin. Some gray patches surround vessels and represent perivascular lymphocytes. There is arbovirus infection in parietal hemispheres flanking the midline.

perivascular cuffs of most viruses do not produce classic vasculitis, exceptions being the herpesviruses, particularly Herpes simplex and Herpes zoster (Fig. 20). Necrosis or hemorrhage may result from this vasculitis (Fig. 21).

Seen in nonischemic neurons along with perivascular cuffs or microglial nodules, neuronophagia confirms encephalitis with few exceptions. Neuronophagia alone may simply reflect selective vulnerability of neurons to a toxic, metabolic, or other disease that targets neurons. The most common of these is ischemia. Lack of red, dead ischemic neurons and single-cell or patchy destruction of neurons favors encephalitis (see Figs. 17–19).

Microglial nodules strongly suggest encephalitis. However, in isolation, they do not necessarily indicate viral disease or a disease that targets neurons. Other infectious agents and autoimmune reactions can produce microglial nodules.

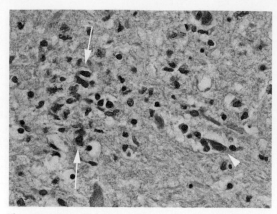

Fig. 17. Microglial nodule (*arrows*) and neuronophagia (*arrowhead*) in the same viral encephalitis as shown in Fig. 16.

Enterovirus infections (eg, coxsackievirus, echovirus) cause between 60% and 90% of cases of acute viral meningitis and meningoencephalitis, and arbovirus infections (eg, eastern equine, St Louis, West Nile) comprise many of the remaining cases.[13] These are without any characteristic light microscopic inclusion. A variety of specific tests for such viruses may be found at reference laboratories or the Center for Disease Control (http://www.cdc.gov).

Because viruses can diffusely involve the brain with variable regional severity, seasonal epidemics and serologies often provide better clues than signs and symptoms about the type of viral disease. West Nile virus is an example of an arbovirus, none of which have signs, symptoms, or pathology that are unique. From mosquito vectors and bird hosts, West Nile virus has infected people.[14] Transmission by blood transfusion and organ transplantation can also occur. Up to 80%

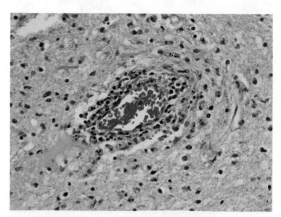

Fig. 16. Perivascular cuff of inflammation in viral encephalitis.

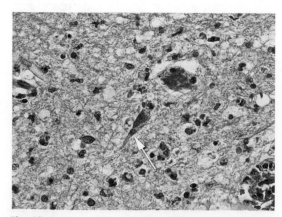

Fig. 18. Neuronophagia in the same viral encephalitis as shown in Fig. 16. A macrophage has crawled inside this neuron to consume it from within (*arrow*).

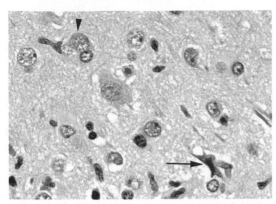

Fig. 19. Neuronophagia in viral encephalitis. Note that the shrunken neuron found by microglia has not lost its purple Nissl substance (*arrow*). Another neuron (*arrowhead*) is touched by a microglial cell with an oddly shaped nucleus.

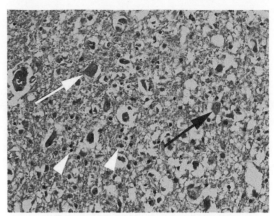

Fig. 21. Tissue edema and neuronal necrosis (*arrows*) may be more prominent than the usual features of perivascular inflammation and microglial nodules in Herpes simplex type 1 infections. Excess lymphocytes and macrophages (*arrowheads*) can be seen in the edematous brain tissue.

of infected people have no symptoms. In others, systemic symptoms are variable and nonspecific, including fever, myalgia, lymphadenopathy, and rash. Neurologic symptoms include headache, encephalopathy, and diffuse weakness or acute flaccid paralysis.[14–16] Fatalities occur principally in the immunosuppressed, diabetic, and elderly with underlying systemic diseases.

Findings include a patchy meningitis, encephalitis, and sometimes polio-like myelitis with variable but, in some cases, severe encephalitis of the substantia nigra, medulla, and cerebellum. Perivascular inflammation, microglial nodules, and neuronophagia can be seen.[15,16] Anterior horn cells are targeted in some patients but not others.[15] Laboratory diagnosis of arboviruses is based predominantly on serology.[17] Additional information on this and other arboviruses is available

from the Arbovirus Diagnostic Laboratory, DRA, CDC/DVBID/ADB, 3150 Rampart Road, Fort Collins, C0 80521; phone: 970-221-6445.

Some viruses produce pink-purple inclusions that can be identified on H&E stain. Many can be identified specifically with immunostains. Neuronal inclusion bodies are in nuclei with most herpesvirus infections and subacute sclerosing panencephalitis (SSPE) of measles (**Fig. 22**). Neuronal inclusions are in the cytoplasm in rabies (**Fig. 23**). Oligodendrocyte nuclear inclusions are seen in progressive multifocal leukoencephalopathy (PML) and SSPE. CMV induces cellular gigantism and inclusions in the nucleus and cytoplasm of endothelial cells, ependymal cells, and glial cells (**Fig. 24**). Many viruses do not manifest inclusions,

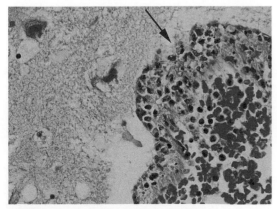

Fig. 20. Necrotizing vasculitis is evident in the empty spaces and inflammatory cells in the vessel wall where collagen and elongated vascular cells are normally located (*arrow*).

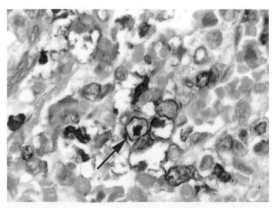

Fig. 22. Cowdry type A nuclear inclusions are seen with immunohistochemical stain for *Herpes simplex* type 1 (*arrow*).

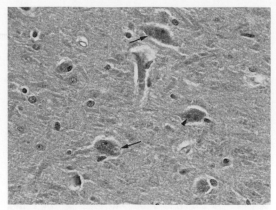

Fig. 23. Negri bodies are round pink inclusions surrounded by clear haloes (*arrows*). Lyssa bodies are less rounded and less clearly defined (*arrowhead*). Both bodies contain particles and debris from the rhabdovirus that causes rabies.

including HIV, poliovirus, and arboviruses including West Nile virus.

Herpes simplex virus (HSV) is the most common cause of nonepidemic encephalitis. Unlike most viruses, HSV encephalitis is usually localized to the temporal and frontal lobes. This distribution may be caused by retrograde viral transmission from cold sores back along peripheral nerves to these parts of the brain. The diagnosis of HSV can be made by biopsy, CSF culture, serology, or PCR evaluation. Perivascular inflammation, composed predominantly of lymphocytes mixed with macrophages, is accompanied by varying degrees of necrosis and hemorrhage. The extent of necrosis and hemorrhage is often profound (see **Fig. 21**). Inclusion bodies can be identified as HSV by in situ hybridization and immunostaining

(see **Fig. 22**). These techniques and PCR are useful in diagnosis of most herpesviruses.

CMV infection in an adult usually represents reactivation of dormant disease.[18,19] Histologic findings vary from cells with typical CMV inclusions and with virtually no associated inflammation to severe necrotizing ependymitis and meningoencephalitis.

Herpesviruses can cause a severe spinal cord inflammation called transverse myelitis, which presents with symptoms that can involve sensory, motor, and autonomic modalities of variable severity.[20]

HIV-1 causes a primary encephalitis that is often manifest as a subacute dementia. Multinucleated giant cells in brain tissue with microglial nodules characterize HIV encephalitis (**Fig. 25**). By immunohistochemistry, the giant cells can contain abundant HIV markers including p23. Neurons and synapses are eventually lost, the blood brain barrier functions poorly, the brain atrophies, and ventricles enlarge. HIV encephalitis is sometimes accompanied by a leukoencephalopathy, vacuolar myelopathy, or lymphocytic meningitis.[21]

Diffuse white matter damage with loss of myelin, gliosis, multinucleated cells, and macrophage infiltrates with few lymphocytes indicate HIV leukoencephalopathy. Highly active antiretroviral therapy (HAART) has changed the presentation of HIV-related CNS diseases, including HIV leukoencephalopathy. Following HAART therapy, the leukoencephalopathy can become more severe, and perivascular macrophage and lymphocyte infiltrates can increase, which may be a response of the revived immune system.[22] HAART therapy has decreased the incidence of primary HIV encephalitis.

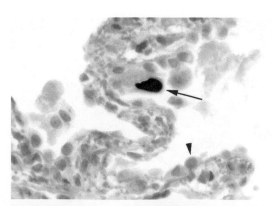

Fig. 24. CMV causes enlargement of cell and nucleus. Immunohistochemical stain for CMV shows huge nucleus positive for viral proteins (*arrow*). Compare with uninfected cell (*arrowhead*).

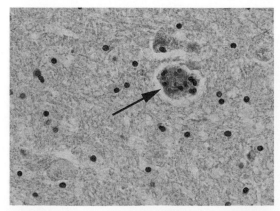

Fig. 25. In the context of encephalitis, a multinucleated giant cell within brain tissue and unaccompanied by a granuloma (*arrow*) is characteristic of HIV encephalitis.

Lymphocytic meningitis of HIV infection causes heavy lymphocytic infiltrates within the leptomeninges and contiguous perivascular spaces. Lymphocytic or multinucleated giant cell infiltration of cerebral vessel walls with necrosis occurs in HIV vasculitis, which is sometimes granulomatous.

The immunocompromised patient is particularly susceptible to CNS infection.[23] Secondary infections are caused by opportunistic organisms that infect the immunodeficient patient with HIV. These organisms include *Toxoplasma*, JC and related viruses, CMV, varicella-zoster virus, *C neoformans*, mycobacteria, and *T pallidum*. These organisms are described with the most common infection that they produce, for example *Toxoplasma* with abscesses, JC virus with PML, *Cryptococcus* with meningitis, and mycobacteria and *T pallidum* with granulomatous meningitis. HAART has decreased the incidence of some secondary diseases. However, PML has not been clearly reduced.[22]

PML is the result of activation in the brain of the papovavirus called JC virus after the patient's initials. The disease is typically seen in the setting of severe immunodeficiency like AIDS, or immunosuppression treatment of lymphoma, organ transplant, and collagen vascular diseases.[24]

PML shows multiple discrete but coalescing foci of demyelination, like puffy clouds in the sky (**Fig. 26**).It may simulate multiple sclerosis or a mass on radiography. Brain biopsy frequently shows an active to subacute process with abundant foamy macrophages, many of which contain myelin. There is often marked gliosis with many astrocytes manifesting bizarre nuclei that can be confused with glioma (**Fig. 27**). Oligodendrocytes have glassy pink-purple nuclear inclusions that enlarge the nucleus and marginate the chromatin. Perivascular infiltrates of mature lymphocytes may occur. Bizarre astrocytes are less frequent, and perivascular inflammatory cells more frequent, in many patients with AIDS. Diagnosis of PML can be confirmed by

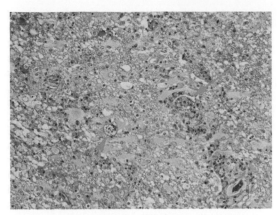

Fig. 27. Perivascular cuffs of lymphocytes and macrophages (*arrow*) within a background busy with reactive macrophages stripping myelin from nerve fibers. An unusual astrocyte has a huge nucleus the size of a small vessel (*arrowhead*).

immunohistochemistry, in situ hybridization, or electron microscopy (**Fig. 28**).[18,23,25]

Subacute sclerosing panencephalitis (SSPE) is a slowly progressive disease, with a high incidence in South America, Asia, and the Middle East. It tends to occur in incompletely vaccinated children. SSPE is caused by an abnormal host-virus interaction that produces persistent infection of the CNS by immune-resistant measles virus. Brain biopsy is rarely performed because antimeasles antibodies, both immunoglobulin (Ig) G and IgM can be found in CSF or serum. Viral encephalitis predominates in gray and white matter with loss of myelin white matter.[18] Nuclear inclusions resembling Cowdry A bodies occur in neurons and oligodendroglial cells.

Acute bacterial, fungal, and parasitic infections that are not sufficiently encapsulated to be an abscess[12,18] cause focal encephalitis in brain

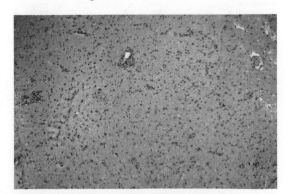

Fig. 26. In cerebral white matter stained blue with Luxol fast blue, pale clouds of demyelination (*arrowhead*) occur in PML.

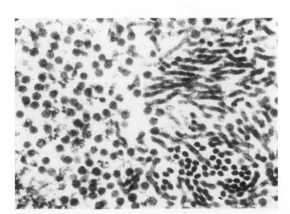

Fig. 28. Viral particles in the nucleus of an oligodendroglial cell show 2 forms: long, round filaments and spheres of slightly larger diameter.

and focal myelitis in spinal cord. In brain, the focal encephalitis is often called cerebritis, but its single characteristic feature, distinguishing it from most viral encephalitis, is its focal nature rather than its frequent cerebral location. This feature probably reflects restricted movement of bacteria, fungi, and larger organisms through brain tissue. Its inflammatory infiltrate is composed of neutrophils, macrophages, lymphocytes, and plasma cells, with or without parenchymal necrosis. Meningitis may precede focal encephalitis. Either fungi or bacteria, commonly originating from an infected heart valve or lung, can produce septic emboli that move to the CNS to cause focal encephalitis and eventually an abscess.

Focal bacterial encephalitis is usually caused by streptococci, staphylococci, or filamentous bacteria (Fig. 29). However, it can also be caused by gram-negative organisms, such as E coli, Pseudomonas, or H influenzae.

Whipple disease causes a subacute to chronic focal encephalitis. The causative bacillus is Tropheryma whippelii. It rarely presents as a primary brain disease, and, even then, usually with concomitant gastrointestinal symptoms. PAS-positive, diastase-resistant bacilli in macrophages are a characteristic feature (Fig. 30). Perivascular lymphocytes, microglial nodules, and reactive microglia can be found. Lesions have a predilection to involve gray matter. Biopsy of the central cingulate gyrus, mediobasal temporal region, and insular cortex may show lesions.

Amoebae can produce severe subacute meningoencephalitis, particularly Naegleria fowleri. Acanthamoeba, Sappinia diploidea, and

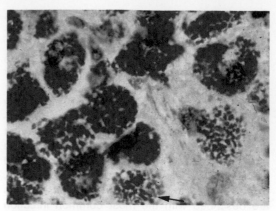

Fig. 30. PAS stain highlights Whipple bacilli (arrow) in macrophages.

Balamuthia are seen mostly in the setting of immunocompromise. They produce a more chronic, granulomatous encephalitis.[26,27] The organisms contain a nucleus, some with a distinct karyosome and chromatin clumping, and they have vacuolated cytoplasm. They may contain ingested red cells. Macrophages can be distinguished from amoebae by the larger and more distinct nuclei and higher nuclear/cytoplasmic ratio in the macrophages (Fig. 31).

Abscess

An abscess can arise from hematogenous spread of organisms from lung or other organs, or can come from infected coverings of the CNS, including meningitis, osteomyelitis, sinusitis, or otitis. Local trauma may be associated with infections that seed an abscess.

Abscesses are typically focal or multifocal. They are preceded by acute and sometimes unnoticed focal encephalitis (cerebritis). Abscesses are often

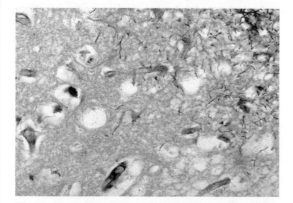

Fig. 29. Nocardia growing in the brain causing bubbly edema. Nocardia is an elongated bacterium that stains with GMS stain (arrow) as if it were a fungus. Most silver stains, including GMS, are not specific for the structures they are known to stain, and must be interpreted by a trained eye. For example, the structure that vaguely resembles a hypha is a capillary (arrowhead) in the brain.

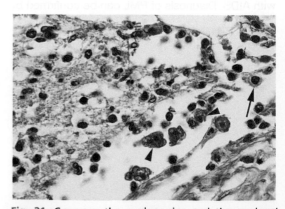

Fig. 31. Compare the nuclear size and the nuclear/cytoplasmic ratio of the macrophage (arrow) with that of amoeba (arrowheads). Amoebic encephalitis.

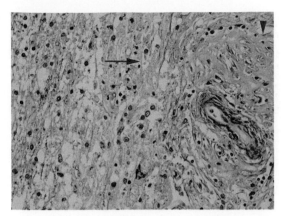

Fig. 32. The blue strands (*arrow*) are collagen made by fibroblasts from hypertrophied vessel walls (*arrowhead*). Trichrome stains collagen blue, and cells and CNS tissue stain light red and gray.

caused by suppurative bacteria or fungi. They take weeks to fully mature, and combine features of inflammation, gliosis, and fibrosis. A mixture of PMN leukocytes, lymphocytes, macrophages, and plasma cells on H&E-stained sections confirms inflammation. Polymorphism of inflammatory components can be verified by finding mixed B-cell and T-cell lymphocytes admixed with CD68-positive macrophages.

The wall of a CNS abscess consists of collagen (Fig. 32), and is surrounded by reactive gliosis. The collagen layer is formed by fibroblasts that migrate out from the surrounding blood vessels. Thus, the thickness of this layer varies depending on the number of viable vessels and their distance from the abscess as well as on the age of the abscess. Because collagen formation is a rare pathologic reaction within the CNS, its presence is an important diagnostic feature of an abscess. Collagen

may be difficult to distinguish from fibrillary gliosis on a slide stained with H&E. Points to remember are the extracellular and often wavy appearance of collagen compared with the intracellular fibrillar character of gliosis. Collagen polarizes yellow-white on sections stained with H&E or Congo red, although gliosis does not. If there is any doubt, it is best to stain histochemically for collagen with trichrome stain or for reticulin with silver stain, or to stain immunohistochemically for collagen type IV.

Bacterial abscess is usually caused by *Streptococcus mileri*, *Bacteroides*, *Nocardia*, actinomycosis, or *Staphylococcus aureus*. Nocardial abscesses of the cerebrum and the spinal cord are increasing in frequency in drug addicts and transplant recipients (Fig. 33). Multiple microabscesses should be considered in the differential diagnosis of encephalopathy in hospitalized patients with chronic disease, immunosuppression, and sepsis.[26]

Toxoplasma gondii causes abscesses with a thin wall and more necrotic brain tissue than pus (Fig. 34A). The associated inflammation varies from mild to severe depending on the host's ability to respond (Figs. 34B–D). Substantial host response can initially produce a necrotizing encephalomyelitis, followed by a granulomatous reaction. Toxoplasmosis is a frequent opportunistic infection in AIDS and other immunosuppressed patients in whom the immune response can be weak. Regardless of response, the abscess always contains macrophages. *T gondii* is present worldwide, and is found in cat feces. Thin-walled cysts are filled with bradyzoites that literally mean slow little animal (Fig. 34E). They contain dark staining dotlike structures representing nuclei. Individual tachyzoites that mean fast little animals are scattered in tissue and in macrophages. Slow and fast terms refer to their

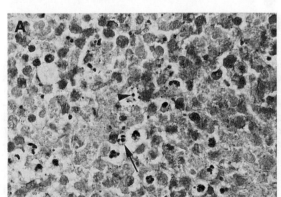

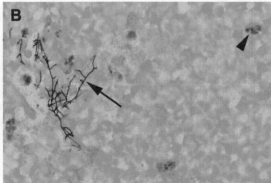

Fig. 33. (*A*, *B*) A frontal lobe biopsy of a patient with a renal transplant a year and a half earlier. (*A*) Central portion of a brain abscess shows purulent material (pus) composed of scattered PMN leukocytes (*arrow*), degenerating PMN (*arrowhead*), and necrotic debris. The small dark dots (*arrowhead*) are remnants of PMN nuclei. Their size is not uniform enough to be bacteria. (*B*) GMS stain shows branching *Nocardia* (*arrow*). The GMS stain is lightly staining (*arrowhead*) 1 of many PMN leukocytes.

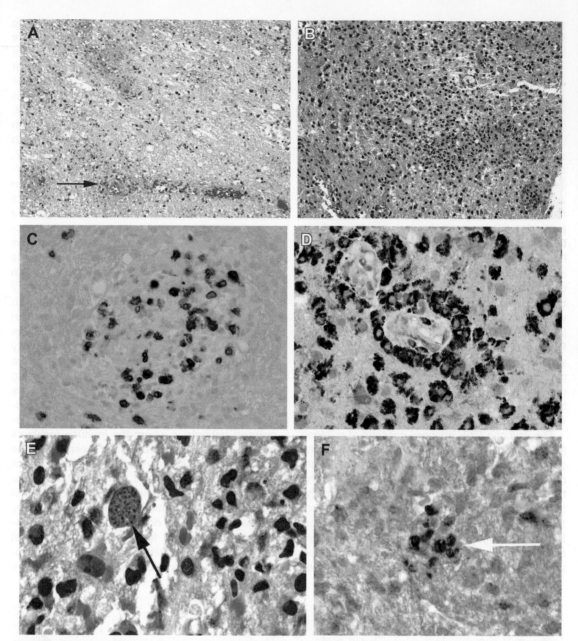

Fig. 34. A 70-year-old heart transplant recipient. (*A*) Preoperative differential was lymphoma, glioma, or infection. A typical lesion of *Toxoplasma* in an immunosuppressed patient is mostly necrotic. Within the necrosis may be remnants of perivascular inflammation (*arrow*). (*B*) A viable region of brain shows chronic active inflammation with neutrophils, macrophages, and lymphocytes. (*C*) Immunohistochemistry for CD3 shows abundant perivascular T-cell lymphocytes. B-cell lymphocytes were rare. (*D*) Immunohistochemistry for CD68 shows abundant parenchymal and perivascular macrophages. (*E*) Cyst (*arrow*) filled with many bradyzoites each with its own purple nucleus is from *T gondii* infecting the heart transplant recipient. (*F*) A cluster of tachyzoites stained brown with an immunohistochemical anti-*Toxoplasma* antibody (*arrow*).

replication and motility. Immunostaining pinpoints the individual organism (**Fig. 34**F), which is not easily done on routine H&E sections.

Toxoplasma infects many more people than it kills. Toxoplasmosis in an adult likely represents a reactivation of dormant parasites introduced by previous exposure. Clinical differentiation between toxoplasmosis and lymphoma can be difficult, sometimes requiring biopsy for diagnosis.

In perinatal infections, *Toxoplasma* is the T in the TORCH complex of organisms (*Toxoplasma*, other infections, rubella, CMV, and HSV). Other infections include hepatitis B, coxsackievirus, syphilis, varicella-zoster virus, HIV, and parvovirus B19. *Toxoplasma* damages periventricular tissues, and causes small and large regions of necrosis associated with vascular thromboses. Parenchymal calcifications and meningitis may occur.

Various cysts resemble abscesses within the CNS. They have highly variable inflammatory components. These components include parasitic cysts, and cysts that have exuded material foreign to the CNS, such as colloid or squamous epithelial cells. Neurocysticercosis are parasitic cysts that contain the larval form (*Cysticercus cellulosae*) of the pig tapeworm (*Taenia solium*). Neurocysticercosis is a common parasitic infection of the CNS.[28] Specimens with live larvae are tan, firm, nodules containing a cystic cavity with the larva, and surrounded by a thin cyst wall. The characteristic invaginated scolex may be seen (**Fig. 35**A). Hooklets are seen best with special stains (see

Fig. 35B). Pale eosinophilic membranes (see **Fig. 35**C) separate the cavity from gliotic brain parenchyma with little chronic perivascular inflammation. If the larva dies, the cavity contains grumous gray-yellow material that stimulates inflammation and a foreign body giant cell reaction. The tissue reaction to dead larvae more closely resembles a CNS tissue granuloma than an abscess.

Granulomas in CNS Tissue

Organisms that invade CNS parenchyma and grow slowly and relentlessly, or die and release foreign material, tend to produce granulomas in CNS tissue. Parasites, particularly their ova (see **Fig. 35**D) or disintegrating larvae, can cause granulomas. Schistosomiasis ova in the CNS elicit an intense, granulomatous inflammatory response.

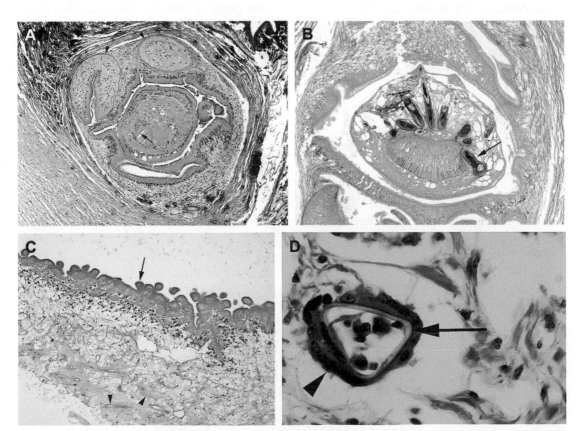

Fig. 35. (*A*) Scolex of cysticercus shows hooklet (*arrow*) in a rostellum, and 2 muscular suckers (*arrowheads*). Hooklets can be hard to see on H&E, but they are revealed by tears in the softer surrounding tissue. (*B*) Hooklets in the rostellum stain well with methenamine silver (*arrow*). (*C*) Wall of cysticercus has a clumped outer cuticle (*arrow*). The inner wall contains canaliculi (*arrowheads*). (*D*) Triangular 60-μm-wide egg and its natural light brown shell (*arrow*) came from a parasitic fluke or trematode. A multinucleated giant cell composed of coalescent macrophages surrounds the egg (*arrowhead*), a cellular reaction called a foreign body giant cell reaction. The macrophages would do the same around a surgical suture.

Syphilitic granulomas in CNS are called gummas. They are rare and more fibrous than tuberculomas.

Hemorrhage and Thrombosis

Intravascular organisms can cause hemorrhage or thrombosis, which is particularly common among fungi that grow hyphae or pseudohyphae in patient hosts, such as *Aspergillus*, zygomycetes (*Mucor*, Rhizopus, Rhizomucor), *Pseudallescheria*, *Fusarium*, *Candida*, and *Coccidioides*. These fungi grow in vessel walls (**Fig. 36**). They can either weaken the wall, causing a mycotic aneurysm; perforate the vessel, causing a hemorrhage; or irritate the vascular lining, causing local thrombosis. The CNS does not respond well to any of these events.

Syphilis causes thickening of vessels and an endarteritis that narrows or occludes vascular lumens. Heubner named this endarteritis obliterans. Fibroblasts and collagen thicken the vascular intima. Although rare, syphilitic arteritis can cause aneurysms and vascular bleeding.

Tuberculosis can cause arterial inflammation and thickening of the vascular intima. This is one explanation for the caseating necrosis found in tuberculous granulomas, although the wax coat of *Mycobacterium* may also contribute to caseation. Other vascular occlusions tend to cause more coagulation and less cheesy caseation.

Infections Without Inflammation

Prions are the only known agent of infection that do not cause inflammation. Prion is a term derived from proteinaceous infectious particle. The counterpart of the pathogenic prion protein is a normal constituent of cells that is probably important to animals because a wide variety of them has been conserved.[29] When an abnormal tertiary structure is present in this protein, it becomes resistant to normal protein degradation and has the capacity to convert the tertiary structure of its normal counterpart to the pathogenic conformation. As this cycle continues, an increasing percentage of normal protein is converted into the pathogenic prion configuration. A rapid dementia from onset to death ensues, and death is certain.

The group of prion diseases that affect people include kuru, the disease that led to the discovery of a transmissible spongiform encephalopathy, and eventually the whole group of prion diseases. Kuru, or laughing disease, was passed from

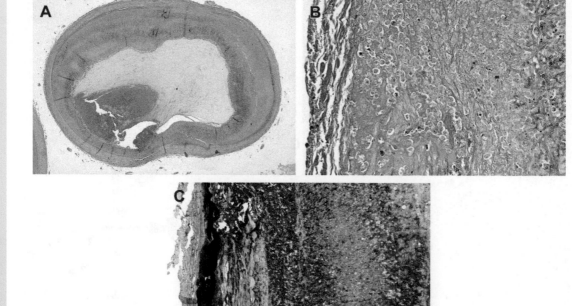

Fig. 36. From the autopsy of an immunodeficient patient. (*A*) Hyphae of *Aspergillus* are growing in the wall of this cerebral artery, eccentrically thickening its wall. (*B*) In this closer view of the cerebral artery, septate hyphae (*arrows*) branch within its necrotic wall. (*C*) Substantial IgM has accumulated in the vessel wall. The deposition of IgM alone does not prove the IgM is targeting the organism. It could simply reflect trapping of large IgM molecules as they leak from plasma through the necrotic vascular wall.

person to person by ceremonial eating of human tissue of dead relatives. Those who ate their relative's CNS tissue were infected first. The most common form of prion disease in patients is Creutzfeldt-Jacob disease (CJD). By its initial transmission to primates, CJD prions have been shown to be infectious agents.[29] Since then, the prion has infected patients receiving growth hormone derived from pooled cadaver pituitaries, contaminated transplanted tissue, and patients exposed to contaminated surgical equipment.[18] Bovine spongiform encephalopathy (BSE) arose in cows fed prion-infected sheep tissue including scrapie-containing brain as cattle feed. BSE spread to a few people in Europe, and is called variant CJD (vCJD). Familial prion diseases include Gerstmann-Sträussler-Scheinker, familial CJD, and fatal familial insomnia. They are caused by germline mutations.

Histologic changes that show evidence of prion disease include a combination of neuropil vacuolation and gliosis (Fig. 37).[30] In cerebrum, vacuolation of the neuropil should not just involve superficial cortical layers that are often vacuolated because of vascular insufficiency or artifact. Vacuolation is more convincing of prion disease if a few vacuoles in the neuropil are lightly eosinophilic rather than clear stained with H&E. Reactive gliosis is abundant in late stages of the prion disease. Perivascular inflammatory infiltrates are not a feature of prion disease.

The histologic appearance of vCJD differs from sporadic CJD by showing stellate plaques composed of prion protein. These plaques can been seen on slides stained with H&E or PAS. Vacuoles of vCJD are more coarse than vacuolation of CJD.

Immunohistochemistry (IHC) after protease predigestion helps to identify protease-resistant prion proteins. The best confirmation of prion disease comes from molecular evaluation for the protease digestion–resistant prion protein by Western blot.[31] This evaluation is performed in a few specialized medical centers and at the National Prion Disease Pathology Surveillance Center in Cleveland, Ohio.

REFERENCES

1. Thomson RB Jr, Bertram H. Laboratory diagnosis of central nervous system infections. Infect Dis Clin North Am 2001;15:1047–71.
2. McKeever PE. Immunohistochemistry of the nervous system. In: Dabbs DJ, editor. Diagnostic immunohistochemistry. 3rd edition. Philadelphia: Churchill Livingstone; 2010. p. 820–89.
3. Fabriek BO, Van Haastert ES, Galea I, et al. CD163-positive perivascular macrophages in the human CNS express molecules for antigen recognition and presentation. Glia 2005;51:297–305.
4. Belluco S, Thibaud JL, Guillot J, et al. Spinal cryptococcoma in an immunocompetent cat. J Comp Pathol 2008;139(4):246–51.
5. Rissi DR, Pierezan F, de Silva MS, et al. Neurological disease in cattle in southern Brazil associated with bovine herpesvirus infection. J Vet Diagn Invest 2008;20(3):346–9.
6. Kreutzberg GW. Microglia: a sensor for pathological events in the CNS. Trends Neurosci 1996;19:312–8.
7. McKeever PE, Balentine JD. Macrophage migration through the brain parenchyma to the perivascular space following particle ingestion. Am J Pathol 1978;93:153–64.
8. McKeever PE. The brain, spinal cord, and meninges. In: Mills SE, Carter D, Greenson JK, et al, editors. Sternberg's diagnostic surgical pathology. 5th edition. Philadelphia: Lippincott; 2010. p. 351–448.
9. Park do Y, Kim JY, Choi KU, et al. Comparison of polymerase chain reaction with histopathologic features for diagnosis of tuberculosis in formalin-fixed, paraffin-embedded histologic specimens. Arch Pathol Lab Med 2000;127:326–30.
10. Frater JL, Hall GS, Procop GW. Histologic features of zygomycosis: emphasis on perineural invasion and fungal morphology. Arch Pathol Lab Med 2001;125:375–8.
11. Johnson PC, Farnie MA. Testing for syphilis. Dermatol Clin 1994;12:9–17.
12. Falcone S, Post MJ. Encephalitis, cerebritis, and brain abscess: pathophysiology and imaging findings. Neuroimaging Clin North Am 2000;10:333–53.

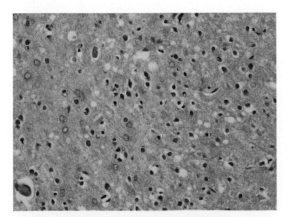

Fig. 37. Cerebral cortex shows spongiform encephalopathy with coalescing vacuoles and gliosis in this case of CJD. There is substantial loss of neurons.

13. Cassady KA, Whitley RJ. Pathogenesis and patho-physiology of viral infections of the central nervous system. In: Scheld WM, Whitley RJ, Durack DT, editors. Infections of the central nervous system. 2nd edition. Philadelphia: Lippincott-Raven; 1997. p. 7–22.

14. Campbell GL, Marfin AA, Lanciotti RS, et al. West Nile virus. Lancet Infect Dis 2002;2:519–29.

15. Leis AA, Fratkin J, Stokic DS, et al. West Nile polio-myelitis. Lancet Infect Dis 2003;3:9–10.

16. Sampson BA, Ambrosi C, Charlot A, et al. The pathology of human West Nile Virus infection. Hum Pathol 2000;31:527–31.

17. Batalis NI, Galup L, Zaki SR, et al. West Nile virus encephalitis. Am J Forensic Med Pathol 2005;26: 192–6.

18. Love SL, Louis DN, Ellison DW. Greenfield's Neuro-pathology. 8th edition. New York: Hodder; 2008.

19. Maschke M, Kastrup O, Diener HC. CNS manifesta-tions of cytomegalovirus infections: diagnosis and treatment. CNS Drugs 2002;16:303–15.

20. Jacob A, Weinshenker BG. An approach to the diag-nosis of acute transverse myelitis. Semin Neurol 2008;28:105–20.

21. Vago L, Bonetto S, Nebuloni M, et al. Pathological findings in the central nervous system of AIDS patients on assumed antiretroviral therapeutic regi-mens: retrospective study of 1597 autopsies. AIDS 2002;16:1925–8.

22. Gray F, Chretien F, Vallat-DeCouvelaere AV, et al. The changing pattern of HIV neuropathology in the HAART era. J Neuropathol Exp Neurol 2003;62:429–40.

23. Burger PC, Scheithauer BW, Vogel FS. Surgical pathology of the nervous system and its coverings. 4th edition. New York: Churchill Livingstone; 2002.

24. McKeever PE, Chronwall BM, Houff SA, et al. Glial and divergent cells in primate central nervous system tumors induced by JC virus isolated from human PML. In: Sever JL, Madden DL, editors. Poly-oma virus and Human Neurological Disease. Prog. Clin. Biol. Res. 1983;105:359–67.

25. Ironside JW, Lewis FA, Blythe D, et al. The identifica-tion of cells containing JC papovavirus DNA in progressive multifocal leukoencephalopathy by combined in situ hybridization and immunocyto-chemistry. J Pathol 1989;157:291–7.

26. Martinez AJ, Visvesvara GS. Free-living, aquatic and opportunistic amebas. Brain Pathol 1997;7:583–98.

27. Gelman BB, Popov V, Chaljub G, et al. Neuropatho-logical and ultrastructural features of amebic encephalitis caused by *Sappinia diploidea*. J Neuropathol Exp Neurol 2003;62:990–8.

28. Carpio A, Escobar A, Hauser WA. Cysticercosis and epilepsy: a critical review. Epilepsia 1998;39: 1025–40.

29. Garcia JH, Budka H, McKeever PE, et al, editors. Neuropathology: the diagnostic approach. Philadel-phia: Mosby; 1997.

30. Ironside JW, Head MW, Bell JE, et al. Laboratory diagnosis of variant Creutzfeldt-Jakob disease. Histopathology 2000;37:1–9.

31. Castellani RJ, Parchi P, Madoff L, et al. Biopsy diag-nosis of Creutzfeldt-Jakob disease by Western blot. Hum Pathol 1997;28:623–6.

Neurosurgical Aspects of Central Nervous System Infections

Jason A. Heth, MD

KEYWORDS

- Cerebral abscess • Meningitis • Subdural empyema • Encephalitis • CNS infection

KEY POINTS

- Intracerebral abscesses can rapidly cause severe neurologic deficits or death and require prompt evaluation, imaging, and treatment.
- Subdural empyema is an uncommon but potentially life-threatening infection that typically requires prompt surgical decompression, culturing, and antibiotics.
- The organisms causing meningitis vary by the age of presentation and require prompt treatment with differing antibiotics.
- Herpes simplex encephalitis requires very rapid recognition, diagnosis, and antiviral treatment to prevent severe neurologic deficits or death.
- Spinal diskitis and spinal epidural abscess are uncommonly a threat to life but may cause paraplegia or quadriplegia without expeditious evaluation, imaging, and treatment.

Infections of the central nervous system (CNS) can be severe, life changing, and potentially fatal. Neurosurgeons play a crucial role in the treatment of certain CNS infections. Imaging is important for appropriate diagnosis, lesion localization, identification of surgical candidates, and performance of surgical procedures. High-quality imaging is therefore crucial to the neurosurgeon. The knowledge of how neurologic imaging is used by the neurosurgeon may be helpful to the interpreting neuroradiologist. This article reviews the most common CNS infections neurosurgeons encounter. Pathogenesis; microbiology; surgical indications; treatment, including surgical procedures; and prognosis are discussed.

INTRACEREBRAL ABSCESS

Brain abscess has been one of the most feared CNS infections. This fear arose from the initial poor outcomes and from the rapid neurologic deterioration that can occur. Although rapid deterioration can still occur, the overall outcomes have improved because of improved antibiotics and imaging, which minimize the delay in diagnosis and treatment.

The brain parenchyma is not prone to parenchymal abscess formation, whereas other events and risk factors are required to set the stage for abscess formation. Inoculation can occur from direct implantation (such as a bullet entering the brain or after neurosurgery) or contiguous spread (such as from adjacent sinusitis or mastoiditis).[1,2] Most commonly, however, infection elsewhere spreads hematogenously to the CNS.[3] A classic example is bacterial endocarditis with septic emboli to the brain resulting in cerebral abscess formation.[4,5] Other common primary sites include dental abscesses,[6] cutaneous abscesses, urinary tract infection, pulmonary infection, and soft tissue infection.[3]

Department of Neurosurgery, University of Michigan, 1500 East Medical Center Drive, Ann Arbor, MI 48103-5338, USA
E-mail address: jheth@umich.edu

Neuroimag Clin N Am 22 (2012) 791–799
doi:10.1016/j.nic.2012.05.005
1052-5149/12/$ – see front matter

Several conditions can predispose to cerebral abscess formation. Systemic immunosuppression is frequently involved. Immunosuppression can occur because of intentional immunosuppression (eg, to prevent organ transplant rejection), immune system destruction (eg, with human immunodeficiency virus [HIV] and AIDS), or other medications that affect the immune system (eg, corticosteroids and chemotherapy agents). Pulmonary arteriovenous malformations, with or without Osler-Weber-Rendu syndrome,[7,8] and congenital cyanotic heart malformations[9,10] are also thought to be risk factors.

> Intracerebral abscesses can rapidly cause severe neurologic deficits or death and require prompt evaluation, imaging, and treatment.

Abscess development occurs in a 3-step process.[11] The early cerebritis phase is marked by an area of poorly demarcated inflammation. The late cerebritis phase is marked by the migration of fibroblasts, which start depositing reticulin. In addition, necrosis begins to appear centrally. The early capsule (abscess) stage is marked by the migration of additional fibroblasts and generation of more reticulin in an attempt to wall off an increasing amount of central necrosis. The late capsule stage is marked by a mature collagen capsule surrounding the central necrotic zone.

The microbiology typically reflects the pathogens from the primary site that seeded the CNS. Therefore, gram-positive cocci (GPC) predominate after intravascular infection. Infections beginning from the urinary tract are more frequently gram-negative rods (GNR). Postsurgical and penetrating injuries typically result in skin-related pathogens—mostly GPC. Abscesses resulting from contiguous sinus spread often may harbor more anaerobic organisms,[3] whereas dental abscesses give rise to polymicrobial or anaerobic cerebral abscess pathogens.

Patients present with a myriad of possible symptoms. The most common symptoms are headache, fever, nausea and vomiting, focal neurologic deficits, abnormal sensorium, and decreased level of consciousness.

Treatment of brain abscess requires accurate microbiological diagnosis and appropriate antibiotic therapy. If a patient is not neurologically deteriorating, has no or minimal deficits; and if a microbiological diagnosis can be obtained from another location, antibiotic therapy may be prescribed without a neurosurgical procedure.

This strategy does require high quality diagnostic imaging to characterize the lesions initially and during follow-up. If the lesions respond to antibiotics by decreasing in size and ultimately resolution, then no neurosurgical procedures are required. If the lesions grow, then biopsy and drainage may be required. Stereotactic biopsy and needle drainage is required when abscess is strongly suspected but no primary sites can be identified to culture and when there is a large lesion or lesions causing mass effect and significant neurologic deficits. Craniotomy for resection of abscess is another surgical alternative if needle drainage is not successful.

The prognosis is related to the initial presentation, response to antibiotic therapy, and any systemic conditions or risk factors that may hinder innate immunologic attempts to clear the infection. Recent mortality ranges from 5 to 50.[3,12–14] Patients with no risk factors and stereotactic aspiration had 5% mortality whereas those with several risk factors had 50% mortality.[12] Negative prognostic factors include worse functional status at presentation, immunocompromise,[12] and older age.[3]

SUBDURAL EMPYEMA

Subdural empyema (SDE) is a very serious but uncommon CNS infection. An empyema is a localized purulent infection in an actual cavity or a potential space. In SDE, the empyema occurs in the subdural space. Several mechanisms explain the development of SDE. SDE can occur as a complication of meningitis,[15] after craniotomy,[16,17] and as a result of extension of paranasal sinus infections[1,18] or otitis media.

> Subdural empyema is an uncommon but potentially life-threatening infection that typically requires prompt surgical decompression, culturing, and antibiotics.

Patients with SDE present with headache, significant neurologic deficits, seizures, decreased level of consciousness, and fever. Empyema can compress the brain focally to cause focal deficits. SDE can cause significant inflammation in the subjacent cortex to cause seizures. If the mass effect, inflammation, and edema are significant enough, midline shift, herniation, and global decline can occur.

The range of microbiological diagnoses is different from that of intracerebral abscess and meningitis because of the direct extension from the paranasal sinuses or mastoid. Gram-negative organisms are frequently reported to predominate.[19,20] In contrast, cultures from postsurgical SDE usually are dominated by gram-positive species.[16,17,21]

Surgical treatment must address 3 issues. The first issue is accurate microbiological diagnosis. On occasion this may be obtained from a primary site such as the paranasal sinuses or mastoid. If no other active site is identified, neurosurgical intervention is required. The second issue is CNS mass effect. Mass effect, midline shift, and parenchymal displacement typically call for surgical intervention. Very significant mass effect and cerebral edema may require craniotomy or craniectomy for decompression and debridement. The third and final issue is the possibility of surgical treatment for purulent loculations that may be too large for antibiotics alone to treat. In such situations, it may be possible to culture, aspirate purulent material, and irrigate the subdural space with antibiotic solution through burr holes.

The prognosis is guarded with SDE. These patients are very ill, both systemically and neurologically. They require close multidisciplinary management among the neurosurgical, infectious disease, and critical care teams. Tsai and colleagues[21] reported 11 of 15 patients having good outcomes (normal to moderate disability) and 4 of 15 patients having poor outcomes (severe disability to death). Hlavin and colleagues[19] reported a mortality rate of 18.5% and an additional 18.5% survived with neurologic morbidity. They also found advanced age and more significant encephalopathy at presentation to portend a worse prognosis as well.

MENINGITIS

Meningitis is one of the most common CNS infections, with an incidence of 3.67 to 12.5/100,000 patients.[22,23] Meningitis is an infection of the cerebrospinal fluid (CSF) and the meningeal layer surrounding the brain. The infection can involve the cerebral ventricles to cause ventriculitis.

> The organisms causing meningitis vary by the age of presentation and require prompt treatment with differing antibiotics.

Meningitis is most frequently treated by neurologists, pediatricians, and infectious disease specialists. However, it is crucial for all physicians to understand and recognize meningitis because meningitis is generally very treatable when promptly diagnosed and treated, whereas meningitis can be devastating if diagnosis and treatment are delayed.

Meningitis presents most commonly with headache, fever, and nuchal rigidity. Other symptoms include seizures and cranial nerve deficits. Loss of consciousness can occur from seizures, inflammation and cerebral edema, or hydrocephalus. Herniation can occur and cause coma and death.

The pathogenesis and range of responsible microbes differ with age groups. Neonatal meningitis occurs due to exposure to pathogens during delivery, particularly with vaginal delivery.[24] Pathogens include Escherichia coli, group B streptococci, and Listeria. Children aged 3 months to 5 years are predominantly affected by Streptococcus pneumoniae and Neisseria meningitidis (meningococcus). Pneumococcus is a colonizer of the nasopharynx that is transmitted via respiratory droplets and secretions. From the nasopharynx, it can spread to cause meningitis. A 7-valent pneumococcal vaccine was licensed for use in the United States which resulted in a decrease in childhood pneumococcal meningitis incidence and mortality.[15] Meningococci are gram-negative commensal bacteria that colonize the nasopharynx. Transmission also occurs through respiratory droplets and secretions. Once colonization has occurred, meningococci can then progress to meningitis, which has a very fulminant and rapid course. This fact makes vaccination strategies much more attractive to prevent meningococcal meningitis.[25] A quadrivalent meningococcal vaccine was licensed for use in 2005, and monitoring is ongoing to assess the decrease in meningococcal meningitis incidence. Haemophilus influenzae type b previously was an important species in this age group; however, routine childhood immunization (Hib) begun in the early 1990's has reduced the incidence of H influenzae meningitis nearly to 0. Patients aged 5 years–50 years continue to experience meningitis caused predominantly by S pneumoniae and meningococci.[24] Spread is facilitated among people living in close quarters, such as dormitories. Patients older than 50 years experience S pneumoniae and meningococcal infections; however, Listeria and gram-negative enteric organisms can also be causative.[24]

The treatment of meningitis requires prompt diagnosis and antibiotic administration. If there is any suspicion about the possible presence of meningitis, especially if a patient is experiencing significant symptoms, a first dose of broad-spectrum antibiotics should be given. The mainstay of diagnosis is the lumbar puncture (LP). Gram's stain and cell count with differential, total protein, and glucose are recommended. Again, antibiotic administration is begun without waiting for these results if concern of meningitis is present.

Neurosurgical intervention is required if hydrocephalus is present. In the setting of meningitis, a ventriculostomy would be placed for ventricular drainage while the infection is treated. Once treated, it may be possible to wean the drainage if the normal CSF outflow can resume. If the normal CSF outflow does not re-establish itself, ventriculo-peritoneal shunt placement is likely required.

Heroic measures such as craniectomies, either supratentorially or in the posterior fossa in the case of trans-foramen magnum herniation are sometimes recommended in severe cases.[26,27] These procedures are more likely to be considered when the deterioration has been very abrupt, observed, brought rapidly to medical attention, and the patient is already in the hospital so that surgery can be rapidly undertaken. When rapid devastating deficits develop before the patient presents in hospital, the time involved in transport, evaluation, transport to operating room, set-up, and start, even when rapidly undertaken, rarely occurs quickly enough to reverse neurologic devastation.

Prognosis for patients with meningitis is variable. Rapid diagnosis and initiation of antibiotics is crucial to improving outcomes; Køster-Rasmussen and colleagues[28] demonstrated a 30% increase in odds of unfavorable outcome per hour of delay before antibiotic administration. Recent mortality ranges from 13% to 18.7%.[13,22] Neonates, the elderly, the immunocompromised, and those presenting with significant neurologic deficits suffer higher mortality rates. Major morbidities occurred in 12.8% of cases and minor morbidities occurred in 8.6% of cases.[29] The most common morbidities were hearing loss (33.6%), seizures (12.6%), and motor deficits (11.6%).[29]

VIRAL, FUNGAL, AND PARASITIC INFECTIONS

Viral and fungal infections can also cause very significant neurologic dysfunction and imaging abnormalities. Antiviral and antifungal agents are the main treatments for these infections; however, neurosurgical treatment is also sometimes required. Such infections include herpes encephalitis (HSE), viral encephalitis, toxoplasmosis, and neurocysticercosis.

HSE

Herpes encephalitis (HSE) is a very serious condition, which is the most common and likely most severe viral encephalitis and therefore will be discussed separately. The herpes virus reactivates and generates a very significant inflammatory reaction that occurs predominantly in the temporal lobes. Viral reactivation sets off a chain of events resulting in necrosis (frequently hemorrhagic) in the temporal lobes. Although a high percentage of the population harbors the herpes virus, HSE is uncommon, occurring in approximately 1 in 250,000 to 500,000 patients per year.[30]

Patients may present with altered mentation, decreasing consciousness, focal neurologic findings, headache, seizures, and fever. HSE occurs in all age ranges.[30]

> Herpes simplex encephalitis requires very rapid recognition, diagnosis, and antiviral treatment to prevent severe neurologic deficits or death.

Effective treatment of HSE depends on rapid recognition and treatment. The presentation, physical examination, imaging, and laboratory results from peripheral blood typically suggest the diagnosis to begin intravenous acyclovir. Early administration of antiviral medication is crucial in halting the process. LP may also be recommended as long as the basal cisterns are patent, and the risk of herniation after LP is thus minimized. CSF is examined to rule out bacterial infection. CSF analysis typically demonstrates a cellular pleocytosis and high protein with normal glucose values. Detection of HSV DNA by polymerase chain reaction (PCR) has a sensitivity of 94% and a specificity of 98%[31] and is now the gold standard of clinical diagnosis of HSV encephalitis.

The primary treatment is the rapid use of acyclovir as first-line therapy.[32] Seizures are aggressively treated. Attentive supportive care is provided. Surgical intervention is rarely undertaken with the possible exception of fulminant HSE with significant mass effect on the brainstem. In this setting, craniectomy may be considered.[33,34]

The prognosis for HSE depends on early diagnosis. Without effective treatment, mortality rate is greater than 70% with only 9% of survivors returning to normal function[30] With acyclovir, the 6-month mortality is 19%.[30] The rate of return to normal function in the setting of acyclovir treatment is 38%.[30]

Viral Encephalitis

Viral encephalitis is a diffuse viral infection, particularly of the cerebrum and cortex. Patients with viral encephalitis present with a range of symptoms, including headaches, behavioral changes, fever, seizures, and altered sensorium.[32,35] Viral pathogens include Varicella; Enteroviruses; Measles; Rubella; Mumps; arthropod-borne viruses, such as West Nile Virus and Japanese encephalitis; rabies; and human herpes virus 6 amongst many others.[36] Diagnosis typically, includes history, physical examination, laboratory studies, imaging, and LP. LP is notable for lack of bacterial growth, normal glucose, high protein, and possibly a high white blood cell count. Frequently, CSF leukocytosis shows a predominance of lymphocytes. CSF from LP can also be subjected to PCR testing to assay for herpes simplex virus (HSV), Varicella zoster virus (VZV), human herpes virus (HHV) 6 and 7, cytomegalovirus (CMV), Epstein-Barr virus (EBV), enteroviruses, and HIV amongst others.[32] Serologic testing for antibodies to HSV, VZV, CMV, HHV6 and HHV7, EBV, HIV, influenza A and B, respiratory syncytial virus, rotavirus, coxsackie B5 and parainfluenza 1 viruses[32] is also available.

The minimum treatment of viral encephalitis is attentive supportive care. Seizures are aggressively treated. Depending on the causative agent, antiviral therapy may be available. For VZV, acyclovir may also be used. Foscarnet or ganciclovir can be used for HHV6. Ganciclovir, foscarnet, cidofovir can be tried for CMV. Corticosteroid treatment is controversial and no definitive recommendations are made for their use in viral encephalitis.

The prognosis is generally variable and depends on the patient's age, systemic condition, and the causative virus. In adults, West Nile Virus encephalitis resulted in death in 13% of cases and 38% discharged to a long-term care facility.[37] Wong and Yeung[38] reported mortality of 28%. Of the survivors, 24% had neurologic sequelae. Wang and colleagues[39] reported 26% mortality in culture-proven enterovirus cases. As these representative reports demonstrate, mortality and morbidity rates can be considerable for viral encephalitis.

Toxoplasmosis

Toxoplasma gondii is an obligate intracellular parasite that is the causative agent of CNS toxoplasmosis. *T gondii* is typically acquired by ingestion of oocysts from contaminated soil or food, or bradyzoites in undercooked meat.[40] In immunocompetent adults, the parasites is typically controlled; however, it can reactivate in the setting of immunosuppression. Two populations may be affected by this parasite: neonates and the immunosuppressed patients (particularly patients with AIDS and transplant patients).[41,42] Risk factors for acquiring *T gondii* include working with meat; having 3 or more cats; eating locally produced cured, dried, or smoked meat; eating rare lamb or raw ground beef; and drinking unpasteurized goat's milk.[43] Neonates may be infected by in utero transplacental transmission of the parasite, which can cause fetal death, CNS calcifications, chorioretinitis, and hydrocephalus. Adult patients

again may present with varying symptoms and signs, including headache, fever, seizures, focal neurologic deficits, and more severely diminished sensorium. PCR and quantitative real time PCR can also be done for the DNA of *Toxoplasma* in the CSF with sensitivity of 79% to 100% and specificity of 92% to 97%.[44,45] In some occasions, when all attempts at diagnosis have failed, stereotactic biopsy of a representative lesion can be performed. This procedure has been an issue in the management of patients with AIDS with abnormal ring-enhancing lesions. The differential diagnosis in this setting includes lymphoma. One strategy to obtain the diagnosis is to treat for toxoplasmosis and assess the response.[46,47] A positive response favors a toxoplasmosis diagnosis whereas no response still leaves a diagnostic dilemma that may require surgical biopsy to resolve.

Toxoplasmosis is treated with antitoxoplasmosis agents. The prognosis is good if treatment is started expeditiously and the immunosuppression can be minimized.

Neurocysticercosis

Neurocysticercosis is a parasitic disease caused by *Taenia solium*. Humans are the definitive hosts in whom the parasite develops into an adult tapeworm, reproduces, and sheds eggs. The eggs can then be ingested by several intermediate hosts. Pigs are the prototypical intermediate host. The cysticerci lodge in the skeletal muscle of pigs; if the meat from infected pigs is not cooked appropriately, the cysts from the ingested meat allow the parasite to complete its life cycle by developing into adult tapeworms,[48] resulting in taeniasis. When a human ingests the parasite eggs, they treat the human host as an intermediate host. The eggs hatch and migrate throughout the body to lodge and develop into cystic larval forms. These cysts can occur in the skeletal muscle, brain, eye, and subcutaneous tissue.[49,50] Neurocysticercosis is endemic in the developing world and is a leading cause of epilepsy worldwide.[49]

Patients with neurocysticercosis may present in different manners based on lesion location. Symptoms depend on cyst location, the number of cysts, and the degree of immune response to the disease.[49] Cysts can occur in the brain parenchyma, the ventricular system, the subarachnoid space, and the spinal cord. Seizures can occur when cysts cause cortical dysfunction. Hydrocephalus can be caused by cysts occluding the CSF outflow pathways and can be symptomatic with headaches, somnolence, or loss of consciousness. Focal neurologic deficits can arise from loss of function caused by a cortical or spinal cyst. Patients may also present with dementia.[51]

The clinical setting and imaging can strongly suggest the diagnosis. Serologic testing on CSF and peripheral blood are very specific and quite sensitive for *T solium* infection.[49,50] Diagnostic biopsy may be obtained from cysts in other locations, such as skeletal muscle. Patients in whom these evaluations cannot solidify the diagnosis, a diagnostic CNS biopsy may be required.

Treatment is directed at the presenting symptoms as well as the parasite itself. Seizures are aggressively treated. Seizure control is very high with appropriate anticonvulsant management although lifelong anticonvulsants may be required. Hydrocephalus must be aggressively treated. Endoscopic treatment can include cyst removal, third ventriculostomy, and septum pellucidum fenestration.[52,53] If endoscopic treatment fails or is not an option, shunt placement can be performed although there is a concern for high rate of failure with neurocysticercosis. If a cyst is large and causing mass effect and neurologic deficits, a cyst resection could be considered. Cysticidal treatment is recommended to treat the parasites themselves.

The prognosis depends on the manner of presentation. Seizures can be readily controlled with good outcomes. Hydrocephalus can also be effectively treated. Intracranial hypertension resulting from mass effect from the cysts or from an aggressive immune response to the cysts can be life threatening.

SPINAL DISKITIS AND SPINAL EPIDURAL ABSCESS

Vertebral diskitis and spinal epidural abscess (SEA) are CNS infections that can affect the spine and spinal cord. They are discussed here, because they are readily treated with good outcomes if promptly recognized and treated. If not promptly recognized and treated, they can cause rapid onset paraplegia and quadriplegia. Diskitis and SEA occur through similar mechanisms. Diskitis can also occur through direct inoculation (even with proper antisepsis), such as LP, diskogram, surgical exposure, and epidural anesthesia. The disk space can be seeded from a primary infection elsewhere, such as a soft tissue infection or endocarditis.

Spinal diskitis and spinal epidural abscess are uncommonly a threat to life but may cause paraplegia or quadriplegia without expeditious evaluation, imaging, and treatment.

SEA can arise from untreated diskitis as well as direct exposure[54,55] as previously mentioned. In one report, as many as 52.6% of SEA cases were associated with neurosurgical procedures or spinal blocks.[56] SEA can also occur from contiguous spread. An example is cervical soft tissue abscess that erodes into the cervical spinal canal.

The main complaint of patients with diskitis is pain appropriate to the spinal level. Diskitis is a very painful condition and responds poorly to first-line medications used to treat degenerative spine disease. Fever can also occur.[56,57] Diskitis in the lumbosacral region can cause radicular symptoms with leg pain and radicular deficits. Stenosis can also occur and cause leg pain that worsens with ambulation. Diskitis in the cervical and thoracic regions can cause radicular symptoms, but most importantly cervicothoracic diskitis can cause spinal cord compression, myelopathy, and quadriparesis/plegia or paraparesis/plegia, respectively. Incontinence can also occur.[57]

Risk factors for diskitis and SEA are similar to previous infectious conditions discussed and include diabetes mellitus, end-stage renal disease, endocarditis, immunosuppression, hepatic cirrhosis, and illicit intravenous drug use.[57,58]

Patients with SEA also can have pain[55] although it is not as uniformly and exquisitely painful as diskitis. The same range of neurologic deficits can occur.

The microbiological species involved vary.[56,57] Staphylococci are the species most commonly isolated.[56–58] If seeding occurs from a primary site, the microbiology of the primary site will dictate the diagnosis. Direct spread from cervical, abdominal, or pelvic abscess increases the possibility of GNR, anaerobic, and polymicrobial infections. Individuals in whom diskitis and SEA occur from direct manipulation, skin flora and GPC dominate. Fungal and candidal diskitis can also occur.[59]

Diagnosis and treatment of diskitis and SEA must address 3 issues. The first issue is microbiological diagnosis, which allows prescription of maximally effective antibiotics. Diagnosis from a primary site may be possible. With diskitis, computed tomography–guided needle biopsy yields the diagnosis in 90% of cases.[59] In some cases, open biopsy may be required if all other diagnostic attempts have failed. The second issue that must be addressed is neural compression. In spinal cord compression with cervical or thoracic myelopathy, emergent decompression is indicated and usually requires laminectomy. If cauda equina symptoms develop from lumbar diskitis or SEA, emergent decompression, usually laminectomy, is required. In cases of radicular symptoms only, nerve root decompression may be considered. The third issue that must be considered is spinal stability. If the infection has destroyed critical spinal elements, then spinal stabilization may be also be required.

The prognosis for diskitis is generally good if promptly diagnosed and the treatment is rapidly begun. Eighty percent of cases can experience a good outcome.[59] Mortality is uncommon and depends more on systemic infection. Similarly, prompt diagnosis is important to overall prognosis in SEA.[56] The prognosis in SEA has been variable in the literature. One group reported 10 of 21 cases deteriorating,[58] whereas another reported 67% to 75% of patients improving after treatment[57] and 5% worsening neurologically. Mortality rate in SEA can be up to 23% and can occur secondary to systemic sepsis or resulting from systemic conditions that predispose to SEA, such as end-stage renal disease.[57]

SUMMARY

CNS infections are very serious conditions, which cause rapidly progressive symptoms and loss of function. Rapid deterioration can also lead to death, which is particularly true of cerebral abscess, SDE, meningitis, and herpes simplex encephalitis. Although perhaps not as frequently life threatening, diskitis and SEA can cause rapid onset of very severe neurologic deficits. In all of these conditions, rapid diagnosis and treatment is crucial. Imaging is important for appropriate localization, diagnosis, and surveillance once treatment has begun. Viral encephalitis, toxoplasmosis, and neurocysticercosis can also cause a myriad of symptoms and disability. Again, imaging plays a crucial role in diagnosis and in treatment of these conditions as well.

REFERENCES

1. Germiller JA, Monin DL, Sparano AM, et al. Intracranial complications of sinusitis in children and adolescents and their outcomes. Arch Otolaryngol Head Neck Surg 2006;32(9):969–76.
2. Isaacson B, Mirabal C, Kutz JW, et al. Pediatric otogenic intracranial abscesses. Otolaryngol Head Neck Surg 2010;142(3):434–7.
3. Chun CH, Johnson JD, Hofstetter M, et al. Brain abscess. A study of 45 consecutive cases. Medicine (Baltimore) 1986;65:415–31.
4. Bitsch A, Nau R, Hilgers RA, et al. Focal neurologic deficits in infective endocarditis and other septic diseases. Acta Neurol Scand 1996;94(4):279–86.
5. Kieran SM, Cahill RA, Sheehan SJ. Mycotic peripheral aneurysms and intracerebral abscesses secondary to infective endocarditis. Eur J Vasc Endovasc Surg 2004;28(5):565–6.
6. Ewald C, Kuhn S, Kalff R. Pyogenic infections of the central nervous system secondary to dental affections—a report of six cases. Neurosurg Rev 2006;29(2):163–6 [discussion: 166–7].
7. Brydon HL, Akinwunmi J, Selway R, et al. Brain abscesses associated with pulmonary arteriovenous malformations. Br J Neurosurg 1999;13(3):265–9.
8. Kawano H, Hirano T, Ikeno K, et al. Brain abscess caused by pulmonary arteriovenous fistulas without Rendu-Osler-Weber disease. Intern Med 2009;48(6):485–7.
9. Ciurea AV, Stoica F, Vasilescu G, et al. Neurosurgical management of brain abscesses in children. Childs Nerv Syst 1999;15(6-7):309–17.
10. Takeshita M, Kagawa M, Izawa M, et al. Current treatment strategies and factors influencing outcome in patients with bacterial brain abscess. Acta Neurochir (Wien) 1998;140:1263–70.
11. Britt RH, Enzmann DR. Clinical stages of human brain abscesses on serial CT scans after contrast infusion. Computerized tomographic, neuropathological, and clinical correlations. J Neurosurg 1983;59(6):972–89.
12. Kondziolka D, Duma CM, Lunsford LD. Factors that enhance the likelihood of successful stereotactic treatment of brain abscesses. Acta Neurochir (Wien) 1994;127(1-2):85–90.
13. Pfister HW, Feiden W, Einhäupl KM. Spectrum of complications during bacterial meningitis in adults. Results of a prospective clinical study. Arch Neurol 1993;50(6):575–81.
14. Yang SY, Zhao CS. Review of 140 patients with brain abscess. Surg Neurol 1993;39(4):290–6.
15. Tsai CJ, Griffin MR, Nuorti JP, et al. Changing epidemiology of pneumococcal meningitis after the introduction of pneumococcal conjugate vaccine in the United States. Clin Infect Dis 2008;46(11):1664–72.
16. Dashti SR, Baharvahdat H, Spetzler RF, et al. Operative intracranial infection following craniotomy. Neurosurg Focus 2008;24(6):E10.
17. McClelland S, Hall WA. Postoperative central nervous system infection: incidence and associated factors in 2111 neurosurgical procedures. Clin Infect Dis 2007;45(1):55–9.
18. Tsai BY, Lin KL, Lin TY, et al. Pott's puffy tumor in children. Childs Nerv Syst 2010;26(1):53–60.
19. Hlavin ML, Kaminski HJ, Fenstermaker RA, et al. Intracranial suppuration: a modern decade of postoperative subdural empyema and epidural abscess. Neurosurgery 1994;34(6):974–80 [discussion: 980–1].
20. Penido Nd O, Borin A, Iha LCN, et al. Intracranial complications of otitis media: 15 years of experience in 33 patients. Otolaryngol Head Neck Surg 2005;132(1):37–42.
21. Tsai YD, Chang WN, Shen CC, et al. Intracranial suppuration: a clinical comparison of subdural

empyemas and epidural abscesses. Surg Neurol 2003;59:191–6 [discussion: 196].

22. Giorgi Rossi P, Mantovani J, Ferroni E, et al. Incidence of bacterial meningitis (2001–2005) in Lazio, Italy: the results of a integrated surveillance system. BMC Infect Dis 2009;9:13.

23. Loughlin AM, Marchant CD, Lett SM. The changing epidemiology of invasive bacterial infections in Massachusetts children, 1984 through 1991. Am J Public Health 1995;85(3):392–4.

24. Williams AJ, Nadel S. Bacterial meningitis: current controversies in approaches to treatment. CNS Drugs 2001;15(12):909–19.

25. Stephens DS. Biology and pathogenesis of the evolutionarily successful, obligate human bacterium *Neisseria meningitidis*. Vaccine 2009;27(Suppl 2): B71–7.

26. Baussart B, Cheisson G, Compain M, et al. Multimodal cerebral monitoring and decompressive surgery for the treatment of severe bacterial meningitis with increased intracranial pressure. Acta Anaesthesiol Scand 2006;50:762–5.

27. Di Rienzo A, Iacoangeli M, Rychlicki F, et al. Decompressive craniectomy for medically refractory intracranial hypertension due to meningoencephalitis: report of three patients. Acta Neurochir (Wien) 2008;150(10):1057–65 [discussion: 1065].

28. Køster-Rasmussen R, Korshin A, Meyer CN. Antibiotic treatment delay and outcome in acute bacterial meningitis. J Infect 2008;57(6):449–54.

29. Edmond K, Clark A, Korczak VS, et al. Global and regional risk of disabling sequelae from bacterial meningitis: a systematic review and meta-analysis. Lancet Infect Dis 2010;10(5):317–28.

30. Whitley RJ. Herpes simplex encephalitis: adolescents and adults. Antiviral Res 2006;71(2-3):141–8.

31. Lakeman FD, Whitley RJ. Diagnosis of herpes simplex encephalitis: application of polymerase chain reaction to cerebrospinal fluid from brain-biopsied patients and correlation with disease. National Institute of Allergy and Infectious Diseases Collaborative Antiviral Study Group. J Infect Dis 1995;171(4):857–63.

32. Steiner I, Budka H, Chaudhuri A, et al. Viral meningoencephalitis: a review of diagnostic methods and guidelines for management. Eur J Neurol 2010;17(8):999–e57.

33. Adamo MA, Deshaies EM. Emergency decompressive craniectomy for fulminating infectious encephalitis. J Neurosurg 2008;174–6.

34. González Rabelino GA, Fons C, Rey A, et al. Craniectomy in herpetic encephalitis. Pediatr Neurol 2008;39(3):201–3.

35. Michael BD, Sidhu M, Stoeter D, et al. Acute central nervous system infections in adults–a retrospective cohort study in the NHS North West region. QJM 2010;103(10):749–58.

36. Huppatz C, Durrheim D, Levi C, et al. Etiology of Encephalitis in Australia, 1990–2007. Emerg Infect Dis 2009;15(9):1359.

37. Tyler KL, Pape J, Goody RJ, et al. CSF findings in 250 patients with serologically confirmed West Nile virus meningitis and encephalitis. Neurology 2006;66(3): 361–5.

38. Wong V, Yeung CY. Acute viral encephalitis in children. Aust Paediatr J 1987;23(6):339–42.

39. Wang SM, Liu CC, Tseng HW, et al. Clinical spectrum of enterovirus 71 infection in children in southern Taiwan, with an emphasis on neurological complications. Clin Infect Dis 1999;29(1):184–90.

40. Walker M, Zunt JR. Parasitic central nervous system infections in immunocompromised hosts. Clin Infect Dis 2005;40(7):1005–15.

41. Denier C, Bourhis JH, Lacroix C, et al. Spectrum and prognosis of neurologic complications after hematopoietic transplantation. Neurology 2006;67(11): 1990–7.

42. Weber C, Schaper J, Tibussek D, et al. Diagnostic and therapeutic implications of neurological complications following paediatric haematopoietic stem cell transplantation. Bone Marrow Transplant 2008;41(3):253–9.

43. Jones JL, Dargelas V, Roberts J, et al. Risk factors for *Toxoplasma gondii* infection in the United States. Clin Infect Dis 2009;49(6):878–84.

44. Alfonso Y, Fraga J, Fonseca C, et al. Molecular diagnosis of *Toxoplasma gondii* infection in cerebrospinal fluid from AIDS patients. Cerebrospinal Fluid Res 2009;6:2.

45. Mesquita RT, Ziegler AP, Hiramoto RM, et al. Real-time quantitative PCR in cerebral toxoplasmosis diagnosis of Brazilian human immunodeficiency virus-infected patients. J Med Microbiol 2010;59(Pt 6):641–7.

46. Portegies P, Solod L, Cinque P, et al. Guidelines for the diagnosis and management of neurological complications of HIV infection. Eur J Neurol 2004; 11(5):297–304.

47. Smego RA, Orlovic D, Wadula J. An algorithmic approach to intracranial mass lesions in HIV/AIDS. Int J STD AIDS 2006;17(4):271–6.

48. Fleury A, Escobar A, Fragoso G, et al. Clinical heterogeneity of human neurocysticercosis results from complex interactions among parasite, host and environmental factors. Trans R Soc Trop Med Hyg 2010;104(4):243–50.

49. Garcia HH, Del Brutto OH, Cysticercosis Working Group in Peru. Neurocysticercosis: updated concepts about an old disease. Lancet Neurol 2005; 4(10):653–61.

50. Mahanty S, Garcia HH, Cysticercosis Working Group in Peru. Cysticercosis and neurocysticercosis as pathogens affecting the nervous system. Prog Neurobiol 2010;91(2):172–84.

51. Ciampi de Andrade D, Rodrigues CL, Abraham R, et al. Cognitive impairment and dementia in

neurocysticercosis: a cross-sectional controlled study. Neurology 2010;74(16):1288–95.

52. Proaño JV, Torres-Corzo J, Rodríguez-Della Vecchia R, et al. Intraventricular and subarachnoid basal cisterns neurocysticercosis: a comparative study between traditional treatment versus neuroendoscopic surgery. Childs Nerv Syst 2009;25(11): 1467–75.

53. Torres-Corzo JG, Tapia-Pérez JH, Vecchia RR, et al. Endoscopic management of hydrocephalus due to neurocysticercosis. Clin Neurol Neurosurg 2010; 112(1):11–6.

54. Green LK, Paech MJ. Obstetric epidural catheter-related infections at a major teaching hospital: a retrospective case series. Int J Obstet Anesth 2010;19(1):38–43.

55. Sethna NF, Clendenin D, Athiraman U, et al. Incidence of epidural catheter-associated infections after continuous epidural analgesia in children. Anesthesiology 2010;113(1):224–32.

56. González-López JJ, Górgolas M, Muñiz J, et al. Spontaneous epidural abscess: analysis of 15 cases with emphasis on diagnostic and prognostic factors. Eur J Intern Med 2009;20(5):514–7.

57. Karikari IO, Powers CJ, Reynolds RM, et al. Management of a spontaneous spinal epidural abscess: a single-center 10-year experience. Neurosurgery 2009;65(5):919–23 [discussion: 923–4.

58. Wang TC, Lu MS, Yang JT, et al. Motor function improvement in patients undergoing surgery for spinal epidural abscess. Neurosurgery 2010;66(5): 910–6.

59. D'Agostino C, Scorzolini L, Massetti AP, et al. A seven-year prospective study on spondylodiscitis: epidemiological and microbiological features. Infection 2010;38(2):102–7.

Index

Note: Page numbers of article titles are in **boldface** type.

Neuroimag Clin N Am 22 (2012) 801–804
http://dx.doi.org/10.1016/S1052-5149(12)00134-7
1052-5149/12/$ – see front matter © 2012 Elsevier Inc. All rights reserved.

neuroimaging.theclinics.com

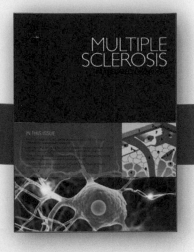

Printed and bound by CPI Group (UK) Ltd, Croydon, CR0 4YY

03/10/2024

01040359-0005